Neuroendoscopy

Spyros Sgouros
Editor

Neuroendoscopy

Current Status and Future Trends

Springer

Editor
Spyros Sgouros
Department of Pediatric Neurosurgery
Mitera Children's Hospital
Athens
Greece

University of Athens Medical School
Athens
Greece

ISBN 978-3-642-39084-5 ISBN 978-3-642-39085-2 (eBook)
DOI 10.1007/978-3-642-39085-2
Springer Heidelberg New York Dordrecht London

Library of Congress Control Number: 2013954879

Printed on acid-free paper

Springer is part of Springer Science+Business Media (www.springer.com)

Preface

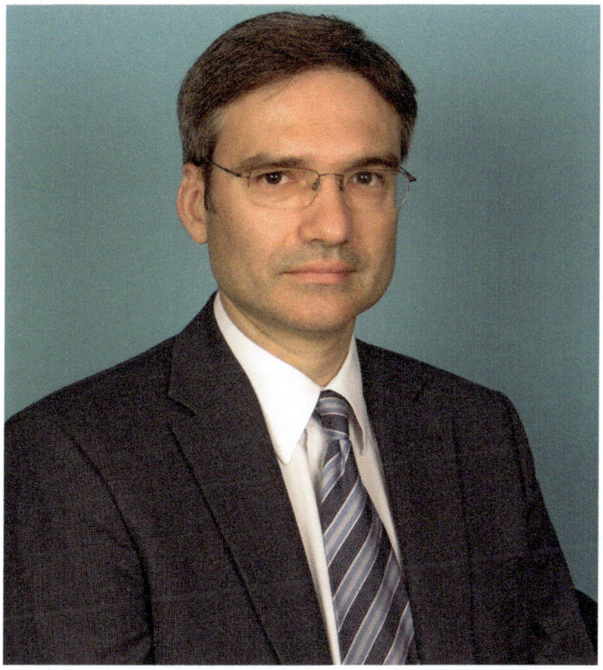

In June 2009, I had the pleasure and honor of hosting the 5th World Congress of Neuroendoscopy in Athens, Greece, under the auspices of the International Federation of Neuroendoscopy (IFNE). The luxurious surroundings and the classical elegance of Hotel "Grande Bretagne," a place synonymous with the history of modern Greece, provided the perfect setting for a rich scientific program, full of innovative ideas, which covered all the aspects of neuroendoscopy. Colleagues from all over the world brought their best work and their most spectacular endoscopy videos and shared them with us all. The social program included a fantastic classical guitar concert by the neurosurgeon Dr. Alvaro Cordoba, who is in fact an accomplished classical guitarist giving concerts in some of the biggest music halls worldwide. Under the heavy shadow of the Acropolis monument, in the courtyard of the first building of the University of Athens, circa 1837, Dr. Cordoba held our breath with his amazing sounds. The Congress was closed with the gala dinner, which was held at the Zappeion Megaron, the place where the ascension treaty of Greece joining the European Community was signed.

This book contains the keynote lectures of the Congress. Each main topic was covered conclusively by a renowned neurosurgeon considered a world authority on the subject. Having listened to these lectures during the meeting, I considered appropriate that they should be collected in a book, which will identify the state-of-the-art standard in neuroendoscopy, at the end of the first decade of the twenty-first century.

I hope that the reader will enjoy reading this book, as much as I enjoyed compiling and editing it.

Athens, Greece Spyros Sgouros

Contents

Historical Trends of Neuroendoscopic Surgery

1

Bernhard L. Bauer

It is a great honour for me to give the laudation on Professor Axel Perneczky, laureate on occasion of the Vth World Congress of IFNE. I hope to succeed in conveying his human and professional dimension. I am well aware that such attempt will fall short of a true reflection.

Professor Axel Perneczky was born November 1, 1945, in Krasnogorsk, Russia, near Moscow (Fig. 1.1). From 1946 to 1965, he lived in Budapest and started studying medicine at the University Medical School of Budapest in 1964. In 1965, he left for Austria and continued his medical studies at the University of Vienna. After graduation from medical school at the University of Vienna in 1971, he spent 2 years at the departments of general surgery and traumatology. In 1973, he started training in neurosurgery at the Neurosurgical University Department in Vienna with Professor Kraus. Because of his very early interest in microsurgery and surgical anatomy, he spent 1 year with Professor G. Yasargil as assistant surgeon in Zürich. In 1980, he became Associate Professor for neurosurgery in Vienna under Professor Koos. In October 1988, he was elected and appointed Professor of Neurosurgery and Chairman of the Neurosurgical Department of the Medical School, University of Mainz, Germany.

Memorial Address: Axel Perneczky 1949–2009

B.L. Bauer, MD, PhD
Department of Neurosurgery,
The Spine Clinic, Celle,
Germany
e-mail: agricola001@t-online.de

His main fields of activity were microsurgical anatomy and the implicating surgical strategies in neurosurgery, aneurysm and angioma surgery and skull base surgery with special consideration of the cavernous sinus. The development of microsurgical strategies resulted in a further refinement of surgical technique, and so since 1989, he was working on the application of endoscopy in neurosurgery. A special technique has been developed for the extended use of the keyhole strategy. He organised the "First International Congress on Minimally Invasive Techniques in Neurosurgery" (Wiesbaden, June 1993), and he was the Editor in Chief of the *International Journal of Minimally Invasive Neurosurgery* (MIN). Hands-on courses on microsurgical planning and neuroendoscopy were held six times per year in Mainz and Tuttlingen. He has been the President of the 1st International Congress on Endoscope-Assisted Microsurgery in June 1998 in Frankfurt. During the last year, his interest was focused on the intraoperative imaging modalities used for surgical planning and navigation.

His published scientific contributions count more than 250 papers. He is co-author of the *Colour Atlas of Microneurosurgery* (Thieme, 1984 and 1993) and *Endoscopic Anatomy for Neurosurgery* (Thieme 1993); he is also the author of the book *Keyhole Concept in Neurosurgery* including *Endoscope-Assisted Microsurgery* (Thieme 1999).

A new centre for "Minimally Invasive Neurosurgery" at the University of Mainz is now

S. Sgouros (ed.), *Neuroendoscopy*,
DOI 10.1007/978-3-642-39085-2_1, © Springer-Verlag Berlin Heidelberg 2014

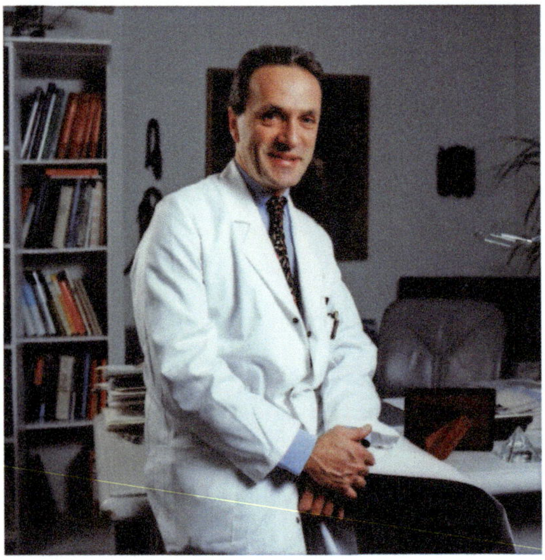

Fig. 1.1 Professor Dr. Med. Axel Perneczky (1949–2009)

under construction, including a special concept for development and application of new concepts and technologies in the neurosurgical operating unit with special innovation in intraoperative visualisation and imaging.

We remember his passion and brilliance as member of the "Skull-Base-All-Stars" band playing jazz guitar. Gifted with talent beyond neurosurgery, we remember him as a painter and last but not least as a sportsman on the tennis court, in the swimming pool and skiing snowy mountains.

Professor Axel Perneczky had a brilliant career in academic neurosurgery, devoting himself to solving many of the problems that existed with microsurgery and neuroendoscopy. He took a truly intellectual approach to these problems, starting with basic laboratory work, devising ingenious surgical methods, carefully applying new concepts and a new technique to previously unmanageable neurosurgical problems in patients and doing all of this with the kindness, compassion and consummate skill of a great physician and surgeon. No one who has met him and has read his writings could not fail to feel a growing respect for his wide knowledge, his directness and his broad cultural background.

He devoted himself to the education of young neurosurgeons; in large numbers, they are his scholars and reside worldwide.

His proposal to reconcile microsurgery and neuroendoscopy as the minimal invasive and tissue-saving procedure called "keyhole surgery" shall be connected forever with his name. He has moulded modern-day neurosurgical practice.

The minor and major setbacks and sad moments in his life did not manage to hinder this man's work and did not influence his character negatively. He was able to control the situation and continue onward both externally as well as with his spirit.

He has given neuroendoscopy worldwide a solid reputation. We, his colleagues and the great family of former scholars are thankful and indebted. His name and his work occupy a worthy and honourable place in the annals of IFNE and a special place in our heart. World Neurosurgery has lost an invaluable teacher and a great master of neurosurgery.

Remembrance of Dr. Philipp Bozzini

Inventor of the Endoscopy 200th Anniversary

Before the end of the last century, there has been little interest in the endoscopic visualisation of the cerebrospinal fluid-filled cavities. CT and MRI scanning had made endoscopy almost obsolete in neurosurgery. Only very special studies on evaluating the nature and degree in internal hydrocephalus by neuroendoscopy were reported. Shunting procedures had overgrown surgical endoscopic technique and procedures. It would seem that endoscopy was about to follow pneumoencephalography, ventriculography and some other techniques to vanish from clinical practice.

When I started neuroendoscopy in 1985, I was convinced that it had a significant potential. The ultimate promise of the technique was the potential of the endoscope to provide a change of paradigms in certain fields of neurosurgical practice. Future applications of neuroendoscopy have the greatest potential to combine both microsurgery and endoscopy. Additionally, the use of virtual reality as a teaching tool promises a revolution in medical education techniques. The virtual clinic trains physicians to perform less invasive surgery without having to practise on animal models or assist other surgeons.

M.L. Apuzzo [1] wrote in 1977: "These technologies will include electronics like neuronavigation, ultrasound, robotics, lasers, and other technologies. So we can approximately attain a precise discipline which can best exploit techniques such as the endoscope. Computer systems coupled to endoscopic surgical instrumentation will make significant future advances possible. Use and incorporation of these techniques into neurosurgical procedures will depend on having access to the know-how necessary to bring these applications into the neurosurgical theatre. Problem is only a few neurosurgeons will have the time and/or the technical knowledge to be truly effective in this area. Therefore, instrument designers and computer scientists must become part with a close affiliation with neurosurgical departments involved in neuroendoscopy. Together they will provide the tools for the future of neuroendoscopy. Surgeons will provide the guidance necessary by telling instrument makers what we need and what is useful".

We must take care not to overwhelm the surgeon with highly sophisticated surroundings which hinder his concentration. Free the neurosurgeon to his true scope to operate on. New instruments like the endo-spatula will offer access to transfrontal, pterional and posterior fossa space-occupying lesions and vascular processes.

Philipp Bozzini [2] a German-Italian physician demonstrating the "Lichtleiter" in 1806 to the Academy of Medicine in Vienna wrote: "Although our eyes can deceive us more than other senses, optical deception rarely prevents real proof of a matter. The eyes lead all the other senses, and guide their impressions to the point of conviction. Rarely do the eyes need their cooperation, and rarely can the other senses do without the eyes help. Even when the other sense of touch has already informed us sufficiently, the sense of sight is more reliable, and the more senses are focused on one object the less the latter is able to deceive us. Until now, we have completely lacked the ability to see into the inner cavities and spaces of the living body; in anatomy the scalpel taught us only about their shape, and conclusions about their functions could only be suspected. This is the main reason why our knowledge of the important laws of motion in the animal organisation is still so retarded, since no change can take place in all of nature other than by increased or decreased motion!"

From the beginning, ventriculoscopy and treatment of hydrocephalus was a domain of intraventricular endoscopy. V.D. L'Espinasse [3, 4] (1878–1946) from Chicago succeeded in carrying out ventriculoscopy with coagulation of the choroid plexus in two infants. One of the patients died 5 years after the operation. The second patient did not survive the operation for reasons that were not clarified. L'Espinasse performed the procedure with a rigid Uroscope. The lens system he used was developed in 1878 by M. Nitze [5] (1849–1906) in collaboration with the instrument builder Josef Leiter [6] (1830–1892) in Vienna, Austria. This system consisted of a metal tube and an appropriate obturator. The incandescent platinum wire light known since 1845 served for illumination. After the discovery of the electric light bulb by T.A. Edison, it could be replaced by the more effective mignon lamp at the distal tip of the endoscope.

On April 3, 1922, Walter Dandy [7] from the Johns Hopkins Hospital reported on occasion of the session of the Medical Society on two diagnostic ventriculoscopies he had carried out. Dandy described the topographic conditions in the lateral ventricles, the location of the interventricular foramen, the pellucid septum and the choroid plexus. His comment was given with discretion: "How useful operating ventriculoscopy will be can scarcely be predicted".

Fay and Grant from the Neurosurgery Division in Philadelphia were the first to combine ventriculoscopy with intraventricular photography. Their case report from 1923 [8] showed that the suggestion to use ventriculoscopy as a means of imaging pathological lesions was already made in September 1921. Unfortunately, only line drawings of the photographs are preserved.

Fay and Grant concluded from their investigations that intraventricular photography is feasible when the ventricles are enlarged. This operation has few complications when it is carried out according to the rules of the medical art. The diagnostic value consists in direct inspection of the ventricles and determination of the location and size of lesions in and surrounding the ventricles.

On February 6, 1923, W.J. Mixter [9] from Boston performed the first ventriculostomy in a baby with congenital hydrocephalus. The floor of the third ventricle was observed and located with a urethroscope and afterwards perforated with a flexible probe. Mixter reported that the operation was not associated with any complications. He recommended therefore ventriculostomy with perforation of the floor of the third ventricle as a means of treating noncommunicating hydrocephalus.

In his paper presented in front of the Society of Neurology and Psychiatry on May 17, 1934, Tracy J. Putnam [10] suggested that this method should be used. He concluded that characteristics such as the focal length of the lens system, the restricted visual field and the size of the endoscopes used at that time were an impediment to plexus coagulation. The coagulation manoeuvre lasted between 5 and 20 min. In one session, the plexus of both lateral ventricles were obliterated as far as possible. In 1938, Putnam presented the results of surgery with communicating hydrocephalus which had been treated by endoscopic plexus coagulation. He rated the outcome as being "overall encouraging".

In 1935 and later, John E. Scarff [11–14] from the Department of Neurological Surgery at the Columbia University Hospital, NY, published his experiences with endoscopic cauterisation of the choroid plexus. The essential feature of his surgical technique was the permanent direct communication between the ventricle and a lavage system with physiological saline attached to the endoscope. This enabled a constant intraventricular pressure to be maintained during the operation so as to prevent a collapse of the ventricle and a potential postoperative complication associated with it. As with Putnam, the duration of the coagulation process was about 15 min. According to Putnam's experience, the most radical cauterization had the most prognostically favourable outcome.

Of 20 babies that were operated endoscopically by Scarff, 3 babies died immediately after the procedure; 7 survived without sustained elimination of the intracranial pressure symptoms. A lasting reduction of intracranial pressure could be achieved by the operation in 10 babies. In his series from 1966, Scarff reported of a further 19 babies that he had operated on in the period from 1946 to 1951. In these cases, the results of surgery were very much better than in the first series from 1936. In 1952, Scarff concluded that this was owed to a greater routine in the application on the new method. What we call "learning by doing" or "learning curve" is coincident with Putnam and Scarff which were involved towards the problems of hydrocephalus. At the same time J.L. Pool [15] focused his whole interest into the spinal endoscope and he succeeded in the endoscopic demonstration of the cauda equina and its roots.

During the time of the Second World War and a long time after, any development in this special field of neuroendosurgery was suspended. The development of the rod lens system by Harold H. Hopkins in 1959 [16] and its installation in a Karl Storz (1911–1996) Endoscope (1965) resulted in a revolution in the field of endoscopy. The introduction of the cold light (1960) and bipolar cutting and coagulation technologies led to a renaissance of endoscopy in neurosurgery in the subsequent years.

The external diameters of the rigid endoscopes were reduced to less than 3 mm with a larger visual angle up to 70° and a ten times greater light conduction. With the introduction of the "cold light source" also by Karl Storz which replaced the Nitze system that had been used up to that time, the new endoscopic system could be optimised. This enabled an extension of the indication spectrum usual up to that time. Until today, the Hopkins lens system has served as a basis for the development and manufacturing of rigid endoscopes.

Ogata et al. [17] from Kyoto presented in 1964 a rigid "encephaloscope". The new details of the system consisted of two components: a glass-fibre light bush and a camera system.

The external diameter of the endoscope was 3.1 mm; the length was 220 mm. The outer trocar had a diameter of 3.6 mm. As a light conductor, 10,000 glass fibres with a diameter of 18 mm were arranged circularly around the lens. For that time, this ultrathin instrument was an excellent construction, but it was to my knowledge tested only in animal experiments.

The next step of importance in the development of the endoscopic technique and indications we owe to G. Guiot [18] from the "Centre National de la Recherche Scientifique" in Paris. He is recognised to have used the endoscope in transphenoidal approach likely for the first time. Guiot used also an external light source adapted to the endoscope and a bi-ventricular approach to the third ventricle in hydrocephalus surgery. In his series from 1973, he successfully operated on nine patients with Mixter's technique and had no serious complications and no deaths. We should remember also the very early (1978) endeavours from Bushe and Halves [19] to use the endoscope in para- and suprasellar pituitary space-occupying lesions.

In a technical note "Ventriculofiberscope: a new technique for endoscopic diagnosis and operation", T. Fukushima [20] from Tokyo University (1973) described for the first time the prototype for a flexible ventriculofibrescope of which the specifications correspond to those of the flexible endoscopes used today in neuroendoscopy. The photographic documentation of ventriculoscopic operations as well as operations on cystic and solid intracerebral space-occupying lesions in 37 cases published in the *Journal of Neurosurgery* was of excellent quality and was a milestone in the development of minimally invasive endoscopic neurosurgery.

Very early in 1977, M.L. Apuzzo contributed to neuroendoscopy in various fields. He recognised the endoscope as a helpful complement to microneurosurgery and practised the combination of endoscopic and stereotaxic neurosurgery for the first time. L.M. Auer [21, 22] from Graz, Austria, extended the spectrum of indications using endoscopic treatment of intracranial haemorrhages and cystic brain lesions and bestowed much care upon the use of the ultrasound in neuroendoscopy.

F. Oppel and G. Mulch [23] in 1979 reported for the first time on endoscopic interventions in the cerebellopontine angle for selective trigeminal root section and endoscopic section of the vestibular nerve by transpyramidal retrolabyrinthine approach in Meniere's disease.

The utilisation of ultrathin flexible-steerable endoscopes and the miniaturisation of instruments as well as the application of laser were introduced in 1980 from DiMagno et al. [24] and Stephen K. Powers [25] from Chapel Hill, University of North Carolina.

Upon this fundament, further development could take place. So the time has come for the first synopsis in minimally endoscopic neurosurgery. H.B. Griffith [26, 27] from Bristol, UK, impresses in his overview "Endoscopic Intracranial Neurosurgery" the term endoneurosurgery.

Robert F.C. Jones [28] from the Prince of Wales Children's Hospital Sydney, Australia, readopted the endoscopic "third ventriculostomy" in treatment of obstructive hydrocephalus. Between 1979 and 1990, he operated on 59 patients with this method. He presented the method of third ventriculostomy in detail in his paper in 1992 on occasion of MIEN II in Marburg, Germany. He specifies the indications for the procedure in detail. His description of the preoperative workup and the surgical technique, as well as the possible complications, is to be regarded as an important contribution to the state of the art in minimal endoscopic neurosurgery.

Alan R. Cohen [29, 30] performed in the years between 1989 and 1990 in Boston endoscopic fenestrations of ventricular cysts and in eight babies with obstructive hydrocephalus pellucid septum fenestration. A flexible endoscope was his instrument. For dissection of the cyst walls and for coagulation of small blood vessels, he used a monopolar dissection needle.

Kim H. Manwaring [31] from the Phoenix Children's Hospital gave with his technical inventions and advices of the "saline torch" (monopolar RF endoscopic dissector) and the "peel-away introducer" new impetus in the development of neuroendoscopy. Besides the content of the publications (1992) mentioned above, Manwaring has also investigated the endoscopic fenestration and dissection of ventricular lesions resulting in compartmentation and septation of the ventricular system. Also to mention is his endeavour with magnetic field guided endoscopic dissection. He perceived with regard to the operative indication the difference between congenital unilateral hydrocephalus, plexus cysts, colloid cysts and septum formation by bacterial and post-hemorrhagic ventriculitis.

At the same time, Lewis and Crone [32] from Cincinnati Children's Hospital Medical Center analysed the problem of the treatment of colloid cysts endoscopically. Remarkable contributions in theory and practice of the development of neuroendoscopy we owe J. Camaert, J. Abdullah and L. Calliauw from Ghent, Belgium [33, 34]. Their reflections on technique and instrumentation in endoscopic diagnosis and treatment of para- and intraventricular cystic lesion should be compulsory lecture for every beginner in neuroendoscopy.

Since the beginning of the 1990s, the spectrum of indications in neuroendoscopy has been extended to cover also the treatment of spinal lesions. To H.M. Mayer and M. Brock from Berlin, Germany [35], the credit is principally due that they have extended the indication of neuroendoscopy in the field of endoscopic discectomy.

The early rudiments of a fundamentally new aspect in the practice of neuroendoscopy is due to A. Perneczky [36] with his "keyhole concept" in neurosurgery. He used the endoscope as an adjunct to the microscopic technique as endoscope-assisted microsurgery. The essence was less brain tissue traumatisation and better outcome concerning morbidity and mortality. That is in contrary to a pure endoscopic approach in which the endoscope is the only device for visualisation and tissue dissection.

This way of approaching the skull base is convincingly demonstrated by E. de Divitiis and P. Cappabianca [37] from Naples. They used the endoscope not only as an additional tool to the microscope. On the contrary, they moved to a pure endoscopic approach. The term "functional endoscopic pituitary surgery" (FEPS) summarised their basic contributions to indication, development of instruments and critical assessment of the outcome after pituitary surgery. Rodziewicz et al. [38] outlined the endoscopic approach to pituitary surgery and stated: "The authors experiences with this technique suggest that, properly used, endoscopes can increase the safety and decrease the postoperative facial discomfort of transphenoidal pituitary surgery". Coincident with the presentation of the keyhole concept, Al Benabid from Grenoble, France [39], opened a new chapter in neuroendoscopy and discussed the potential use of robots in endoscopic neurosurgery.

Bauer and Hellwig [40–45] initiated international workshops on "Minimally Invasive Neurosurgery, MIEN I and II and Minimally Invasive Techniques for Neurosurgery". Neurosurgeons from all over the world interested in neuroendoscopy came together for the first time. New and better understanding of the anatomy of the ventricles and changes in the operative strategy has been focus of discussions. Neurosurgeons demonstrated how highly sophisticated microinstruments, laser equipment, ultrasound guidance and neuronavigation have converted the endoscope from a pure "visualising instrument" into a real "surgical instrument". The results of the meetings have been published in Acta Neurochirurgica and pushed neuroendoscopy towards the forefront of neurosurgical interest. It was already at that time agreement and absolutely clear that endoscopic procedures have to be evaluated according to the standards of classical microneurosurgical operations. Contrasting views of various authors make it difficult to come to a consensus still today because there is a lack of a clear-cut list of indications for endoneurosurgical procedures. We still miss prospective randomised trials for most indications to be compared with the outcomes of the evaluated results of microneurosurgery. Last but not least, it was the aim of the workshops to come to a modest list of basic recommendations for the use of the endoscope in neurosurgery. Minimally invasive endoscopic neurosurgery requires besides new techniques and technologies also a better understanding concerning physiology and pathophysiology of CSF circulation system. The piecemeal resection of intra- and extracerebral space-occupying lesions is not the last attempt to introduce this technology into brain surgery.

Such consideration is to be commended, not least because medical history provides many examples of failed surgical approaches and techniques.

The current extended endoscopic approaches (EEA) are dominated by those who are pushing the frontiers. Some papers of the last years that come forward are of high neurosurgical interest. Only a few of the procedures are convincing in comparison with the established prospective and randomised standards of microneurosurgery. More recently comments given from authors experienced in extended endoscopic skull base surgery (EESS) delineate a careful optimistic glance of the future of EESS and may illustrate the actual discussion.

Some papers of the last year deal with the extended endoscopic skull base surgery. Surgical and nonsurgical problems should be emphasised in the context of pure endonasal endoscopic tumour resection. As with all new techniques that come forward for analysis when compared with the established microsurgical procedures a prospective critical review of the complications must be undertaken. Should extended endoscopic transphenoidal surgery be left in expert surgeon's hand? Is it surgery for every neurosurgeon? Is this approach (method) for the virtuosi only? Questions are up to now not answered. We have to keep in mind that space-occupying lesions of the skull base and processes in and surrounding the brain decide the fate and the destiny of the patient and not only the surgeon.

In most publications, EEA and EESS is a well-tolerated procedure, and the vast majority of the patients do well after tumour resection. Fewer papers published are about ophthalmological and endocrine functions; functions were reasonably well preserved and/or maintained. The problem not solved up to now concerns the rate of CSF leakage and its management.

> Well selected midline lesions that may be amenable to endonasal surgery will be treated in this way with a decrease in morbidity, it must be emphasized that this procedure should only be considered once the surgical team and surrounding equipment has acquired the appropriate experience (Kassam et al. [46]).

> In well selected cases this technique may provide an adjustive method for microsurgeon. It must be emphasized, however, that principles of microsurgical repair were strictly followed (Kassam et al. [47]).

> The majority of the patients underwent planned complete resection. In these patients, 73% had a gross-total resection without recurrency during a mean follow up of 34 months. No patient in this series experienced visual worsening. Postoperative rate of permanent diabetes insipidus (DI) was 8%. CSF leaks were documented in 58 % of patients. In 1 patient, a stroke occurred from a perforating vessel from a posterior cerebral artery injury. The authors conclude the Expended Endonasal Approach (EEA) for the resection of craniopharyngeomas provides acceptable results and holds the potential to improve outcomes (Gardener et al. [48]).

> Years ago I would have thought such an approach to the "retrochiasmatic" craniopharyngeoma would have been impossible. Now, with the advent of the techniques that have been uniquely shared by Neuroendoscopists and ENT surgeons craniopharyngeomas of most types can be the target of EEA. The EEA in this series was performed in adults. As craniopharyngeomas commonly occur in children, it would be interesting to use this approach in the child with a craniopharyngeoma. Limitations are small nares, nonpneumatized sella, smaller midline corridor between the carotid arteries. One can argue that the EEA may be a beneficial approach over craniotomy and subfrontal or pterional approaches to craniopharyngeomas (Rutka [49]).

> Limitations should not be underestimated. He emphasized the need for an incremental acquisition of skills before becoming confident with the peculiar anatomy and the manipulation of all structures. Necessity for dedicated instruments, all of which as yet are not available. Lack of initial skill, which makes the operative times longer.
>
> In the meantime there will be those who will be playing the role to push the frontiers and others who will move in subsequent advancements, trying to be at the same time in the game and in the posse, which is not always easy or even possible. We have to keep in mind sometimes it is the lesion and not the surgeon that decides the course of the disease and the destiny of the patient" (Cappabianca [50]).

> Endoscopic resection may be technically feasible for intraparenchymal brain tumors. Minimizing both corticotomy volume and white-matter dissection required to resect the tumor. Using dynamic retraction of the port and piecemeal extirpation, tumors much larger than the conduit itself can be effectively removed. In appropriately selected patients the port may offer a valuable option to achieve the goals of surgery – that is cytoreduction or radical tumor removal with an acceptable level of morbidity. Further prospective, randomized studies are essential and will help to delineate the applicability and safety of the procedure (Kassam et al. [51]).

Tabaee et al. in 2009 [52] summarised in their clinical article: "The results of this meta-analysis support the safety and short-term efficacy of endoscopic pituitary surgery. Future studies with long-term follow-up are required to determine tumor control".

So far up to the turning point of the millennium, the basic development of modern minimal endoscopic neurosurgery (MIEN) was far from being complete. Unresolved problems require future provision of well-organised workshops and meetings. Planning well-designed prospective, randomized trials to establish the results against standardised and proved outcomes of microneurosurgery is mandatory. The foundation of the "International Study Group on Neuroendoscopy" ISGNE in 2001 and since 2009 International Federation of Neuroendoscopy IFNE serves as an international platform for teamwork and development last but not least as a forum for international discussions and interchange of ideas.

Bernard of Chartres († 1124 a.c.), the Scholasticist, can clarify our actual standing: "We are dwarfs, sitting on the shoulders of giants. We can see more and further than they can, not because we have a superior vision or a superb conformation, but because their size causes, that we are lifted and carried".

References

1. Apuzzo ML (1977) Neurosurgical endoscopy using the side-viewing telescope. J Neurosurg 46(3): 398–400
2. Bozzini P (1806) Lichtleiter, eine Erfindung zur Anschauung innerer Theile und Krankheiten nebst der Abbildung. In: Hufeland CW (ed) Neues Journal der praktischen Heilkunde und Wundarzneykunst. Commission bei LW Wittich, Berlin, pp 108–124
3. Grant JA (1996) Victor Darwin Lespinasse: a biographical sketch. Neurosurgery 39(6):1232–1233
4. L'Espinasse VD (1936) Hydrocephalus and Spina bifida. In: Davis L (ed) The principles of neurological surgery. Lea et Febiger, Philadelphia, p 405
5. Nitze MCF (1998) Das Zystoskop mit distaler Beleuchtung als Schrittmacher der Endoskopie. In: Reuter MA (ed) Geschichte der Endoskopie. K. Krämer Verlag, Stuttgart, pp 170–222, 238
6. Leiter J (1998) Nachruf. In: Reuter MA (ed) Geschichte der Endoskopie. K. Krämer Verlag, Stuttgart, p 194
7. Dandy WE (1922) Cerebral ventriculoscopy – an operative procedure for hydrocephalus. Johns Hopkins Hosp Bull 33:189–190
8. Fay T, Grant F (1923) Ventriculostomy and intraventricular photography in internal hydrocephalus. JAMA 80:461–463
9. Mixter WJ (1923) Ventriculoscopy and puncture of the floor of the third ventricle. Boston Med Surg J 188:277–278
10. Putnam T (1934) Treatment of hydrocephalus by endoscopic coagulation of the choroid plexus. N Engl J Med 210:1373–1376
11. Scarff JE (1935) Third ventriculoscopy as the rational treatment of obstructive hydrocephalus. J Pediatr 6: 870–871
12. Scarff JE (1952) Nonobstructive hydrocephalus; treatment by endoscopic cauterization of the choroid plexus; long term results. J Neurosurg 9(2):164–176
13. Scarff JE (1963) Treatment of hydrocephalus: an historical and critical review of methods and results. J Neurol Neurosurg Psychiatry 26:1–26
14. Scarff JE (1966) Third ventriculostomy by puncture of the lamina terminalis and the floor of third ventricle. J Neurosurg 24(5):935–943
15. Pool JL (1938) Myeloscopy, diagnostic inspection of the cauda equina by means of an endoscope. Bull Neurol Inst N Y 7:178–189
16. Hopkins HH (1976) Optical principles of the endoscope. In: Berci G (ed) Endoscopy. Appleton Century Crofts, New York, pp 3–27
17. Ogata M, Ishikawa T et al (1965) Encephaloscope: basic study. J Neurosurg 22:288–291
18. Guiot G (1973) Ventriculo-cisternostomy for stenosis of the aqueduct of Sylvius. Puncture of the floor of the third ventricle with a leucotome under television control. Acta Neurochir (Wien) 28(4):275–289
19. Bushe KA, Halves E (1978) Modified technique in transsphenoidal operations of pituitary adenomas. Technical note (author's transl). Acta Neurochir (Wien) 41(1–3):163–175
20. Fukushima T, Ishijima B et al (1973) Ventriculofiberscope: a new technique for endoscopic diagnosis and operation. Technical note. J Neurosurg 38(2): 251–256
21. Auer LM (1985) Endoscopic evacuation of intracerebral haemorrhage. High-tech-surgical treatment – a new approach to the problem? Acta Neurochir (Wien) 74(3–4):124–128
22. Auer LM (1992) Ultrasound stereotaxic endoscopy in neurosurgery. Acta Neurochir Suppl (Wien) 54:34–41
23. Oppel F, Mulch G (1979) Selective trigeminal root section via an endoscopic transpyramidal retrolabyrinthine approach. Acta Neurochir Suppl (Wien) 28(2):565–571
24. DiMagno EP, Buxton JL et al (1980) Ultrasonic endoscope. Lancet 1(8169):629–631
25. Powers SK (1986) Fenestration of intraventricular cysts using a flexible, steerable endoscope and the argon laser. Neurosurgery 18(5):637–641

26. Griffith HB (1975) Technique of fontanelle and persutural ventriculoscopy and endoscopic ventricular surgery in infants. Childs Brain 1(6):359–363
27. Griffith HB (1986) Endoneurosurgery: endoscopic intracranial surgery. Adv Tech Stand Neurosurg 14:2–24
28. Jones RF, Kwok BC et al (1994) Neuroendoscopic third ventriculostomy. A practical alternative to extracranial shunts in non-communicating hydrocephalus. Acta Neurochir Suppl 61:79–83
29. Cohen AR (1993) Images in clinical medicine. Endoscopic laser third ventriculostomy. N Engl J Med 328(8):552
30. Cohen AR (1993) Endoscopic ventricular surgery. Pediatr Neurosurg 19(3):127–134
31. Manwaring KH (1992) Endoscopic ventricular fenestration. In: Manwaring KH, Crone K (eds) Neuroendoscopy. Mary Ann Liebert, New York, pp 121–152
32. Lewis AI, Crone KR et al (1994) Surgical resection of third ventricle colloid cysts. Preliminary results comparing transcallosal microsurgery with endoscopy. J Neurosurg 81(2):174–178
33. Caemaert J, Abdullah J (1993) Diagnostic and therapeutic stereotactic cerebral endoscopy. Acta Neurochir (Wien) 124(1):11–13
34. Caemaert J, Abdullah J et al (1994) A multipurpose cerebral endoscope and reflections on technique and instrumentation in endoscopic neurosurgery. Acta Neurochir Suppl 61:49–53
35. Mayer HM, Brock M (1993) Percutaneous endoscopic discectomy: surgical technique and preliminary results compared to microsurgical discectomy. J Neurosurg 78(2):216–225
36. Perneczky A, Fries G (1998) Endoscope-assisted brain surgery: part 1 – evolution, basic concept, and current technique. Neurosurgery 42(2):219–224; discussion 224–225
37. Cappabianca P, Alfieri A et al (1998) Endoscopic endonasal transsphenoidal approach to the sella: towards functional endoscopic pituitary surgery (FEPS). Minim Invasive Neurosurg 41(2):66–73
38. Rodziewicz AS, Kelley RT (1998) Endoscopic pituitary surgery: present and future. In: Hellwig D, Bauer BL et al (eds) Minimally invasive techniques for neurosurgery. Springer, Berlin/Heidelberg, pp 121–152
39. Benabid AL, Lavallee S et al (1992) Potential use of robots in endoscopic neurosurgery. Acta Neurochir Suppl (Wien) 54:93–97
40. Hellwig D, Bauer BL (1991) Endoscopic procedures in stereotactic neurosurgery. Acta Neurochir Suppl (Wien) 52:30–32
41. Hellwig D, Bauer BL (1992) Minimally invasive neurosurgery by means of ultrathin endoscopes. Acta Neurochir Suppl (Wien) 54:63–68
42. Bauer BL, Hellwig D (1994) Minimally invasive endoscopic neurosurgery – a survey. Acta Neurochir Suppl 61:1–12
43. Bauer BL, Hellwig D (1995) Intracranial and intraspinal endoscopy. In: Schmidek HH, Sweet WH (eds) Operative neurosurgical techniques. Indication, methods and results. W.B. Saunders Company, Philadelphia, pp 695–713
44. Hellwig D, Bauer BL (1998) Three-dimensional-endoscopy: a useful tool for neuroendoscopy? An anatomical study using MRI and three–dimensional endoscopy. In: Minimally invasive techniques for neurosurgery. Springer, Berlin/Heidelberg, pp 37–45
45. Hellwig D, Grotenhuis JA et al (2005) Endoscopic third ventriculostomy for obstructive hydrocephalus. Neurosurg Rev 28(1):1–34; discussion 35–38
46. Kassam AB, Mintz AH et al (2006) The expanded endonasal approach for an endoscopic transnasal clipping and aneurysmorrhaphy of a large vertebral artery aneurysm: technical case report. Neurosurgery 59(1 Suppl 1):ONSE162–ONSE165; discussion ONSE162–165
47. Kassam AB, Gardner PA et al (2007) Endoscopic endonasal clipping of an unsecured superior hypophyseal artery aneurysm. Technical note. J Neurosurg 107(5):1047–1052
48. Gardner PA, Kassam AB et al (2008) Outcomes following endoscopic, expanded endonasal resection of suprasellar craniopharyngiomas: a case series. J Neurosurg 109(1):6–16
49. Rutka JT (2008) Endonasal resection of craniopharyngiomas. J Neurosurg 109:1
50. Cappabianca P, Cavallo LM et al (2008) Craniopharyngiomas. J Neurosurg 109:1–3
51. Kassam AB, Engh JA et al (2009) Completely endoscopic resection of intraparenchymal brain tumors. J Neurosurg 110(1):116–123
52. Tabaee A, Anand VK et al (2009) Endoscopic pituitary surgery: a systematic review and meta-analysis. J Neurosurg 111(3):545–554

2 The Application of Neuroendoscopic Techniques in Improving Altered CSF Physiology

Yavor P. Enchev and Shizuo Oi

2.1 CSF Dynamics (Production, Flow, and Absorption)

The study of CSF dynamics is scientific area of interest of both basic researchers and clinicians with many still existing problems to be solved associated with significant expectations for improvement of the clinical outcome [2, 6, 10, 15, 16, 18, 19, 48–50, 53–55, 57, 61, 62, 75, 76, 84].

Cerebrospinal fluid (CSF) represents the natural optimal environment for the central nervous system (brain and spinal cord). CSF dynamics, being an integrated part of the intracranial dynamics, is reciprocally dependent on the dynamics of the brain and the intracranial blood (arterial and venous). The continuum of CSF dynamics includes three simultaneous and continuous processes: CSF production, CSF flow, and CSF absorption [10].

CSF is produced mainly (50–70 %) by the choroid plexus in both lateral ventricles as well as in the third and fourth ventricles. The remainder is produced by the ventricular ependyma, pia-arachnoid capillaries, and brain parenchyma. The overall rate of daily CSF production is about 500 ml or 0.35 ml/min, with three to four times turnover of the persistent CSF volume in man, which is about 140 ml with 25 ml intraventricular and 115 ml extraventricular volumes.

CSF flows from the lateral ventricles through the foramina of Monro (interventricular foramens) into the third ventricle. Then the CSF circulates consecutively through the aqueductus sylvii (cerebral aqueduct) into the fourth ventricle and leaves the intraventricular space through the foramina of Luschka (lateral apertures) and through the foramen of Magendie (medial aperture). After entering the cisterns of subarachnoid space, the CSF reaches the arachnoid granulations in the regions adjacent to the superior sagittal sinus.

CSF absorption or transfer from the subarachnoid space to the venous system is mainly realized by the arachnoid villi. The extra-arachnoid sites for CSF absorption include ventricular ependyma (subependymal veins), leptomeninges (cortical veins), pia-arachnoid capillaries, choroid plexus, and perineural space (lymphatic channels).

2.2 Disorders of CSF Dynamics

The pathophysiology of altered CSF dynamics is subject of numerous scientific studies [48–50, 53–55, 57, 62, 75, 76].

2.2.1 Disorders of the CSF Production

The only one known, clinically significant disorder of the CSF production is the CSF

Y.P. Enchev, MD, PhD, FRCS (✉)
Department of Neurosurgery, University Hospital Sv. Marina, Medical University – Varna, Varna, Bulgaria
e-mail: dr.y.enchev@gmail.com

S. Oi, MD, PhD
President, St. Thomas University, Amagasaki, Hyogo, Japan

S. Sgouros (ed.), *Neuroendoscopy*,
DOI 10.1007/978-3-642-39085-2_2,

overproduction by choroid plexus papilloma. Usually, in these cases the CSF flow and CSF absorption are intact initially but excessively overloaded. However, later due to the tumor growth and CSF metastases, the risk for obstruction of the CSF flow increases.

Abnormal, clinically significant CSF hypoproduction is not described in the literature up to date.

2.2.2 Disorders of the CSF Flow

The disorders of the CSF flow could be classified according to the point of obstruction. The critical points of potential obstruction are four: foramen of Monro, aqueductus sylvii, fourth ventricle foramina, and the transition between spinal and cranial subarachnoid space. The obstruction could be as a result of congenital atresia or stenosis; ventriculitis; tumor; subarachnoid hemorrhage; choroid plexus hyperplasia or cyst; AVM of the choroid plexus; basilar artery aneurysms or ectasia; functional changes following ventriculoperitoneal, ventriculoatrial, or lumbo-peritoneal CSF shunts; and Arnold-Chiari malformation.

2.2.3 Disorders of the CSF Absorption

Disorders of CSF absorption are caused by obstruction of the arachnoid granulations/villi as a consequence of infection or hemorrhage or by venous hypertension due to sinus thrombosis and pseudotumour cerebri.

2.3 Neuroendoscopic Treatment of the Disorders of CSF Dynamics (Table 2.1)

2.3.1 Neuroendoscopic Treatment of the Disorders of CSF Production

Currently neuroendoscopic treatment of the disorders of CSF production does not exist.

2.3.2 Neuroendoscopic Treatment of Disorders of CSF Flow

The historical trends of neuroendoscopic surgical technique in the treatment of hydrocephalus were thoroughly discussed by the authors in a previous paper [17].

2.3.2.1 Neuroendoscopic Treatment of Obstruction of Foramen of Monro: Unilateral or Bilateral

Neuroendoscopic Foraminoplasty of Foramen of Monro (NEFPFMO)

Indications. NEFPFMO, although infrequently applied in clinical practice, represents the most physiologic surgical approach in the treatment of isolated obstruction or stenosis of foramen of Monro caused by membranous occlusion of the interventricular foramen, leading to restoration of the natural CSF flow. In cases with unclear ventricular landmarks and difficult intraoperative orientation, neuronavigation is extremely valuable in defining the margins of obstructed foramen of Monro and the neighboring eloquent neurovascular structures, thus preventing procedure-related injuries.

Operative technique. The surgical technique of NEFPFMO is straightforward without any significant nuances. The burr hole for NEFPFMO is usually positioned 2–3 cm laterally to the midline and 2–3 cm in front of the coronal suture. After penetration of the dilated lateral ventricle, the obstructed foramen of Monro could be found by tracing up the choroid plexus from the body of the lateral ventricle to its passage to the third ventricle, just behind the fornix. Another landmark is the junction point of the choroid plexus, the thalamostriate vein and the septal vein. However, in complicated cases neuronavigation could be a very useful adjunct. The fenestration of the membrane is usually bluntly performed with or without prior coagulation of the ependyma. The next step is the dilatation with a micro balloon catheter. In patients with high risk of re-occlusion, the implantation of interventricular stent is reasonable and must be judged.

Clinical experience. NEFPFMO is not frequently reported in the literature.

Table 2.1 Neuroendoscopic techniques in the treatment of the altered CSF dynamics

Disorder of the CSF dynamics	Cause	Neuroendoscopic treatment								
			Neuroendoscopic techniques							
		Yes/no	Neuro-endoscopic foramino-plasty of foramen of Monro (NEFPFMO)	Neuro-endoscopic septostomy (NESS)	Neuro-endoscopic aqueducto-plasty (NEAP)	Neuro-endoscopic third ventri-culostomy (NETV)	Neuro-endoscopic lamina terminalis fenestration (NELTF)	Neuro-endoscopic foramino-plasty of foramen of Magendie (NEFPFMA)	Neuro-endoscopic foramino-plasty of foramen of Luschka (NEFPFL)	Neuro-endoscopic fourth ventri-culostomy (NEFV)
Disorder of the CSF production										
Hyperproduction	Choroid plexus papilloma	No								
Hypoproduction		No								
Disorder of the CSF flow										
Obstruction of foramen of Monro	Congenital atresia or stenosis; ventriculitis; tumor; subarachnoid hemorrhage; choroid plexus hyperplasia or cyst; AVM of the choroid plexus; basilar artery aneurysms or ectasia; functional changes following ventriculoperitoneal, ventriculoatrial, or lumbo-peritoneal CSF shunts; post-NETV; Arnold-Chiari malformation	Yes	(+)	(+)	0	0	0	0	0	0
Obstruction of aqueductus sylvii		Yes	0	0	(+)	(+)	(+)	0	0	0
Obstruction of fourth ventricle foramina		Yes	0	0	0	(+)	(+)	(+)	(+)	(+)
Obstruction of the transition between spinal and cranial subarachnoid space		Yes				(+)	(+)			
Disorder of the CSF absorption										
Obstruction of the arachnoid villi	Infection or hemorrhage	No								
Venous hypertension	Sinus thrombosis or pseudotumour cerebri	No								

In 1996, Mohanty et al. [42] reported a case of unilateral hydrocephalus caused by membranous occlusion of the ipsilateral foramen of Monro. NEFPFMO was successfully performed simultaneously with fenestration of septum pellucidum.

In 1999, S. Oi et al. [58] in their series described one case with post-shunt monoventricular unilateral hydrocephalus handled effectively by NEFPFMO and neuroendoscopic septostomy (NESS). S. Oi, first in the literature, introduced the term "foraminal plasty of foramen of Monro."

In 2000, T.T. Wong and and L.S. Lee [85] reported two cases of membranous occlusion of the foramen of Monro with a consequent lateral ventricle dilatation as a complication of ventriculoperitoneal CSF drainage. The patients underwent NEFPFMO of the affected foramen of Monro (in one case NEFPFMO of both foramina of Monro) and neuroendoscopic third ventriculostomy (NETV). The result was excellent in one case, and shunt insertion followed in the other.

In 2001, J. Javier-Fernandez et al. [33] described an adult patient with isolated monoventricular unilateral hydrocephalus due to the obstruction of the foramen of Monro by a thin membrane. NEFPFMO was performed successfully.

In 2007, H. Moriet al. [43] described a case of endoscopic stent placement for treatment of secondary bilateral occlusion of the Monro foramina following endoscopic third ventriculostomy in a patient with aqueductal stenosis. From the very beginning of her clinical history, the patient was treated by ventriculoperitoneal shunt for tri-ventricular hydrocephalus due to aqueductal stenosis. Six years later an MR imaging demonstrated slit-like ventricle with the ventricular catheter and dilated contralateral and third ventricles. NESS and NETV were performed with excellent postoperative clinical recovery and with restoration of the normal ventricle configuration on control postoperative MR images. However, 2 years later the patient's complaints reappeared and MRI revealed dilatation of both lateral ventricles with a patient stoma on the third ventricle floor. The patient underwent re-NESS and NEFPFMO by fiberscope as well as implantation of stent through one of the foramina of Monro with excellent clinical and radiological recovery at 3-year follow-up.

In 2008, S. Oi and and Y. Enchev [52] in their detailed study of NEFPFMO in the treatment of isolated unilateral hydrocephalus presented two personal cases, thoroughly reviewed the literature, and analyzed the applied surgical techniques. S. Oi and Y. Enchev described the first neuronavigational NEFPFMO performed alone without any additional neuroendoscopic procedure. The neuronavigation was used to point the most appropriate entry point and to outline the borders of the obstructed foramen of Monro (Fig. 2.1).

In 2008, De Bonis et al. [13] presented an adult patient with idiopathic occlusion of the foramina of Monro. NEFPFMO was performed unilaterally due to the observed wide fenestration of septum pellucidum. At the end of the procedure, an intraventricular catheter with subcutaneous Rickham reservoir was inserted. Six months later the patient was without any complaints and follow-up MRI demonstrated gradually decreasing ventricular size.

In 2010, Sharifi et al. [74] described a case of adult post-shunt bilateral occlusion of foramina of Monro treated successfully by simultaneous NESS and bilateral NEFPFMO.

In 2011, S. Kalhorn et al. [36] reported a case of an idiopathic bilateral stenosis of the foramen of Monro treated effectively by image-guided NEFPFMO and NESS. The authors approached the narrower lateral ventricle in order to enable a safer penetration into the contralateral frontal horn during NESS.

In 2012, El Refaee et al. [14] published a unique case of bilateral occlusion of the foramina of Monro as a consequence of third ventriculostomy performed with clinical success 30 months ago. Since the septum pellucidum was perforated as a result of chronic hydrocephalus, the patient underwent unilateral NEFPFMO together with implantation of a silicon stent through the restored interventricular foramen. To prevent the intraventricular stent migration, it was fixed to

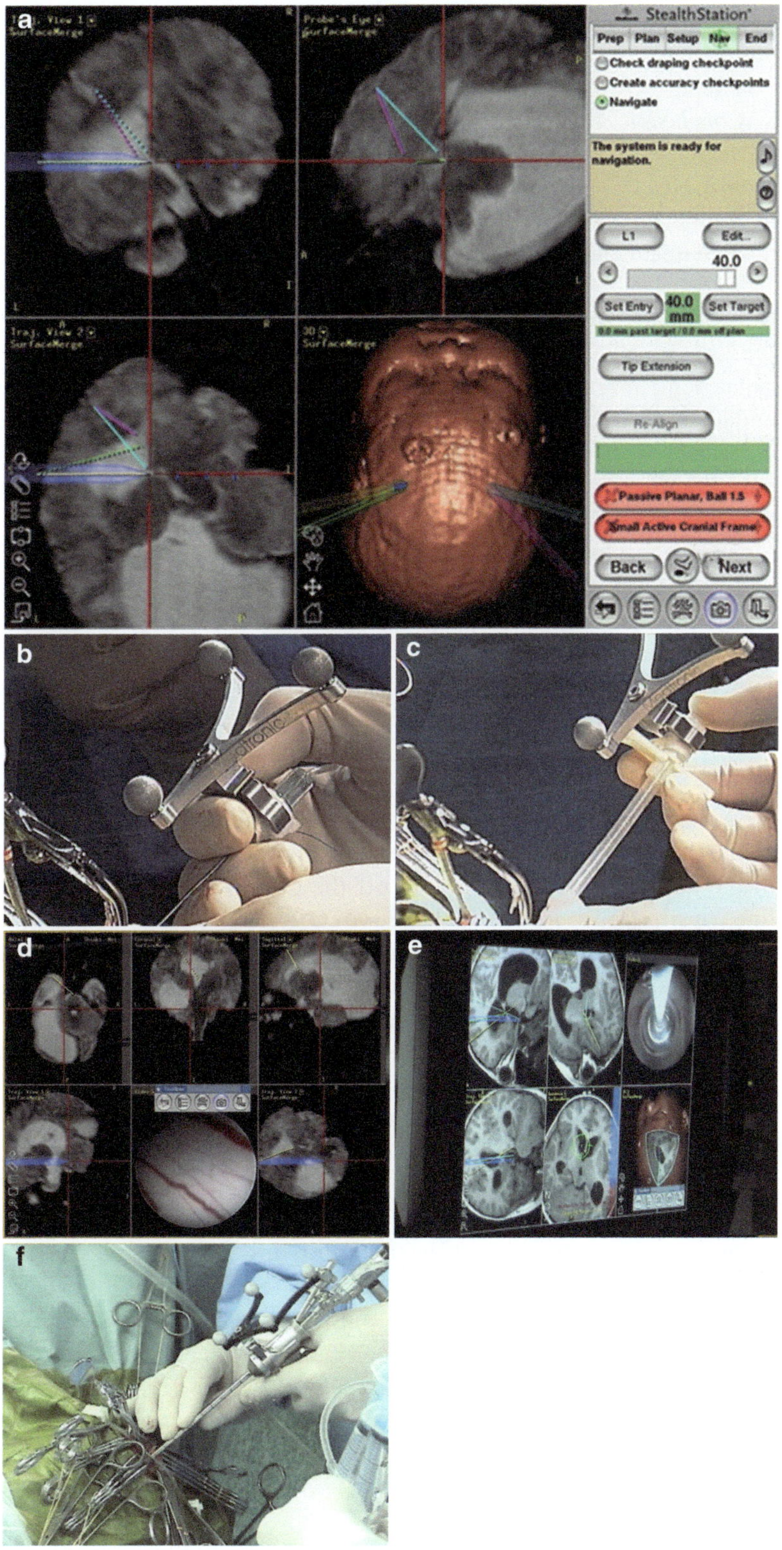

Fig. 2.1 Navigational neuroendoscopic foraminal plasty of foramen of Monro, clinical case. (**a**, **d**, **e**) Navigational guidance to the occluded foramen of Monro. (**b**, **c**) The ventricular puncture needle and the transparent peel-away sheath with the navigational reference star. (**f**) Freehand maneuver of a small-diameter rigid-rod neuroendoscope [56] with the navigational reference (Reproduced with permission from Enchev and Oi [17])

subcutaneous Rickham reservoir. Ten months postoperatively, the clinical and image result was excellent.

Conclusion. In the cases with unilateral or bilateral obstruction or stenosis of foramen of Monro, NEFPFMO as a stand-alone procedure or in combination with NESS represents safe and reliable treatment option.

Neuroendoscopic Septostomy (NESS)

Indications. NESS is indicated in patients with isolated monoventricular hydrocephalus due to unilateral obstruction of the foramen of Monro associated with distorted intraventricular anatomy landmarks of the effaced foramen and thus expected risky NEFPFMO. If both foramina of Monro are occluded and septum pellucidum is intact, NESS is preferable to bilateral foraminoplasty because the former procedure is technically easier and the latter has the risk of bilateral fornix injury. In symptomatic cavum septum pellucidum, NESS is the treatment of choice.

Operative technique. NESS could be performed as a single procedure or simultaneously with NEFPFMO. In cases indicated for NESS alone, the burr hole is usually positioned in front of the coronal suture and 5–6 cm off the midline, ipsilaterally to the enlarged ventricle. Frameless stereotaxy could be useful in defining the optimal position of the entry point, in guiding the trocar through the parenchyma and in selecting the most secured fenestration site. Usually, the septostomy is performed bluntly in a thin avascular part followed by balloon dilatation. The eventual bleeding from septum pellucidum vessels could be controlled by continuous irrigation or by bipolar cautery. The resulted communication between both lateral ventricles must be wide enough to reduce the risk for re-occlusion.

Clinical experience. NESS is more frequently reported in the literature than NEFPFMO.

In 1991, C. Heilman and A. Cohen [30] described two NESS performed by the so-called saline torch. In the follow-up period, no additional treatment was required.

In 1994, M. Walker et al. [82] reported a series of nine NESS. Unsatisfactory results, in long follow-up period, were attained in only two patients.

In 1998, M. R. Gaab and H. W. Schroeder [22] described 4 patients with NESS. In 10 months mean follow-up reduced ventricular volumes were observed in all cases.

In 1999, three series of NESS were published. In the study of M. Gangemi et al. [24], five patients with monoventricular hydrocephalus underwent NESS. Within a follow-up period of almost 3 years, the clinical results were excellent in all cases, which were asymptomatic.

S. Oi et al. [58] reported five cases with different forms of hydrocephalus successfully treated by NESS (with clinical and radiological improvement at follow-up).

J. U. Choi et al. [7] described ten patients with NESS for obstructed ventricles due to various pathologies. The authors found that NESS makes shunting possible and reasonable in all cases.

In 2002, M. Fritsch and M. Mehdorn [20] in their paper "Endoscopic intraventricular surgery for treatment of hydrocephalus and loculated CSF space in children less than 1 year of age" presented a case of failed NESS with a consequent CSF shunt insertion.

In 2003, H. Hamada et al. [29] reported a series of 20 patients with isolated monoventricular hydrocephalus treated by NESS. NESS was unsuccessful in two adult patients due to thick septum pellucidum and limited working space. NESS was repeated in two children. In the remaining patients, good results were achieved without septostomy-related morbidity.

In 2003, P. Aldana et al. [1] published their experience with 43 NESS in 32 patients. During the mean follow-up of 2.5 years, the primary septostomies persisted in more than half of the cases. Ten patients underwent second NESS following the re-occlusion of their initial septal fenestration, with clinical success in 9 of them. The repeat NESS on the last follow-up revealed septostomy failure rate of less than 20 %. Based on these results, it was summarized that NESS represents effective and reliable treatment option for both initial and recurrent isolated lateral ventricle hydrocephalus, preventing insertion of CSF shunts.

In 2004, T. Beems and J. Grotenhuis [3] in their study of long-term complications of neuroendoscopic procedures presented a series of 21 NESS with or without NETV with 95 % success rate. Procedure-related complications were 10 % and mortality rate 0 %.

In 2008, S. Oi and Y. Enchev [52] described a case of congenital isolated unilateral hydrocephalus successfully treated by NESS in combination with NEFPFMO.

In 2009, J. Oertel et al. [45] in their series of 134 neuroendoscopic procedures in children presented 13 NESS in 12 patients. NESS was associated with NETV in five cases, with tumor biopsy in 3, with stent insertion in 2, with cystoventriculostomy in 1, and with aqueductoplasty in one. Clinical and radiological benefit was achieved in 6 patients. Four patients became shunt dependent. Clinical and radiological success rate was worst in children younger than 6 months of age.

In the same year, same authors [46] described a series of 32 NESS performed in 30 patients. The CSF flow disorder was caused by neoplasm (16 cases), multiloculated cystic hydrocephalus (8 cases, including 2 revisions), septum pellucidum cysts (3 cases), membranous or inflammatory isolated lateral ventricles (3 cases), and giant aneurysms (2 cases). NESS was combined in one stage with 13 endoscopic tumor biopsies/resections, 9 NETV, and 9 other neuroendoscopic procedures. During the mean follow-up period of 26 months, 26 patients improved clinically.

In 2011, F. Vaz-Guimaraes Filho et al. [80] reported seven adult patients with unilateral hydrocephalus, selected out of their almost 800 neuroendoscopic procedures in a 15-year period. All but one case (6/7) were with intraventricular cysticercosis and one (1/7) with congenital stenosis of foramen of Monro. NESS restored the CSF flow in all seven patients with uneventful postoperative period and excellent clinical outcome during the mean follow-up of 66 months.

In 2012, G. Tamburrini et al. [77] described a series of 63 patients (50 adults and 13 children) which underwent NESS during the period of 10 years. In 46 of the patients, all adults, hydrocephalus was due to neoplasm; in 11 the etiology was postinfectious and/or posthemorrhagic; and in the remaining 6 patients, hydrocephalus was malformative. The authors succeeded to perform NESS in all but 2 posthemorrhagic cases, presenting with a dense multilayered septum; 37 out of 63 patients underwent simultaneously one or more additional neuroendoscopic procedures. During the mean follow-up of 2 years, all but one patient demonstrated clinical and radiological improvement.

Conclusion. NESS is a reasonable treatment option for selected cases of isolated lateral ventricle with negligible procedure-related morbidity and mortality. Hence, NESS as a stand-alone procedure or in combination with NEFPFMO must be the treatment of choice of these forms of disordered CSF dynamics. Neuronavigation is usually dispensable. Difficulties in performing NESS could be expected in postinfectious ventricle causing thickening of the septum.

2.3.2.2 Neuroendoscopic Treatment of Obstruction of Aqueductus Sylvii

Neuroendoscopic Aqueductoplasty (NEAP)

Indications. NEAP with or without aqueductal stenting is indicated in cases with membranous aqueductal stenosis. NEAP could be performed alone or in combination with NETV.

Operative technique. The position of the entry point is selected based on detailed analysis of CT and especially MR images or with the aid of neuronavigation. Most frequently its coordinates are about 2 cm off the midline and 3–5 cm in front of the coronal suture, depending on the width of the foramen of Monro. Following the inspection of the floor of the third ventricle and the proximal part of the aqueduct, the NEAP is performed by the tip of Fogarty balloon catheter. If it is necessary a delicate dilatation of the perforation could be accomplished by inflation of the micro balloon. Further inspection of the distal aqueductal part and the foramina of the fourth ventricle could be performed by flexible neuroendoscope but with substantial risk for iatrogenic injury of the tectal region.

Clinical experience. NEAP is one of the infrequent neuroendoscopic procedures in treatment of disordered CSF flow. The idea for aqueductoplasty belonged to Dandy [11] as he was the first to perform aqueductal reconstruction by open surgery in 1920.

In 1993, Oka et al. [60] described a series of seven anterograde NEAP, performed by flexible neuroendoscope, simultaneously with NETV in patients with obstructive hydrocephalus due to aqueductal stenosis. Procedure-related complications were not observed. All but one patient did not require CSF shunt insertion during the follow-up period.

In 1999, Oi et al. [58] reported the first 2 cases with NEAP as a stand-alone procedure for distal membranous aqueductal stenosis. One of the patients underwent anterograde and the other retrograde NEAP. However, subsequent restenosis occurred.

In 1999, H. W. Schroeder and M. R. Gaab [70] presented a heterogeneous series of 17 NEAP: NEAP as a stand-alone procedure, NEAP in combination with NETV, and NEAP plus subsequent aqueductal stenting. In 6 of the patients diplopia was observed as a procedure-related complication. Within the mean follow-up of 1.5 years, the clinical results were satisfactory in all but 6 of the cases.

In 1999, C. Teo et al. [78] described their experience with neuroendoscopic treatment of trapped fourth ventricle, including 4 NEAP, one of them via suboccipital approach. In two of the cases restenosis was successfully treated by combination of NEAP and aqueductal stenting.

In 2004, M. Fritsch et al. [21] reported 8 patients with NEAP as a stand-alone procedure and 5 patients with NEAP plus aqueductal stent implantation. In the first group 6 restenoses were observed. However, in the second group no complications were found.

In 2004, H. Schroeder et al. [72] described a series of 39 NEAP in 33 patients with noncommunicating hydrocephalus due to aqueductal stenosis. NEAP was combined with NETV in 13 patients and with aqueductal stenting in 1. The success rate in the whole group was 76 % and higher (82 %) in the group with NEAP alone. In 22 patients radiological improvement was noticed. During the follow-up period of 40 months, aqueductal restenosis occurred in seven cases. The authors concluded that even the initial success rate of NEAP was comparable to that of NETV; with longer follow-up the aqueductal restenosis rate became higher.

In 2005, J. Sansone and B. Iskandar [65] presented 11 NEAP by trans-foramen magnum trans-fourth ventricle approach in 9 patients with membranous aqueductal stenosis. At the end of the almost 2-year-long follow-up period, all the patients were symptom-free. One case underwent two subsequent re-NEAP procedures as an attempt to treat the restenosis. However, aqueductal stenting was needed ultimately. The authors recommended their technique to be applied by experienced neuroendoscopist for selected cases.

In 2005, Gavish et al. [25] reported a series of 5 NEAP through a "tailored craniocervical approach." The selected patients presented with a distal membranous aqueductal stenosis. The postoperative course was uneventful with excellent clinical and radiological outcome in all patients. Based on these excellent results, the authors advocated their approach as a reliable alternative to other neuroendoscopic techniques.

In 2006, G. Cinalli et al. [9] described 7 complicated cases with posthemorrhagic and postinfectious loculated hydrocephalus previously treated by CSF shunting and in 5 of them by other neuroendoscopic procedures for supratentorial isolated compartments. Three of the patients underwent NEAP alone and the remaining 4 NEAP plus aqueductal stenting. Supratentorial approach was used in 5 cases and infratentorial in 2. All patients improved clinically and radiologically. Two of the patients without aqueductal stent experienced restenosis.

In 2009, J. Oertel et al. [45] reported 14 NEAP in 14 children. NEAP was combined with NETV (9 cases), aqueductal stenting (5 cases), NESS (1 case), and tumor removal (1 case). Excellent outcome was achieved clinically in 57 % and radiologically in 43 %. Restenosis of the cerebral aqueduct was confirmed in 3 patients. During the follow-up period, 53 % needed CSF shunting. Permanent procedure-related complications were observed in 2 patients.

Conclusion. NEAP is a tricky procedure with significant potential hazards for the fornix, the floor of the third ventricle, and especially for the periaqueductal parenchyma. NEAP is indicated in cases with short or membranous proximal (anterograde NEAP) or distal (retrograde NEAP) aqueductal stenosis as well as in cases in whom NETV is contraindicated due to a dense and thick third ventricle floor or to an atypical position of the basilar tip at the prospective fenestration site. In most of the cases, if available, neuronavigation could be useful for planning and guiding. Aqueductal stenting as an addition of NEAP most probably reduces the restenosis rate.

Neuroendoscopic Third Ventriculostomy (NETV)

Indications. NETV is indicated in any case of obstruction of the CSF flow distal to the floor of the third ventricle, including the patients with aqueductal stenosis and occlusion.

Operative technique. The preoperative analysis of sagittal and coronal MR images is of utmost importance for the precise planning of the burr hole position in a trajectory line with the foramen of Monro and the optimal position of the ventriculostomy. Important consideration is full awareness of the relation between the third ventricle floor and the basilar artery. Neuronavigation is highly recommended if it is available. The entry point is usually 2–3 cm off the midline and in front of the coronal suture. After entering the lateral ventricle, the endoscope is advanced through the foramen of Monro. The floor of the third ventricle is inspected, and the infundibular recess and mamillary bodies are identified (Fig. 2.2). According to the individual anatomical peculiarities, the best position of the stoma is defined in order to prevent neurovascular injury. Usually, the safest perforation site is in the center of the triangle with angles of the mamillary bodies and infundibular recess, just behind the clivus [73]. The blunt perforation by rigid instrument is the preferred method. Schroeder et al. [73] recommend avoidance from perforation of the floor by the tip of balloon catheter, because of the risk of slippage of the tip and eventual consequent neurovascular damage (Fig. 2.3). In cases with dense thick floor in which the blunt perforation could be associated with significant hypothalamic traction, the reasonable approach is the bipolar cauterization. The initial perforation is dilated by Fogarty balloon catheter, inflated with fluid, to dimensions of 3–6 mm in diameter [73]. The underlying interpeduncular and pontine cisterns could be inspected and the Liliequist membrane is perforated.

Clinical experience. Currently, NETV is the most frequently performed neuroendoscopic procedure.

The first NETV in history was performed by William Mixter, a urologist, in 1923 [41], using a urethroscope. Despite the technical imperfections, the postoperative course in his child patient with noncommunicating hydrocephalus was uneventful, and the clinical result was excellent.

The next reports of NETV were 12 years later in 1935 and 1936, by J. Scarff [66, 67]. Scarff used a sophisticated endoscope equipped with an electrode for coagulation, system for irrigation, and special tip for performing the third ventriculostomy. Based on his clinical results and autopsy studies, Scarff concluded that simple puncture fenestration was not functionally enough and that further dilatation of perforation was necessary.

In the 1960s, J. Scarff published his long-term results with NETV and choroid plexus coagulation [68, 69].

In 1968, G. Guiot reported NETV by leucotome with ventriculographic guidance with satisfying results [28].

In 1976, H. J. Hoffman described a series of NETV under stereotactic guidance and made extensive review of the literature with 797 cases of NETV [32]. Hoffman found that stereotactic NETV was a reliable minimal invasive treatment option of obstructive hydrocephalus.

In 1978, J. Vries [81] reported the first hydrocephalic patients who underwent NETV by flexible fiberscope. Unfortunately, all five cases later became CSF shunt dependent.

In 1990, R. Jones et al. [34] presented a series of NETV in 24 patients with different forms of hydrocephalus. Half of the patients did not require CSF shunt insertion. In 1994, R. Jones reported clinically successful NETV in 61 % of 103 patients [35].

In 1996, A. Rieger et al. [63] described ultrasound-guided NETV for noncommunicating

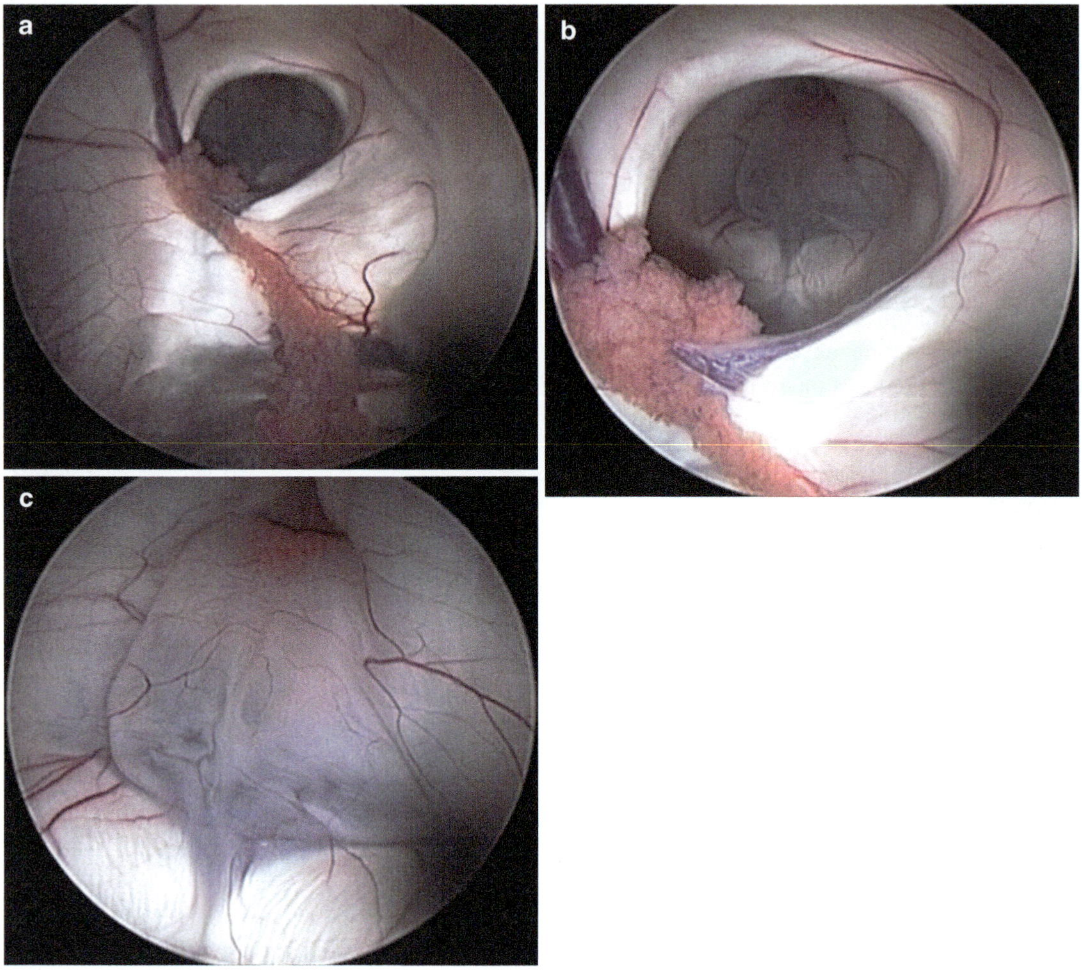

Fig. 2.2 High-resolution neuroendoscopic surgical field approach to the floor of the third ventricle. (**a**) Note the choroid plexus, septal vein, and the foramen of Monro. (**b**) Note the landmarks of the third ventricle floor. (**c**) The floor of the third ventricle with the mamillary bodies and the infundibular recesses. Note the partial transparency of the floor (Reproduced with permission from Enchev and Oi [17])

hydrocephalus in 12 patients. Intraoperative ultrasound guidance was sufficiently effective and reliable tool in defining the optimal trajectory through the foramen of Monro. The method was equally accurate to stereotaxy but more rapid and intuitive. No procedure-related complications were reported. The clinical outcome was excellent in 75 % of the patients and acceptable in the rest. During the long-term follow-up, MR examinations demonstrated the existence of ventriculostomy.

In 1998, V. Rohde et al. [64] reported neuronavigational NETV in ten patients with hydrocephalus. The entry point, the target point, and the optimal trajectory through the foramen of Monro were neuronavigationally preplanned. The neuronavigational NETV was performed frameless but arm based. In all but one patient with very small third ventricle, NETV were successfully performed without any procedure-related complications. In that series neuronavigational guidance was safe, reliable, and effective. The authors summarized that neuronavigational guidance of neuroendoscope ensured intraoperative neurovascular protection.

In 1999, G. Cinalli et al. [8] presented 119 cases of NETV compared with 94 cases of third ventriculostomy performed by the aid of ventriculographic guidance for the treatment of aqueductal stenosis. The success rate of whole series was 72 % (6-year follow-up period) as 29 patients became shunt dependent and re-NETV was performed in 9 cases.

In 1999, M. Gangemi et al. [23] described a series of 125 NETV for obstructive hydrocephalus, using flexible neuroendoscope. The overall success rate (shunt independency) was 86 % with rare and frequently transient procedure-related complications and absent mortality. The authors suggested widened indications of NETV in every case of distorted CSF flow distally to the third ventricle floor and preserved CSF absorption.

In 2000, S. Oi et al. [59] defined a new form of hydrocephalus, "long-standing overt ventriculomegaly in adults" ("LOVA"). Eight patients with LOVA underwent NETV and one aqueductoplasty (Fig. 2.4). During follow-up of 6 months to 13 years, all cases demonstrated clinical improvement in different degree independently of the

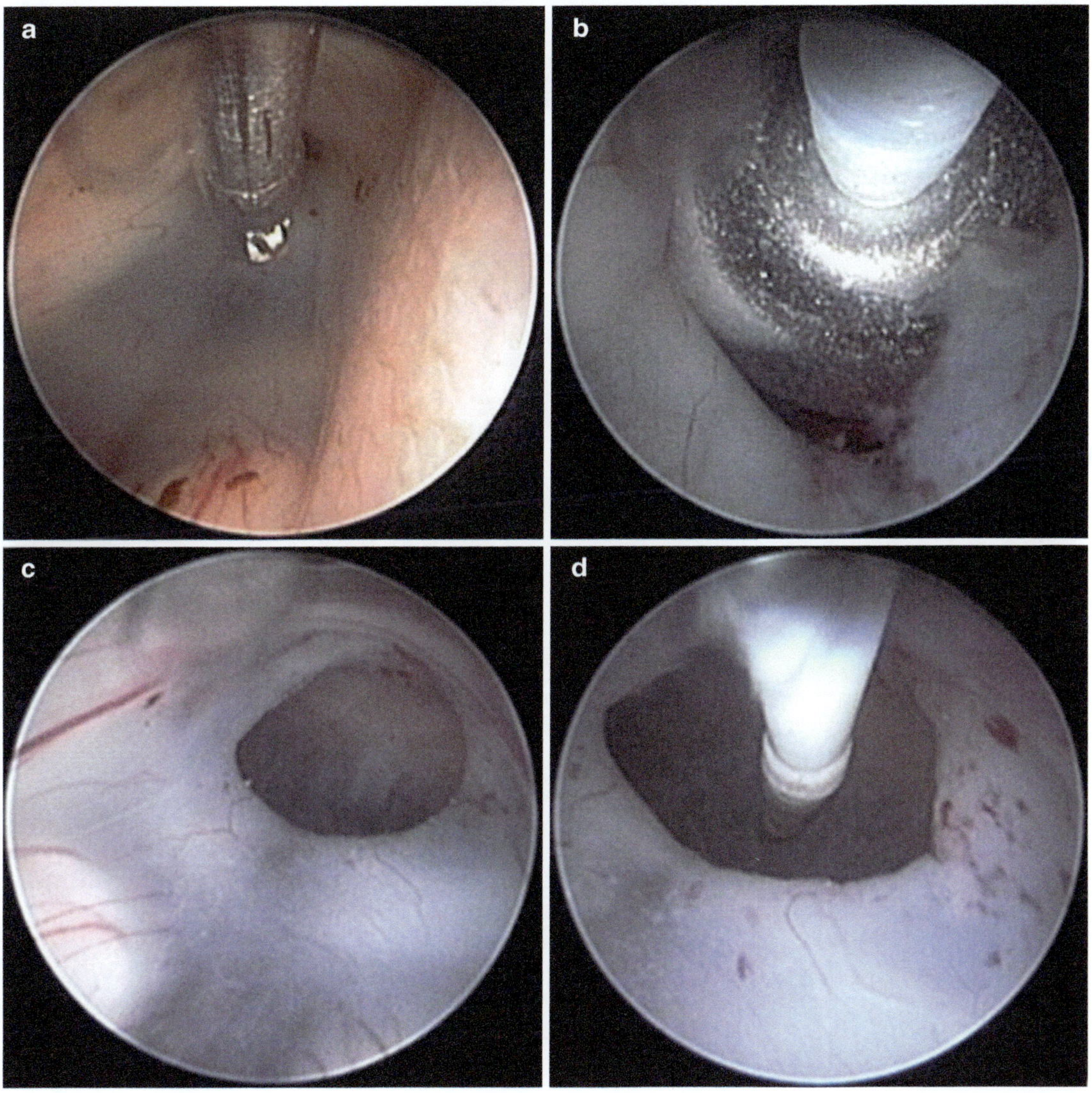

Fig. 2.3 Neuroendoscopic third ventriculostomy (NETV). Note the fenestration of Liliequist membrane (**c**–**f**) as additional and separated procedure after NETV (**a**, **b**) (Reproduced with permission from Enchev and Oi [17])

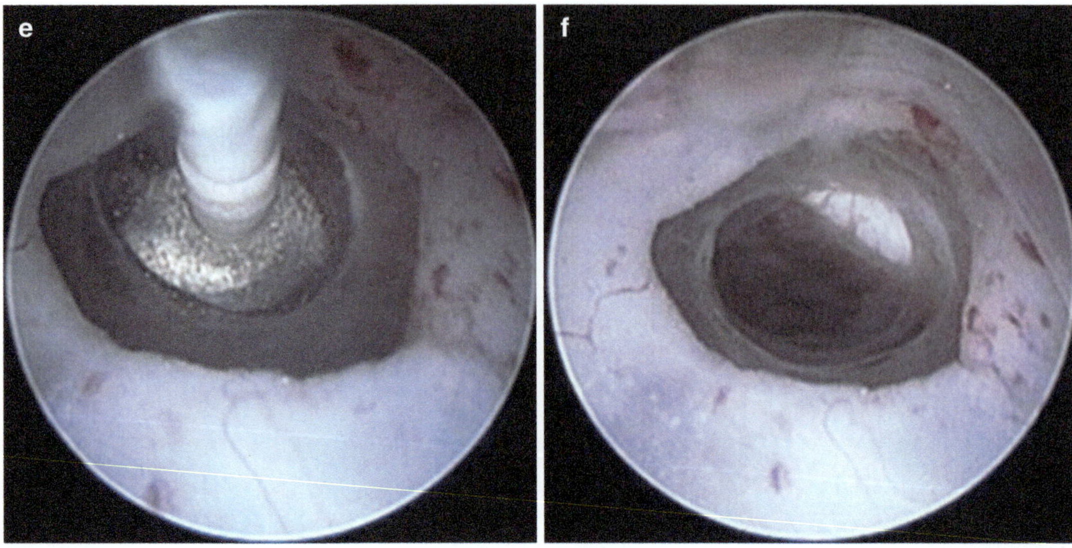

Fig. 2.3 (continued)

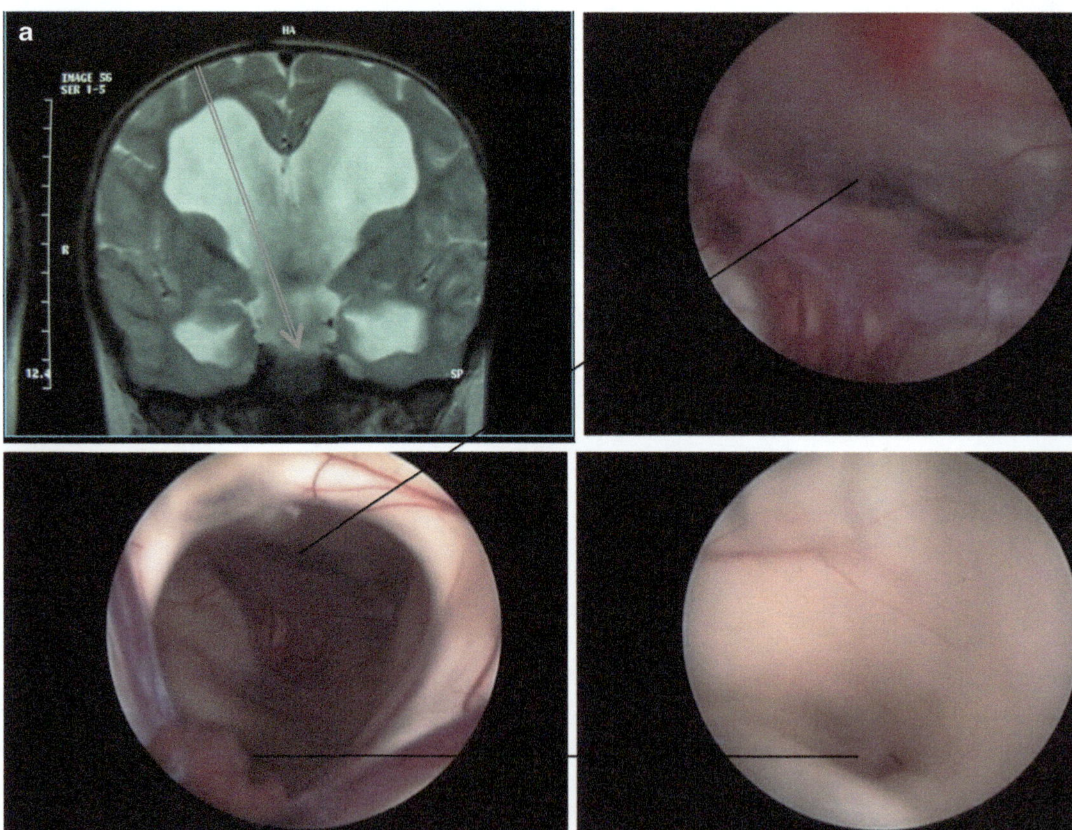

Fig. 2.4 NETV in "LOVA" [59]. (**a**), Bottom right: the inlet of the cerebral aqueduct, with membranous occlusion; Top right: the transparent floor of the third ventricle. (**b**), NETV by Fogarty balloon catheter

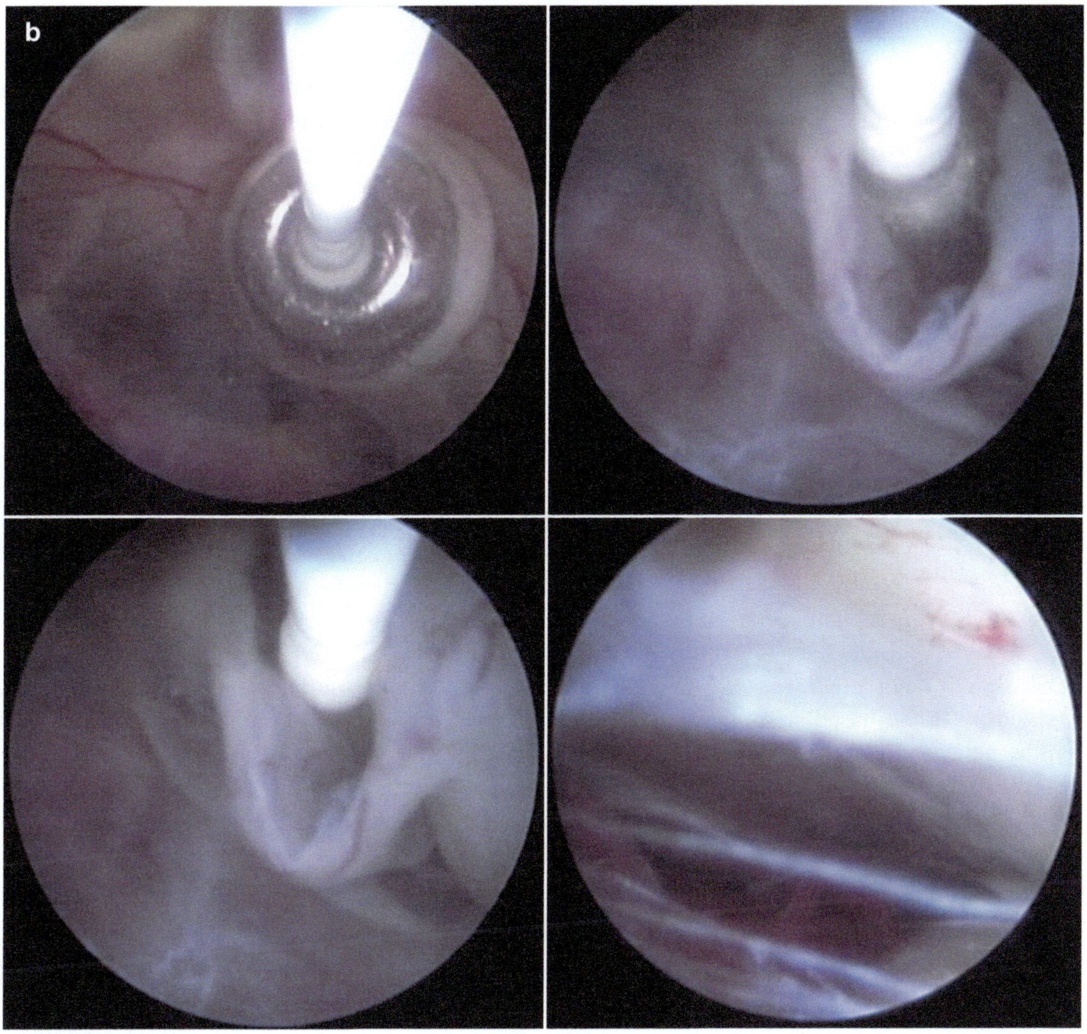

Fig. 2.4 (continued)

radiologically persistent ventriculomegaly as arrested hydrocephalus.

In 2000, J. Burtscher et al. [5] introduced the virtual endoscopy for planning of 10 NETV procedures in 9 patients with tumors and idiopathic aqueductal stenosis. The virtual endoluminal MR views perfectly corresponded with the real-time intraoperative neuroendoscopic images of the ventriculoscope in all but one patient who underwent NETV. Virtual neuroendoscopy demonstrated the relations between the landmarks of the anterior part of the floor of the third ventricle, the underlying major arteries, and the clivus. Thus, preoperative virtual endoscopy planning increased neurosurgeon's safety and comfort.

In 2002, H. Schroeder et al. [71] presented a series of 193 NETV in 188 patients. The success rate was 66 % and the mortality rate 1 % (1 SAH and one 1 infection). The authors concluded that a steep learning curve of NETV existed, because of the predominance of the serious procedure-related complications in their early cases. The incorrect positioning of the fenestration site was the leading cause for the significant complications.

In 2002, A. Krombach et al. [39] reported combined application of neuronavigational guidance and virtual neuroendoscopy (MR ventriculoscopy) for performing NETV. NETV trajectory was planned by neuronavigation. Virtual endoscopy was successfully accomplished in most of the cases retrospectively. Obvious advantage of virtual neuroendoscopy was the demonstration of the relation between the neurovascular structures at risk. However, its important drawback was that septum pellucidum and the floor of the third ventricle were not well visualized. Hence, eventual anomalies could not be evaluated properly. An advantage of neuronavigation was the ability to modify the trajectory simulated by virtual endoscopy in accordance with the anatomical reality and in this way to reduce additionally the risk of neurovascular injury.

In 2003, P. Grunert et al. [27] described a series of 171 NETV in 159 patients with obstructive hydrocephalus, caused by aqueductal stenosis, tumors, cysts, intraventricular hemorrhages, and other reasons. NETV was assisted by frame-based stereotaxy in 31 cases and by neuronavigation in 4 patients. The success rate was 71 %, worse results were achieved in children younger than 1 year. The clinical outcome was not influenced by the stereotaxy. Complications were observed in 6 patients and all but one was not permanent. No procedure-related mortality was found out during the follow-up period.

In 2003, K. Nishiyama et al. [44] demonstrated a series of 15 shunt-dependent patients with occlusive hydrocephalus, whose shunt malfunctions were treated by NETV and consequent removal of the CSF shunt system. Within 1 week after NETV, the shunt-dependent CSF dynamics transformed to a shunt-independent state. However, simultaneous reduction of ICP was not demonstrated in all cases.

In 2004, T. Beems and J. Grotenhuis [3] presented a series of 339 NETV as a stand-alone procedure with 80 % success rate within a follow-up period longer than 5 years. Procedure-related complications were 8 % and mortality was 0 %. In a separate group of 41 NETV in combination with biopsy of intraventricular/paraventricular neoplasm, the complication rate was much higher, 20 %. The authors summarized that the majority of post-NETV complications are transient and the mortality rate is very low.

In 2004, M. Zimmerman et al. [86] first reported robot-assisted NETV in a series of 6 patients with aqueductal stenosis. The robot-assisted NETV were successfully performed without any device-related and/or procedure-related complications. The advantages of the robot assistance were the secure guiding and precise movement of the neuroendoscope. Notable disadvantage of the technique was the additional time needed for setting of the robot, which decreased during the learning curve. However, the duration of the procedure alone was comparable to that of the standard freehand NETV.

In 2005, Oi et al. [56] presented a newly designed rigid-rod neuroendoscope and proposed a new neuroendoscopic surgical technique as "frameless freehand maneuver" combined with high-resolution imaging. The device and the technique were initially applied in 20 cases of NETV with excellent clinical and radiological results and without device and/or procedure-related morbidity or mortality [56].

In 2005, B. Warf [83] reported a large series of 550 NETV as a primary treatment of hydrocephalus of various etiologies in African children. In 284 patients NETV was performed as a stand-alone procedure, and in the remaining 266 cases, neuroendoscopic cauterization of the choroid plexus (NECCP) was simultaneously done along with NETV. The data pointed the superiority of the combined NETV and NECCP procedures over the NETV alone in patients younger than 1 year of age, especially for those with myelomeningocele or noninfectious origin of hydrocephalus.

In 2005, D. Hellwig et al. [31] published a thorough review on all aspects of NETV. NETV indications, operative techniques, and technological adjuncts, surgical series, clinical and radiological outcomes, and postoperative complications were discussed and analyzed in depth.

In 2006, S. Oi and C. Di Rocco [51] published a milestone paper for the CSF dynamics (Fig. 2.5). In an attempt to explain the higher failure rate of NETV in neonates and infants with obstructive hydrocephalus, they hypothesized that the CSF dynamics evolve from a predominance of the

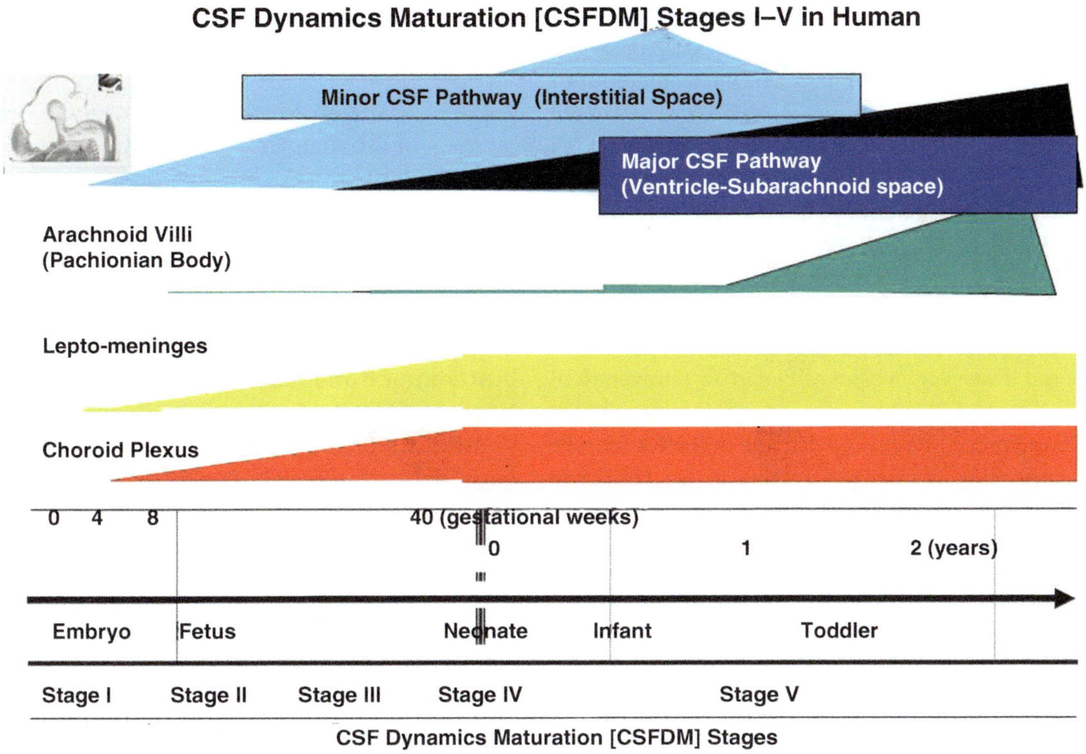

Fig. 2.5 The "evolution theory in CSF dynamics" [51]

minor CSF pathways in the immature brain to a predominance of the major CSF pathways in the matured brain. Their evolutional theory of CSF dynamics was supported by the ventriculo-cisternography data which confirmed the predominance of the minor CSF pathways (intraparenchymal pattern) over the major one in neonates and infants. Thus, the authors proposed that the hydrocephalus in this age group be called "minor pathways hydrocephalus."

In 2009, J. Oertel et al. [45] reported a series of 76 NETV in 73 children. NETV was performed simultaneously with NESS (5 cases), NEAP (9 cases), NEFPFMO (1 case), tumor excision (11 cases), cysts fenestration (4 cases), and removal of blood clot (1 case). The NETV success rate was clinically 70 % and radiologically 56 %. Re-NETV was applied in 4 %. During the follow-up period in 26 % of the patients, CSF shunt insertion was needed, most frequently in the age group less than 6 months. The permanent procedure-related complications were 3 %.

In 2011, T. Bouras and S. Sgouros [4] presented a systematic Medline-based meta-analysis of NETV-related complications. The authors reviewed 34 series of NETV, with 2985 NETV procedures in 2884 patients of all age groups and with heterogeneous etiology of obstructive hydrocephalus. The procedure-related complications were 8.5 %, the permanent morbidity rate 2.38 %, mortality rate 0.21 %, and the frequency of delayed "sudden death" 0.07 %.

Conclusion. NETV represents the most frequently performed neuroendoscopic procedure in the treatment of disordered CSF flow. Generally, NETV is the neuroendoscopic treatment of choice in cases with distal to the third ventricular floor CSF obstruction and reasonable alternative of CSF shunts. The technological assistance of NETV by virtual neuroendoscopy, neuronavigation, and robotic devices is obviously beneficial for the clinical outcome and for the patients' safety. New findings in the CSF physiology would be able to change our attitude for NETV in neonates and infants.

Neuroendoscopic Lamina Terminalis Fenestration (NELTF)

Indications. NELTF is a surgical method of choice in the cases in which NETV is indicated but not feasible or functionally insufficient. A *conditio sine qua non* is the visibility of the neighboring anterior cerebral arteries through lamina terminalis. The decision to perform NELTF as a rule is intraoperative.

Operative technique. In patients with wide foramen of Monro, rigid neuroendoscope could be used. However, in cases with narrow intraventricular foramen, flexible neuroendoscope is required to avoid procedure-related damage of the fornix. The entry point is usually the same as for NETV, in front of the coronal suture and 2–3 cm off the midline. After entering the lateral ventricle, the endoscope is advanced through the foramen of Monro. The floor of the third ventricle is inspected, and if NETV is too risky, lamina terminalis is examined. The fenestration is bluntly performed and subsequently dilated by Fogarty micro balloon catheter.

Clinical experience. NELTF is sporadically mentioned in the literature.

In 1922, W. Dandy [12] reported for the first time perforation of lamina terminalis for the treatment of noncommunicating hydrocephalus. The procedure was performed nonedoscopically by craniotomy and trans-frontal approach.

In 2007, H. Schroeder et al. [73] described the operative technique of NELTF as a vital option of the endoscopic treatment of CSF flow obstruction.

In 2012, J. Torres-Corzo et al. [79] reported a series of 25 NELTF in patients with obstructive hydrocephalus caused by neurocysticercosis (11 cases), tumors (6 cases), aqueductal stenosis (3 cases), and other (5 cases). The decision to perform NELTF was taken intraoperatively due to risky or non-applicable ETV, insufficient basal subarachnoid cisterns, and adhesions in the third ventricle. Within the mean follow-up period of more than 5 years, the clinical and radiological success rate was 76 % (19 cases). The rest 6 patients became shunt dependent. The authors concluded that adequate intraoperative assessment was crucial to identify the patients that would benefit.

Conclusion. NELTF represents valuable alternative of NETV in selected cases.

2.3.2.3 Neuroendoscopic Treatment of Obstruction of Fourth Ventricle Foramina

Neuroendoscopic Foraminoplasty of Foramen of Magendie (NEFPFMA) (Anterograde and Retrograde), Neuroendoscopic Foraminoplasty of Foramen of Luschka (NEFPFL) (Anterograde and Retrograde), and Neuroendoscopic Fourth Ventriculostomy (NEFV)

Indications. Neuroendoscopic techniques for treatment of obstruction of the 4th ventricle foramina are indicated in cases with their membranous occlusion.

Operative technique. The restoration of the CSF flow through the foramina of the fourth ventricle could be performed in both anterograde and retrograde manner. In the anterograde mode, a flexible neuroendoscope is needed and the approach is via the lateral ventricle, the foramen of Monro, the third ventricle, and the cerebral aqueduct. The retrograde method being quite less complicated and less risky is accomplished by rigid neuroendoscope and transcerebellar approach.

Clinical experience. These techniques are the most rarely reported in the literature.

In 1999, S. Oi et al. [58] presented 3 cases of "disproportionately enlarged fourth ventricle" unsuccessfully treated by NEFPFMA. Two cases underwent NEFPFMA plus fourth ventriculostomy and one patient NEFPFMA simultaneously with NETV and fourth ventriculostomy.

In 2006, P. Longatti et al. [40] reported a case of endoscopic opening of membranous obstruction of the foramen of Magendie using transaqueductal navigation. The procedure was performed by flexible neuroendoscope, introduced through a precoronal burr hole, the foramen of Monro, and the cerebral aqueduct to the fourth ventricle. After identification of the obstructed foramen of Magendie, the membrane was perforated by monopolar cautery and dilated by Fogarty balloon. The postoperative course was without complications with excellent clinical outcome. The authors suggested that the proposed technique is indicated in cases of distorted CSF flow due to obstructed 4th ventricle foramina associated with collapse of the prepontine cistern and therefore with eventual risky NETV.

In 2011, A. Giannetti et al. [26] described a case of transcerebellar neuroendoscopic fourth ventriculostomy (NEFV) for treatment of hydrocephalus caused by atresia of the fourth ventricle foramina and shunt malfunction. The entry point was positioned in the suboccipital paramedian region. The rigid endoscope was introduced into the fourth ventricle, and the anatomical landmarks of the fourth ventricle floor were inspected. The membranes obstructing the foramina of Luschka and the foramen of Magendie were bluntly perforated by the tip of the monopolar cautery and subsequently dilated by Fogarty balloon. CSF flow was restored. Within the follow-up period of 3 years, excellent clinical and radiological result was accounted. The transcerebellar neuroendoscopic opening of the 3 foramina of the fourth ventricle, termed by the authors as NEFV, surpass the technique suggested by Longatti et al. [40] in being less risky for the neurovascular structures and more feasible for application.

Conclusion. The neuroendoscopic techniques for restoration of the CSF flow through the obstructed foramina of the fourth ventricle represent potentially valuable surgical techniques, which need further evaluation in larger clinical series.

Neuroendoscopic Third Ventriculostomy (NETV)

NETV most frequently is the treatment of choice of obstructed fourth ventricle foramina if the cerebral aqueduct is passable.

In 2003, C. Karachi et al. [37] reported a series of three patients with idiopathic stenosis of foramina of Magendie and Luschka and consequent four-ventricular hydrocephalus, treated by NETV. All patients became asymptomatic postoperatively, and the 3-year follow-up term was uneventful.

2.3.2.4 Neuroendoscopic Treatment of Obstruction of the Transition Between Spinal and Cranial Subarachnoid Space

Neuroendoscopic Third Ventriculostomy (NETV)

In 2003, U. Kehler and J. Gliemroth [38], in attempt to explain the successful NETV in communicating hydrocephalus, proposed a hypothesis for the existence of extraventricular intracisternal obstructive hydrocephalus. Their series included five cases with patent CSF flow in the ventricles to cisterna magna. MRI demonstrated dilated ventricular system, caudal displacement of the third ventricular floor, anterior displacement of lamina terminalis, and unchanged basal cisterns. All the patients underwent NETV with clinical success. Based on these results, the authors suggested the existence of intracisternal obstruction in such patients that could not be directly visualized up to date.

In 2010, J. Oertel et al. [47] reported their experience with endoscopic diagnosis and treatment of far distal obstructive hydrocephalus. In 20 patients with obstruction of the CSF flow distal to the fourth ventricle were performed 20 NETV in combination with transaqueductal inspection of the posterior fossa by flexible neuroendoscope in 16 cases. The overall success rate was 75 % with significant difference between the pediatric (50 %) and adult (83 %) group. A radiological benefit was observed in 50 %. Five patients became shunt dependent.

2.3.3 Neuroendoscopic Treatment of the Disorders of CSF Absorption

Unfortunately, up to date noneuroendoscopic treatment options exist for the disorders of CSF absorption.

2.4 Future Perspectives

The future trends of neuroendoscopic treatment of altered CSF dynamics are most probably associated with refined neuroendoscopic devices and sophisticated integration with intraoperative imaging, neuronavigation, and neurosurgical robots in an attempt to develop completely automated operating theaters allowing the performance of robotic tele-neuroendoscopic procedures [2, 15, 16]. The fetal neuroendoscopic treatment is another direction with a significant clinical potential if the concomitant surgical complications are limited.

References

1. Aldana PR, Kestle JR, Brockmeyer DL, Walker ML (2003) Results of endoscopic septal fenestration in the treatment of isolated ventricular hydrocephalus. Pediatr Neurosurg 38:286–294
2. Balmer B, Bernays RL, Kollias SS, Yonekawa Y (2002) Interventional MR-guided neuroendoscopy: a new therapeutic option for children. J Pediatr Surg 37:668–672
3. Beems T, Grotenhuis J (2004) Long-term complications and definition of failure of neuroendoscopic procedures. Childs Nerv Syst 20:868–877
4. Bouras T, Sgouros S (2011) Complications of endoscopic third ventriculostomy. J Neurosurg Pediatr 7: 643–649
5. Burtscher J, Dessl A, Bale R, Eisner W, Auer A, Twerdy K, Felber S (2000) Virtual endoscopy for planning endoscopic third ventriculostomy procedures. Pediatr Neurosurg 32:77–82
6. Bussarsky A, Marinov M, Enchev Y, Kalionsky R, Genov P, Bussarsky V (2005) Impact of virtual endoscopy and frameless stereotaxy on the safety of neuroendoscopic interventions. In: Proceedings of the 13th world congress of neurological surgery, Marrakesh, Morocco, 19–24 June 2005, pp 1189–1194
7. Choi JU, Kim DS, Kim SH (1999) Endoscopic surgery for obstructive hydrocephalus. Yonsei Med J J40:600–607
8. Cinalli G, Sainte-Rose C, Chumas P, Zerah M, Brunelle F, Lot G, Pierre-Kahn A, Renier D (1999) Failure of third ventriculostomy in the treatment of aqueductal stenosis in children. J Neurosurg 90(3):448–454
9. Cinalli G, Spennato P, Savarese L, Ruggiero C, Alberti F, Cuomo L, Cianciulli E, Maggi G (2006) Endoscopic aqueductoplasty and placement of a stent in the cerebral aqueduct in the management of isolated fourth ventricle in children. J Neurosurg 104(1 Suppl Pediatrics):21–27
10. Cohen B, Voorhees A, Vedel S, Wei T (2009) Development of a theoretical framework for analyzing cerebrospinal fluid dynamics. Cerebrospinal Fluid Res 6:12
11. Dandy WE (1920) The diagnosis and treatment of hydrocephalus resulting from strictures of the aqueduct of Sylvius. Surg Gynecol Obstet 31:340–358
12. Dandy WE (1922) An operative procedure for hydrocephalus. Johns Hopkins Hosp Bull 33:189–190
13. De Bonis P, Anile C, Tamburrini G, Tartaglione T, Mangiola A (2008) Adult idiopathic occlusion of the foramina of Monro: diagnostic tools and therapy. J Neuroimaging 18(1):101–104
14. El Refaee E, Baldauf J, Schroeder HW (2012) Bilateral occlusion of the foramina of Monro after third ventriculostomy. J Neurosurg 116(6):1333–1336
15. Enchev Y (2009) Neuronavigation: genealogy, reality, and prospects. Neurosurg Focus 27(3):E11
16. Enchev Y (2013) Neuronavigational neuroendoscopy-to be or not to be? An international pilot questionnaire-based study. World Neurosurg 79(2 Suppl):S16.e15–S16.e21
17. Enchev Y, Oi S (2008) Historical trends of neuroendoscopic surgical techniques in treatment for hydrocephalus. Neurosurg Rev 31(3):249–262
18. Enchev Y, Bussarsky A, Romansky K, Marinov M, Bussarsky V (2005) Neuronavigation-intraoperative experience in 156 patients. In: Proceedings of the 13th world congress of neurological surgery, Marrakesh, Morocco, 19–24 June 2005, pp 885–890
19. Enchev Y, Karakostov V, Bussarsky A, Romansky K, Marinov M, Bussarsky V (2005) Cranial neuronavigation-application, accuracy, errors. In: Proceedings of the 14th meeting of the world society for stereotactic and functional neurosurgery, Rome, 13–17 June 2005, pp 53–58
20. Fritsch MJ, Mehdorn M (2002) Endoscopic intraventricular surgery for treatment of hydrocephalus and loculated CSF space in children less than one year of age. Pediatr Neurosurg 36(4):183–188
21. Fritsch MJ, Kienke S, Manwaring KH, Mehdorn HM (2004) Endoscopic aqueductoplasty and interventriculostomy for the treatment of isolated fourth ventricle in children. Neurosurgery 55:372–379
22. Gaab MR, Schroeder HWS (1998) Neuroendoscopic approach to intraventricular lesions. J Neurosurg 88: 496–505
23. Gangemi M, Donati P, Maiuri F, Longatti P, Godano U, Mascari C (1999) Endoscopic third ventriculostomy for hydrocephalus. Minim Invasive Neurosurg 42(3):128–133
24. Gangemi M, Maiuri F, Donati PA, Signorelli F, Basile D (1999) Endoscopic surgery for monoventricular hydrocephalus. Surg Neurol 52:246–250
25. Gavish I, Reisch R, Perneczky A (2005) Endoscopic aqueductoplasty through a tailored craniocervical approach. J Neurosurg 103:778–782
26. Giannetti AV, Malheiros JA, daSilva MC (2011) Fourth ventriculostomy: an alternative treatment for hydrocephalus due to atresia of the Magendie and Luschka foramina. J Neurosurg Pediatr 7(2): 152–156

27. Grunert P, Charalampaki P, Hopf N, Filippi R (2003) The role of the third ventriculostomy in the management of obstructive hydrocephalus. Minim Invasive Neurosurg 46(1):16–21
28. Guiot G, Derome P, Hertzog E, Bamberger C, Akerman M (1968) Ventriculocisternostomie sous controle radioscopique pour hydrocéphalie obstructive [in French]. Presse Med 40:1923–1926
29. Hamada H, Hayashi N, Kurimoto M, Umemura K, Hirashima Y, Endo S (2003) Neuroendoscopic septostomy for isolated lateral ventricle. Neurol Med Chir 43:582–588
30. Heilman CB, Cohen AR (1991) Endoscopic ventricular fenestration using a "saline torch". J Neurosurg 74:224–229
31. Hellwig D, Grotenhuis J, Tirakotai W, Riegel T, Schulte D, Bauer B, Bertalanffy H (2005) Endoscopic third ventriculostomy for obstructive hydrocephalus. Neurosurg Rev 28:1–34
32. Hoffman HJ (1976) The advantages of percutaneous third ventriculostomy over other forms of surgical treatment for infantile obstructive hydrocephalus. In: Morley TP (ed) Current controversies in neurosurgery. W.B. Saunders, Philadelphia, pp 691–703
33. Javier-Fernandez J, Garcia-Cosamalon PJ, Vinuela J, Ibanez FJ, Mostaza A, Heres S, Ortega F (2001) Endoscopic fenestration as a treatment for asymmetrical hydrocephalus due to obstruction of the foramen of Monro [in Spanish]. Neurocirugia (Astur) 12: 513–515
34. Jones RF, Stening WA, Brydon M (1990) Endoscopic third ventriculostomy. Neurosurgery 26:86–92
35. Jones RF, Kwok BC, Stening WA, Vonau M (1994) Neuroendoscopic third ventriculostomy. A practical alternative to extracranial shunts in non-communicating hydrocephalus. Acta Neurochir Suppl 61:79–83
36. Kalhorn SP, Strom RG, Harter DH (2011) Idiopathic bilateral stenosis of the foramina of Monro treated using endoscopic foraminoplasty and septostomy. Neurosurg Focus 30(4):E5
37. Karachi C, Le Guérinel C, Brugières P, Melon E, Decq P (2003) Hydrocephalus due to idiopathic stenosis of the foramina of Magendie and Luschka. Report of three cases. J Neurosurg 98(4):897–902
38. Kehler U, Gliemroth J (2003) Extraventricular intracisternal obstructive hydrocephalus – a hypothesis to explain successful 3rd ventriculostomy in communicating hydrocephalus. Pediatr Neurosurg 38(2): 98–101
39. Krombach A, Rohde V, Haage P, Struffert T, Kilbinger M, Thron A (2002) Virtual endoscopy combined with intraoperative neuronavigation for planning of endoscopic surgery in patients with occlusive hydrocephalus and intracranial cysts. Neuroradiology 44:279–285
40. Longatti P, Fiorindi A, Feletti A, Baratto V (2006) Endoscopic opening of the foramen of Magendie using transaqueductal navigation for membrane obstruction of the fourth ventricle outlets. Technical note. J Neurosurg 105(6):924–927
41. Mixter WJ (1923) Ventriculostomy and puncture of the floor of the third ventricle. Boston Med Surg J188:277–278
42. Mohanty A, Das BS, Sastry-Kolluri VR, Hedge T (1996) Neuro-endoscopic fenestration of occluded foramen of Monro causing unilateral hydrocephalus. Pediatr Neurosurg 25:248–251
43. Mori H, Koike T, Fujimoto T, Nishiyama K, Yoshimura J, Tanaka R (2007) Endoscopic stent placement for treatment of secondary bilateral occlusion of the Monro foramina following endoscopic third ventriculostomy in a patient with aqueductal stenosis. Case report. J Neurosurg 107(2): 416–420
44. Nishiyama K, Mori H, Tanaka R (2003) Changes in cerebrospinal fluid hydrodynamics following endoscopic third ventriculostomy for shunt-dependent noncommunicating hydrocephalus. J Neurosurg 98: 1027–1031
45. Oertel JM, Baldauf J, Schroeder HW, Gaab MR (2009) Endoscopic options in children: experience with 134 procedures. J Neurosurg Pediatr 3(2): 81–89
46. Oertel JM, Schroeder HW, Gaab MR (2009) Endoscopic stomy of the septum pellucidum: indications, technique, and results. Neurosurgery 64(3): 482–491
47. Oertel J, Mondorf Y, Schroeder H, Gaab M (2010) Endoscopic diagnosis and treatment of far distal obstructive hydrocephalus. Acta Neurochir 152: 229–240
48. Oi S (1996) Recent advances in neuroendoscopic surgery: the realistic indication and clinical achievement. Crit Rev Neurosurg 6:64–72
49. Oi S (2011) Classification of hydrocephalus: critical analysis of classification categories and advantages of "Multi-categorical Hydrocephalus Classification" (Mc HC). Childs Nerv Syst 27:1523–1533
50. Oi S, Abbott R (2004) Loculated ventricles and isolated compartments in hydrocephalus: their pathophysiology and the efficacy of neuroendoscopic surgery. Neurosurg Clin N Am 15:77–87
51. Oi S, Di Rocco C (2006) Proposal of "evolution theory in cerebrospinal fluid dynamics" and minor pathway hydrocephalus in developing immature brain. Childs Nerv Syst 22:662–669
52. Oi S, Enchev Y (2008) Neuroendoscopic foraminal plasty of foramen of Monro. Childs Nerv Syst 24(8):933–942
53. Oi S, Matsumoto S (1985) Slit ventricles as a cause of isolated ventricles after shunting. Childs Nerv Syst 1:189–193
54. Oi S, Matsumoto S (1985) Pathophysiology of nonneoplastic obstruction of the foramen of Monro and progressive unilateral hydrocephalus. Neurosurgery 17:891–896

55. Oi S, Matsumoto S (1986) Pathophysiology of aqueductal obstruction in isolated IV ventricle after shunting. Childs Nerv Syst 2:282–286
56. Oi S, Samii A, Samii M (2005) Frameless free-hand maneuvering of a small-diameter rigid-rod neuroendoscope with a working channel used during high-resolution imaging. J Neurosurg (Pediatrics 1) 102: 113–118
57. Oi S, Honda Y, Hidaka M, Sato O, Matsumoto S (1998) Intrauterine high-resolution magnetic resonance imaging in fetal hydrocephalus and prenatal estimation of postnatal outcomes with "perspective classification". J Neurosurg 88:685–694
58. Oi S, Hidaka M, Honda Y, Togo K, Shinoda M, Shimoda M, Tsugane R, Sato O (1999) Neuroendoscopic surgery for specific forms of hydrocephalus. Childs Nerv Syst 15:56–68
59. Oi S, Shimoda M, Shibata M, Honda Y, Togo K, Shinoda M, Tsugane R, Sato O (2000) Pathophysiology of long-standing overt ventriculomegaly in adults. J Neurosurg 92:933–940
60. Oka K, Yamamoto M, Ikeda K, Tomonaga M (1993) Flexible endoneurosurgical therapy for aqueductal stenosis. Neurosurgery 33:236–243
61. Rangel-Castilla L, Hwang SW, Jea A, Torres-Corzo J (2012) Efficacy and safety of endoscopic transventricular lamina terminalis fenestration for hydrocephalus. Neurosurgery 71(2):464–473
62. Rekate H (2011) A consensus of the classification of hydrocephalus: its utility in the assessment of abnormalities of cerebrospinal fluid dynamics. Childs Nerv Syst 27:1535–1541
63. Rieger A, Rainov NG, Sanchin L, Schopp G, Burkert W (1996) Ultrasound-guided endoscopic fenestration of the third ventricular floor for non-communicating hydrocephalus. Minim Invasive Neurosurg 39:17–20
64. Rohde V, Reinges MH, Krombach GA, Gilsbach JM (1998) The combined use of image-guided frameless stereotaxy and neuroendoscopy for the surgical management of occlusive hydrocephalus and intracranial cysts. Br J Neurosurg 12:531–538
65. Sansone JM, Iskandar BJ (2005) Endoscopic cerebral aqueductoplasty: a trans-fourth ventricle approach. J Neurosurg 103(5 Suppl):388–392
66. Scarff JE (1935) Third ventriculostomy as the rational treatment of obstructive hydrocephalus. J Pediatr 6: 870–871
67. Scarff JE (1936) Endoscopic treatment of hydrocephalus. Description of a ventriculoscope and preliminary report of cases. Arch Neurol Psychiatry 35: 853–861
68. Scarff JE (1963) Treatment of hydrocephalus: an historical and critical review of methods and results. J Neurol Neurosurg Psychiatry 26:1–26
69. Scarff JE (1966) Evaluation of treatment of hydrocephalus. Results of third ventriculostomy and endoscopic cauterization of choroid plexuses compared with mechanical shunts. Arch Neurol 14:382–391
70. Schroeder HWS, Gaab MR (1999) Endoscopic aqueductoplasty: technique and results. Neurosurgery 45: 508–518
71. Schroeder H, Niendorf W, Gaab M (2002) Complications of endoscopic third ventriculostomy. J Neurosurg 96(6):1032–1040
72. Schroeder H, Oertel J, Gaab M (2004) Endoscopic aqueductoplasty in the treatment of aqueductal stenosis. Childs Nerv Syst 20:821–827
73. Schroeder H, Oertel J, Gaab M (2007) Endoscopic treatment of cerebrospinal fluid pathway obstructions. Neurosurgery 60(2 Suppl 1):ONS44–ONS51
74. Sharifi G, Alavi E, Rezaee O, Jahanbakhshi A, Faramarzi F (2010) Neuroendoscopic foraminoplasty for bilateral idiopathic occlusion of foramina of Monro. Turk Neurosurg 22(2):265–268
75. Surchev JK, Georgiev KD, Enchev Y, Avramov RS (2002) Ventriculoperitoneal shunts in children – our 14-year experience. Childs Nerv Syst 18:259 (abstr)
76. Surchev J, Georgiev K, Enchev Y, Avramov R (2002) Extremely rare complications in cerebrospinal fluid shunt operations. J Neurosurg Sci 46:100–102
77. Tamburrini G, Frassanito P, Massimi L, Caldarelli M, Di Rocco C (2012) Endoscopic septostomy through a standard precoronal ventricular access: feasibility and effectiveness. Acta Neurochir (Wien) 154(8):1517–1522
78. Teo C, Burson T, Misra S (1999) Endoscopic treatment of the trapped fourth ventricle. Neurosurgery 44:1257–1262
79. Torres-Corzo JG, Rangel-Castilla L, Jea A, Wei-Hung Hwang S (2012) Efficacy and safety of endoscopic transventricular lamina terminalis fenestration for hydrocephalus. Neurosurgery 71(2):464–473
80. Vaz-Guimarães Filho FA, Ramalho CO, Suriano ÍC, Zymberg ST, Cavalheiro S (2011) Neuroendoscopic surgery for unilateral hydrocephalus due to inflammatory obstruction of the Monro foramen. Arq Neuropsiquiatr 69(2A):227–231
81. Vries J (1978) An endoscopic technique for third ventriculostomy. Surg Neurol 9:165–168
82. Walker ML, Petronio J, Carey CM (1994) Ventriculoscopy. In: Cheek WR, Marlin AE, McLone DG, Reigel DH, Walker ML (eds) Pediatric neurosurgery: surgery of the developing nervous system. W.B. Saunders, Philadelphia, pp 572–581
83. Warf BC (2005) Comparison of endoscopic third ventriculostomy alone and combined with choroid plexus cauterization in infants younger than 1 year of age: a prospective study in 550 African children. J Neurosurg 103(6 Suppl):475–481
84. Westerlund U, Svensson M, Moe MC, Varghese M, Gustavsson B, Wallstedt L, Berg-Johnsen J, Langmoen IA (2005) Endoscopically harvested stem cells: a putative method in future auto transplantation. Neurosurgery 57:779–784
85. Wong TT, Lee LS (2000) Membranous occlusion of the foramen of Monro following ventriculoperitoneal shunt insertion: a role for endoscopic foraminoplasty. Childs Nerv Syst 16:213–217
86. Zimmermann M, Krishnan R, Raabe A, Seifert V (2004) Robot-assisted navigated endoscopic ventriculostomy: implementation of a new technology and first clinical results. Acta Neurochir (Wien) 146:697–704

3 Neuroendoscopy in Infants and the International Infant Hydrocephalus Study (IIHS)

Shlomi Constantini, Spyros Sgouros, and Abhaya V. Kulkarni

3.1 Introduction: Hydrocephalus, VPS, and ETV

Pediatric hydrocephalus is one of the most common neurosurgical conditions. It is the leading cause of brain surgery for children in the USA. The ventriculoperitoneal shunt (VPS) is the classic treatment for pediatric hydrocephalus since the early 1960s. Shunts are the "bread and butter" of pediatric neurosurgery. Shunts have modified the prognosis of hydrocephalus from a lethal disease to a curable disease with a relatively good prognosis according to etiology [1–4].

Hydrocephalus is a heterogeneous disease. Shunts are able to resolve almost all cases of hydrocephalus, whatever the etiology, with almost no contraindications. Many different types of shunts have been developed and are in use, including pressure-regulated, volume-regulated, externally regulated, shunt assistants, and dual-switch valves [5–24]. When shunts first appeared in our field, the advantages were clear and far outweighed the disadvantages; they enabled a relatively normal life with a relatively simple procedure.

It took some time to realize and acknowledge that the shunt failure rate is significant, that complications are common, and that children with shunts are dependent upon surgical maintenance throughout their lives [1, 25–34].

Shunt complication rates are unacceptably high. Children with shunts have an increased likelihood of seizures, they can develop *slit ventricle syndrome*, and some of them suffer from under- or over-shunting [35–53].

With all these complications in mind, the arrival of neuroendoscopy on the scene was greeted with great enthusiasm. Neuroendoscopy was seen as a means of solving the challenges of hydrocephalus without the issues of the hardware.

Endoscopic third ventriculostomy (ETV) was designed primarily for hydrocephalus cases in which there is a blockage at the level of the aqueduct of Sylvius. In these cases, the endoscope is guided to the floor of the third ventricle, and an opening is created between the third ventricle and the interpeduncular cistern. This is a straightforward diversion procedure; no hardware is usually left in place, and fluid can egress from the third ventricle to the base of skull and ultimately arrive at the normal absorption sites at the convexity of the brain.

S. Constantini, MD, MSc
Department of Pediatric Neurosurgery, Dana Children's Hospital, Tel Aviv Medical Center, Tel Aviv, Israel

S. Sgouros, MD, FRCS (SN) (✉)
Department of Pediatric Neurosurgery, Mitera Children's Hospital, Athens, Greece

University of Athens Medical School, Athens, Greece
e-mail: sgouros@med.uoa.gr, ssgouros@mitera.gr

A.V. Kulkarni, MD, PhD, FRCSC
Division of Neurosurgery, Hospital for Sick Children, University of Toronto, Toronto, ON, Canada

S. Sgouros (ed.), *Neuroendoscopy*,
DOI 10.1007/978-3-642-39085-2_3, © Springer-Verlag Berlin Heidelberg 2014

3.2 Technical Challenges of ETV

There is no single standardized technique defined for ETV. The same basic procedure is implemented with considerable technical variability in different medical centers. Technical nuances include the use of rinsing fluid, use of navigation, scope types (rigid or flexible), techniques for creating and widening the hole in the base of the third ventricle, and even basic concepts of how to close the skin and open the bone [54–57].

Endoscopic third ventriculostomy and all other neuroendoscopic operations are advanced procedures that are heavily dependent on sophisticated technology. ETVs require a learning curve, substantial experience, and careful coaching of young neurosurgeons. Every case should be carefully discussed between the participating neurosurgeons, analyzing the indications and contraindications, following a close inspection of the specific microanatomical details on the MR. The professional discussions must be accompanied by a discussion with the family of the available alternatives, their advantages, and disadvantages.

Morbidity from endoscopic third ventriculostomy may be underreported. The nightmare of every neuroendoscopist is massive bleeding, mainly arterial, during the procedure. Perforation of the basilar artery has been reported from even the best of medical centers [58–72]. Smaller bleeds, mainly of venous origin, usually stop by themselves with either simple rinsing or a short burst of mono- or bipolar coagulation. Tissue damage during insertion and manipulation of the endoscope, subdural hematomas, endocrinological abnormalities, infections, cranial neuropathies, and other complications are also reported [60, 71, 73–82].

Although most failures from endoscopic third ventriculostomy occur in the early period after the procedure, late obstruction of the stoma may lead to increased ICP and even sudden death [83–92]. It is therefore strongly advised that patients who undergo a successful ETV should be clearly told that they are not *cured* from the hydrocephalus and that symptoms can reappear and may have dangerous consequences [93]. These patients should be followed on an ongoing basis, and the medical center should have an open door policy that encourages the patients to call or come back if any related symptoms are appearing. It is still not known if those patients with no flow void at the third ventricle stoma on postoperative MRI may be at a higher risk to develop a clinical syndrome and should be followed even more closely.

3.3 ETV: Meeting the Standard of Evidence-Based Medicine

Series on the results of ETV in the pediatric age group started to appear in the 1980s, developed during the 1990s, and continue to appear in the literature to this day [56, 60, 91, 94–118].

However, even with all the series that have been published to date, it is hard to extract meaningful research data or operative guidelines. There are too many inconsistencies in the basic "ground rules" used by these researchers [119]. For example, success rates of endoscopic third ventriculostomy are usually defined as one or more of the following factors: the disappearance of hydrocephalus symptoms, no signs of intracranial hypertension evident, and/or a technically successful procedure. Perhaps partially as a result of this wide range of definitions for the term "success," large disparities are found when looking at the results of ETV in children. Success rate varies widely, ranging from a low 35 % success rate in a series from Toronto [116] up to a high of 83–89 % in other series [106, 108, 120, 121].

Analyzing the differences between successful series and series with less promising results shows that most of the differences can be traced to a gap in the early failure rate. Early ETV failures could be due to wrong technique, different selection criteria in recruiting the patients or in defining failure, and also the multifactorial etiology of the hydrocephalic process itself [122, 123]. It is essential, therefore, to define a uniform set of selection and failure criteria in order to objectively and meaningfully compare results among different centers.

Since the 1990s, ETV has been recognized as a valid alternative to shunt implants, mainly for patients with obstruction at the level of the aqueduct, the tectal plate, and the pineal region. ETV quietly developed into a mainstream, common procedure in pediatric neurosurgery without *any* prospective randomized trials (and certainly no multicenter trials) proving its efficacy compared to shunt procedures. Unfortunately, it seems apparent today that a classic randomized trial is no longer possible, since most of us treating these patients would not agree to expose a classic candidate for ETV to randomization between two alternatives.

As ETV technology continues to evolve and improve, and as we collectively accumulate more experience and confidence with ETV, indications for ETV have broadened, introducing more challenges in understanding the pathophysiology of hydrocephalus and in proving the efficacy of a new procedure (ETV) over the more standard alternative (shunts).

This was one of the reasons that in 2001 we established the International Study Group for Neuroendoscopy (ISGNE). The goal of this organization (more recently transformed into the International Federation for Neuroendoscopy (IFNE)) is to promote neuroendoscopy research and education.

There are many pathologies for which treatment with ETV is debatable. These include hydrocephalus in infants, patients with meningomyelocele and Chiari, Dandy-Walker malformation, fourth ventricular outlet obstruction, during tumor surgery, and patients who have had a hemorrhage or an infection in their past [39, 124–171].

Over the course of 10 years of collaboration within the IFNE, we have learned to appreciate the advantages of cooperative multicenter studies. Our first attempt was with a study on repeat ETV for those patients for whom the original ETV initially succeeded. We pooled our experiences with 20 patients recruited from four centers [114]. Another collaboration involved a multicenter study on the efficacy of ETV in patients who had previously experienced an infection and/or hemorrhage. For this study, we pooled our experiences with 101 patients from seven medical centers around the world [161]. We are currently analyzing the results of the International Neuroendoscopy Biopsy Study (INEBS) which included 293 patients from 13 medical centers (submitted for publication). In addition to these clinical series, our group has led several major multicenter epidemiological papers that have recently been published. These papers analyzed meta-results obtained by merging data from the very large number of patients recruited through a combination of other series, focusing on specific variables and how they affect success or failure in pediatric ETV [55, 93, 100, 109, 110, 172, 173].

3.4 Uncertainty Regarding ETV in Infants

For infants, the potential benefit of ETV is substantial, due to the admittedly high complication rate of shunting. Common complications include a high rate of mechanical failure, high rate of infection, slit ventricle syndrome, and seizures. Shunt complication rate (both mechanical and infectious) is age-dependent. Infants usually have more complications compared to older patients. Shunted infants generally require many surgical revisions. Twenty to forty percent of infants require revisions in the first year following insertion and, in subsequent years, generally add another 10–15 % per year [28].

There are other concerns regarding ETV in infants. Is ETV more dangerous for infants? Safety concerns fall into three areas: *short term* (during the surgery itself), *intermediate term* (e.g., postoperative leaks or infections), and *long term* (e.g., perhaps due to unforeseen risks to development or stoma closure leading to a sudden hydrocephalus emergency). Another unresolved concern is whether the CSF absorption mechanism in infants with aqueductal stenosis is mature enough to handle the CSF after the obstruction is bypassed.

Even if all the technical/physiological issues were resolved, another major concern is that some of the infants considered to have been successfully treated with ETV may actually have been transformed from *active* hydrocephalus to an *arrested* type. We might be paying a neurological price for such "successes" by adversely affecting their long-term development. This theory is based on the observation that children who have had their hydrocephalus treated with ETV almost always have ventricles considerably larger than children who were treated with VPS [174]. At least one study has shown a direct correlation between decreased ventricular volume and clinical improvement [175]. Unfortunately, nobody, so far, has been reviewing systematically the relevant developmental variables in children following ETV. No study has attempted to correlate the size of the ventricles to any neurodevelopmental measurement. So this belief has not been scientifically proven or refuted.

Conversely, other surgeons advocating ETV are concerned with the long-term complications of *shunting* on the developing brain, especially the cumulative risk of shunt infections due to multiple operations. The theory for this correlation is based on the observed link between shunt infection and reduction of IQ, as well as measured memory deficits among shunted children [94, 169, 176–186]. Advocates for ETV also claim that it is a more "physiological solution" and therefore is better for the infant brain.

Having reviewed the papers that appeared on this subject over the last 10 years, 32 papers reported an average success rate from 50 to 55 %. However, this "average" success rate does not really reflect the wide range of results found when analyzing the studies to date.

Results from around the world ranged from 25 % shunt independence [108, 126, 187–190] up to 89 % shunt independence [59, 191–197].

Two-thirds of the studies reviewed concluded that age is a significant predictor of success, suggesting that for infants up to 1 year of age, the ETV success rate is strongly age-dependent [27, 55, 79, 80, 99, 100, 106, 108, 113, 116, 149, 167, 191, 198–203]. On the other hand, one-third of the studies found no correlation between age and success rates [97, 132, 134, 150, 168, 192, 197, 204].

There is also a very wide range of failure definition after ETV in this age group. Some would shunt every post-ETV infant who still has a full fontanel, while others would wait for more overt signs of high ICP before declaring a failure [22, 55, 59, 60, 78–80, 82, 93, 94, 96, 97, 100, 102, 106–113, 116–118, 126, 132, 134, 141, 149, 150, 152, 156, 161, 166–169, 172, 173, 177, 185, 187–256].

With all these very plausible theories and beliefs, *there has never been a direct controlled comparison of the two types of treatment, studying their impact on the intellectual development of children*, and certainly not of infants.

3.5 The International Infant Hydrocephalus Study (IIHS)

Because ETV in infants is so controversial, with strong, plausible arguments on both sides of the divide, we concluded that a randomized prospective study in this group would be morally justified and well accepted by our community. This was why more than 4 years ago we initiated the International Infant Hydrocephalus Study (IIHS).

IIHS is a multicenter prospective randomized study on infants up to 2 years of age with no flow at the level of the aqueduct. IIHS represents a major departure from most published works on the value of neuroendoscopy in the treatment of hydrocephalus. Whereas most studies focus on the survival of the created stoma or implanted shunt and surgical complications, this study focuses primarily on the effect of treatment on the neurodevelopmental outcome at 5 years, including a comprehensive assessment of relevant risks and benefits [257].

IIHS is the first randomized study of the long-term outcome for patients with infantile hydrocephalus due to aqueductal stenosis. Due to the lack of clear superiority of either surgical technique, it became obvious that randomization to shunt or ETV groups, in the clearly defined population of infants under 2 years of age with obstructive hydrocephalus due to pure aqueductal stenosis, is not only ethical but also a duty for all medical personnel involved in the management of such patients. Nevertheless, families who are presented with both options in a non-biased way and elect to choose one, possibly on the basis of information that they have already gathered on their own, are also included in the study. This option (termed "parental preference") does not violate the statistical validity of the study and is built into the study design, based on a comprehensive cohort design model [257, 258].

Given the complexity of the study outcomes, it is possible that there might not be a single, clear, unambiguous set of findings. For example, it may well prove that one type of treatment enjoys a considerably better neurodevelopmental outcome but possibly at the "cost" of a higher complication rate. Ultimately, we may decide that in the future, it may be up to the parents, together with the treating neurosurgeon, to choose one or the other treatment, with full awareness and understanding of the facts and details. With this in mind, IIHS is also analyzing other factors as secondary outcome measures, such as complication rates, hospitalization time, the need for repeat surgeries, and imaging use. This dual-level approach will ultimately provide a unique opportunity to directly compare, under controlled circumstances, the management consequences of ETV and VPS.

Until now, such a comparison has not been possible. Currently, when neurosurgeons counsel patients and their families before surgery, we quote complication rates from different studies. Unfortunately, the studies available to date are not even directly comparable because, at the very least, they are not based on comparable patient populations. And of course, the reality is that with all the uncertainty surrounding the question of ETV vs. VPS, we all have our own personal beliefs and biases. It is only human nature for the neurosurgeon to choose, perhaps subconsciously, the statistics most supportive of a preferred choice. Hopefully, one of the outcomes of the IIHS will be to provide a more objectively balanced set of data to discuss with the families.

3.6 How Does the IIHS Work?

Information about the IIHS administrative and organizational details, (steering committee, study coordinator, etc.), as well as the study principles, is provided on the study web site www.IIHStudy.org. IIHS principles are also presented in a paper by Sgouros, Kulkarni, and Constantini [257].

Participating medical centers must meet a stiff set of inclusion criteria. IIHS participation requires medical centers have strong neuroendoscopic orientations with at least five infant ETV operations per surgeon annually and a philosophical acceptance of the underlying principles of the study. IIHS demands a strong commitment to timely patient follow-up and data submissions, combined with the ability to follow patients for at least 5 years. Research ethics requirements are per institutional rules.

Recruited infants must meet their own set of inclusion criteria. Children must be under 2 years of age, the product of a full-term pregnancy, and newly diagnosed with untreated obstructive hydrocephalus. Ventricular enlargement and no flow at the aqueductal level must be clearly visible on the MR. Local logistics and social complexities must be considered – it must be possible for the medical center to follow the child and schedule follow-up exams for at least 5 years. Exclusion criteria include children who are either prematurely born or have other major structural neurological and brain abnormalities.

Eligible patients and their families must have a long discussion with the treating neurosurgeon. After an explanation of the study and the different arms, they may be either randomized or categorized according to "parental preference." All children are subject to continuous follow-up until they reach the age of 5 years. The 5-year outcome measurements are based on a complete test battery, including three questionnaires completed by the parents and two questionnaires completed by professionals. These tests have being translated and validated in eight different languages. A number of secondary variables reflecting more standard secondary outcome measures will also be documented.

3.7 What Has the IIHS Achieved So Far?

IIHS patient recruitment began about 4 years ago, following a major design process. Forty-three international centers have joined the IIHS. The majority (27) are from Europe, with other participants from

North America, Latin America, and other continents. Twenty-five centers have already contributed over 150 patients. Most of our patients were recruited at under 1 year of age. An interim analysis showed a similar rate of adverse surgical affects between the two arms. Our monitoring committee therefore authorized continuing the recruitment process. Outcome results will be analyzed only after study recruitment is completed. Patient recruitment will probably continue for another 3 years and follow-up for another 5 years after that.

Four years into the IIHS, we can conclude the following: We are dealing with a rare disease. Even very busy centers usually recruit no more than two to four patients yearly. So maintaining a high recruitment rate is an ongoing challenge. Randomization of a surgical procedure is a difficult challenge as well. This is a culture change and requires time and effort from the participating centers. Since our study is only modestly funded, a strong determination and certain "idealism" is part of the participation motivation.

One more point is as follows: While it *is* important to try to provide informative, objective, prospective data, the significance of the IIHS is much more than that of a single important study. The fact that we have the commitment of so many colleagues around the world, who are all equally passionate about treating and hydrocephalus, is very encouraging. This group of centers and investigators can be used for other collaborative hydrocephalus studies in the future. IIHS is, therefore, laying the groundwork for a future of global collaborative studies that may just change the way medical research is conducted.

3.8 Other Challenges in Infant Neuroendoscopy

ETV in infants with aqueductal stenosis is only one of the scientific and clinical dilemmas facing us today. Several other controversial indications exist.

ETV combined with Choroid Plexus Coagulation (ETV/CPC) has been rejuvenated by Benjamin Warf, who has contributed enormously to the body of research through his Uganda experience. He and others have reported on the use of CPC, mainly in post-meningitis hydrocephalus and in those with MMC [22, 141, 166, 168, 169, 200, 253, 254, 259–261]. In the coming years, the challenge will be to see if the huge African experience can be extrapolated to developed nations. It has been proposed that ETV/CPC can play an important role in post-hemorrhagic hydrocephalus, for example. This condition is rarely seen in sub-Saharan Africa, but very common in developed nations. A prospective study designed to advance our knowledge in this direction is about to start soon.

ETV for Dandy-Walker syndrome is a valid option, but only small series are available in the literature [124, 126, 146, 148, 150, 164, 262–268].

ETV for obstruction of the outlet of the fourth ventricle is another clinical front. Theoretically, ETV should work to bypass such an obstruction. Nevertheless, several obstacles in defining this entity and the role of ETV exist. First, the MR criteria to differentiate those who have a combined obstruction of the Luschka and the Magendie vs. those with "communicating" hydrocephalus are not clear. Most clinicians will not expose their patients to invasive preparatory imaging such as a dynamic ventriculography. When performing this study on several candidates, we realized the low predictive ability of MR in selecting the right candidates for this procedure. While initial results are promising [39, 53, 128, 129, 131, 133, 136, 138–140, 143, 147, 149, 153, 155], the jury is out on the indication for ETV in this situation.

ETV for hydrocephalus in dysraphic patients is also an option. Although it makes sense in selected patients, it has not yet become too popular as a first measure to control hydrocephalus in infants following closure of their MMC [127, 132, 134, 137, 141, 142, 145, 154, 163, 166–170, 269].

Conclusion

Neuroendoscopy in infants poses a special clinical research challenge. Available data is accumulating rather slowly. The IIHS offers some hope of providing more reliable data in infants with aqueductal stenosis. Other indications for endoscopy in this age group need to be better studied to expand our understanding of the indications, dangers, and benefits.

References

1. Aschoff A, Kremer P, Hashemi B, Kunze S (1999) The scientific history of hydrocephalus and its treatment. Neurosurg Rev 22(2–3):67–93; discussion 94–95
2. Beni-Adani L, Biani N, Ben-Sirah L, Constantini S (2006) The occurrence of obstructive vs absorptive hydrocephalus in newborns and infants: relevance to treatment choices. Childs Nerv Syst 22(12):1543–1563
3. Golden JA, Bonnemann CG (2007) Developmental structural disorders. In: Goetz CG (ed) Textbook of clinical neurology, 3rd edn. Saunders/Elsevier, Philadelphia, p ch. 28
4. Kinsman SL, Johnston MV (2007) Congenital anomalies of the central nervous system. In: Kliegman RM, Behrman RE, Jenson HB, Stanton BF (eds) Nelson textbook of pediatrics, 18th edn. Saunders/Elsevier, Philadelphia, p 592
5. Czosnyka ZH, Cieslicki K, Czosnyka M, Pickard JD (2005) Hydrocephalus shunts and waves of intracranial pressure. Med Biol Eng Comput 43(1):71–77
6. Davis SE, Levy ML, McComb JG, Sposto R (2000) The delta valve: how does its clinical performance compare with two other pressure differential valves without antisiphon control? Pediatr Neurosurg 33(2):58–63
7. Drake JM, Kestle J (1996) Rationale and methodology of the multicenter pediatric cerebrospinal fluid shunt design trial. Pediatric hydrocephalus treatment evaluation group. Childs Nerv Syst 12(8):434–447
8. Drake JM, Kestle J (1996) Determining the best cerebrospinal fluid shunt valve design: the pediatric valve design trial. Neurosurgery 38(3):604–607
9. Drake JM, Kestle JT (1998) Determining the best cerebrospinal fluid shunt valve design: the pediatric valve design trial. Neurosurgery 43(5):1259–1260
10. Drake JM, Kestle JR, Milner R, Cinalli G, Boop F, Piatt J Jr, Haines S, Schiff SJ, Cochrane DD, Steinbok P, MacNeil N (1998) Randomized trial of cerebrospinal fluid shunt valve design in pediatric hydrocephalus. Neurosurgery 43(2):294–303; discussion 303–305
11. Drake JM, Kestle JR, Tuli S (2000) CSF shunts 50 years on – past, present and future. Childs Nerv Syst 16(10–11):800–804
12. Hanlo PW, Cinalli G, Vandertop WP, Faber JA, Bogeskov L, Borgesen SE, Boschert J, Chumas P, Eder H, Pople IK, Serlo W, Vitzthum E (2003) Treatment of hydrocephalus determined by the European Orbis Sigma Valve II survey: a multicenter prospective 5-year shunt survival study in children and adults in whom a flow-regulating shunt was used. J Neurosurg 99(1):52–57
13. Jain H, Sgouros S, Walsh AR, Hockley AD (2000) The treatment of infantile hydrocephalus: "differential-pressure" or "flow-control" valves. A pilot study. Childs Nerv Syst 16(4):242–246
14. Jain H, Natarajan K, Sgouros S (2005) Influence of the shunt type in the difference in reduction of volume between the two lateral ventricles in shunted hydrocephalic children. Childs Nerv Syst 21(7):552–558
15. Lundkvist B, Eklund A, Koskinen LO, Malm J (2003) An adjustable CSF shunt: advices for clinical use. Acta Neurol Scand 108(1):38–42
16. Mangano FT, Menendez JA, Habrock T, Narayan P, Leonard JR, Park TS, Smyth MD (2005) Early programmable valve malfunctions in pediatric hydrocephalus. J Neurosurg 103(6 Suppl):501–507
17. Meier U, Zeilinger FS, Reyer T, Kintzel D (2000) Clinical experience with various shunt systems in normal pressure hydrocephalus. Zentralbl Neurochir 61(3):143–149
18. Meier U, Kintzel D (2002) Clinical experiences with different valve systems in patients with normal-pressure hydrocephalus: evaluation of the Miethke dual-switch valve. Childs Nerv Syst 18(6–7):288–294
19. Ringel F, Schramm J, Meyer B (2005) Comparison of programmable shunt valves vs standard valves for communicating hydrocephalus of adults: a retrospective analysis of 407 patients. Surg Neurol 63(1):36–41; discussion 41
20. Tuli S, O'Hayon B, Drake J, Clarke M, Kestle J (1999) Change in ventricular size and effect of ventricular catheter placement in pediatric patients with shunted hydrocephalus. Neurosurgery 45(6):1329–1333; discussion 1333–1335
21. Udayakumaran S, Roth J, Kesler A, Constantini S (2010) Miethke DualSwitch Valve in lumboperitoneal shunts. Acta Neurochir (Wien) 152(10): 1793–1800
22. Warf BC (2005) Comparison of 1-year outcomes for the Chhabra and Codman-Hakim Micro Precision shunt systems in Uganda: a prospective study in 195 children. J Neurosurg 102(4 Suppl):358–362
23. Xenos C, Sgouros S, Natarajan K, Walsh AR, Hockley A (2003) Influence of shunt type on ventricular volume changes in children with hydrocephalus. J Neurosurg 98(2):277–283
24. Zeilinger FS, Reyer T, Meier U, Kintzel D (2000) Clinical experiences with the dual-switch valve in patients with normal pressure hydrocephalus. Acta Neurochir Suppl 76:559–562
25. Hoppe-Hirsch E, Laroussinie F, Brunet L, Sainte-Rose C, Renier D, Cinalli G, Zerah M, Pierre-Kahn A (1998) Late outcome of the surgical treatment of hydrocephalus. Childs Nerv Syst 14(3):97–99
26. Kestle J, Milner R, Drake J (1999) The shunt design trial: variation in surgical experience did not influence shunt survival. Pediatr Neurosurg 30(6):283–287
27. Kestle J, Milner R, Drake D (1999) An assessment of observer bias in the shunt design trial. Pediatr Neurosurg 30(2):57–61
28. Kestle J, Drake J, Milner R, Sainte-Rose C, Cinalli G, Boop F, Piatt J, Haines S, Schiff S, Cochrane D, Steinbok P, MacNeil N (2000) Long-term follow-up data from the Shunt Design Trial. Pediatr Neurosurg 33(5):230–236

29. Kestle JR (2003) Pediatric hydrocephalus: current management. Neurol Clin 21(4):883–895, vii
30. Kestle JR, Drake JM, Cochrane DD, Milner R, Walker ML, Abbott R 3rd, Boop FA (2003) Lack of benefit of endoscopic ventriculoperitoneal shunt insertion: a multicenter randomized trial. J Neurosurg 98(2):284–290
31. Renier D, Sainte-Rose C, Pierre-Kahn A, Hirsch JF (1988) Prenatal hydrocephalus: outcome and prognosis. Childs Nerv Syst 4(4):213–222
32. Sainte-Rose C, Piatt JH, Renier D, Pierre-Kahn A, Hirsch JF, Hoffman HJ, Humphreys RP, Hendrick EB (1991) Mechanical complications in shunts. Pediatr Neurosurg 17(1):2–9
33. Simon TD, Riva-Cambrin J, Srivastava R, Bratton SL, Dean JM, Kestle JR (2008) Hospital care for children with hydrocephalus in the United States: utilization, charges, comorbidities, and deaths. J Neurosurg Pediatr 1(2):131–137
34. Williams MA, McAllister JP, Walker ML, Kranz DA, Bergsneider M, Del Bigio MR, Fleming L, Frim DM, Gwinn K, Kestle JR, Luciano MG, Madsen JR, Oster-Granite ML, Spinella G (2007) Priorities for hydrocephalus research: report from a National Institutes of Health-sponsored workshop. J Neurosurg 107 (5 Suppl):345–357
35. Bourgeois M, Sainte-Rose C, Cinalli G, Maixner W, Malucci C, Zerah M, Pierre-Kahn A, Renier D, Hoppe-Hirsch E, Aicardi J (1999) Epilepsy in children with shunted hydrocephalus. J Neurosurg 90(2):274–281
36. Bruce DA, Weprin B (2001) The slit ventricle syndrome. Neurosurg Clin N Am 12(4):709–717, viii
37. Bryant MJ, McEniery J, Walker DG, Campbell R, Lister B, Sargent P, Withers TK, Baker J, Guazzo E, Rossato R, Anderson D, Tomlinson F (2004) Preliminary study of shunt related death in paediatric patients. J Clin Neurosci 11(6):614–615
38. Buchhalter JR, Dichter MA (1990) Migraine/epilepsy syndrome mimicking shunt malfunction in a child with shunted hydrocephalus. J Child Neurol 5(1):69–71
39. Dollo C, Kanner A, Siomin V, Ben-Sira L, Sivan J, Constantini S (2001) Outlet fenestration for isolated fourth ventricle with and without an internal shunt. Childs Nerv Syst 17(8):483–486
40. Drake J (2005) Slit-ventricle syndrome. J Neurosurg 102(3 Suppl):257–258; discussion 258–259
41. Epstein F, Lapras C, Wisoff JH (1988) 'Slit-ventricle syndrome': etiology and treatment. Pediatr Neurosci 14(1):5–10
42. Fattal-Valevski A, Beni-Adani L, Constantini S (2005) Short-term dexamethasone treatment for symptomatic slit ventricle syndrome. Childs Nerv Syst 21(11):981–984
43. Klepper J, Busse M, Strassburg HM, Sorensen N (1998) Epilepsy in shunt-treated hydrocephalus. Dev Med Child Neurol 40(11):731–736
44. Kramer U, Kanner AA, Siomin V, Harel S, Constantini S (2001) No evidence of epilepsy following endoscopic third ventriculostomy: a short-term follow-up. Pediatr Neurosurg 34(3):121–123
45. Oi S, Matsumoto S (1987) Infantile hydrocephalus and the slit ventricle syndrome in early infancy. Childs Nerv Syst 3(3):145–150
46. Olson S (2004) The problematic slit ventricle syndrome. A review of the literature and proposed algorithm for treatment. Pediatr Neurosurg 40(6):264–269
47. Piatt JH Jr, Carlson CV (1996) Hydrocephalus and epilepsy: an actuarial analysis. Neurosurgery 39(4):722–727; discussion 727–728
48. Rekate HL (2004) The slit ventricle syndrome: advances based on technology and understanding. Pediatr Neurosurg 40(6):259–263
49. Roth J, Biyani N, Udayakumaran S, Xiao X, Friedman O, Beni-Adani L, Constantini S (2011) Modified bilateral subtemporal decompression for resistant slit ventricle syndrome. Childs Nerv Syst 27(1):101–110
50. Sato O, Yamguchi T, Kittaka M, Toyama H (2001) Hydrocephalus and epilepsy. Childs Nerv Syst 17(1–2):76–86
51. Saukkonen AL, Serlo W, von Wendt L (1988) Electroencephalographic findings and epilepsy in the slit ventricle syndrome of shunt-treated hydrocephalic children. Childs Nerv Syst 4(6):344–347
52. Saukkonen AL, Serlo W, von Wendt L (1990) Epilepsy in hydrocephalic children. Acta Paediatr Scand 79(2):212–218
53. Udayakumara S, Biyani N, Rosenbaum DP, Ben-Sira L, Constantini S, Beni-Adani L (2011) Posterior fossa craniotomy for trapped fourth ventricle in shunted hydrocephalic children - long term outcome. J Neurosurg Pediatr 7(1):52–63
54. Constantini S, Roth J (2010) Endoscopic third ventriculostomy (ETV). In: Jallo G, Kothbauer K, Padilla G (eds) Controversies in pediatric neurosurgery. Thieme Medical & Scientific Publishers, New York
55. Kulkarni AV, Drake JM, Mallucci CL, Sgouros S, Roth J, Constantini S (2009) Endoscopic third ventriculostomy in the treatment of childhood hydrocephalus. J Pediatr 155(2):254–259, e251
56. Roth J, Bo X, Beni-Adani L, Elran H, Constantini S (2007) Endoscopic third ventriculostomy – a physiological alternative to shunts as treatment for obstructive hydrocephalus in children. Harefuah 146(9): 660–665, 735
57. Siomin VC, Constantini S (2004) Basic principles and equipment in neuroendoscopy. In: Abbott R (ed) Clinical neuroendoscopy. WB Saunders, Philadelphia
58. Abtin K, Thompson BG, Walker ML (1998) Basilar artery perforation as a complication of endoscopic third ventriculostomy. Pediatr Neurosurg 28(1):35–41
59. Baykan N, Isbir O, Gercek A, Dagcnar A, Ozek MM (2005) Ten years of experience with pediatric neuroendoscopic third ventriculostomy: features and perioperative complications of 210 cases. J Neurosurg Anesthesiol 17(1):33–37
60. Brockmeyer D, Abtin K, Carey L, Walker ML (1998) Endoscopic third ventriculostomy: an outcome analysis. Pediatr Neurosurg 28(5):236–240
61. Cartmill M, Vloeberghs M (1999) The use of transendoscopic Doppler ultrasound as a safety-enhancing

measure during neuroendoscopic third ventriculostomy. Eur J Pediatr Surg 9(Suppl 1):50–51

62. Darbar A, Kim PD, Yusopov I, Krishnamurthy S (2008) Use of Grotenhuis perforator in endoscopic third ventriculostomy and cyst fenestration. Minim Invasive Neurosurg 51(2):126–129
63. Edwards RJ, Pople IK (2003) Death and third ventriculostomy. J Neurosurg 98(3):649–650; author reply 650–651
64. Horowitz M, Albright AL, Jungreis C, Levy EI, Stevenson K (2001) Endovascular management of a basilar artery false aneurysm secondary to endoscopic third ventriculostomy: case report. Neurosurgery 49(6):1461–1464; discussion 1464–1465
65. Kehler U, Gliemroth J, Knopp U, Arnold H (1998) How to perforate safely a resistant floor of the 3rd ventricle? Technical note. Minim Invasive Neurosurg 41(4):198–199
66. McLaughlin MR, Wahlig JB, Kaufmann AM, Albright AL (1997) Traumatic basilar aneurysm after endoscopic third ventriculostomy: case report. Neurosurgery 41(6):1400–1403; discussion 1403–1404
67. Peretta P, Ragazzi P, Galarza M, Genitori L, Giordano F, Mussa F, Cinalli G (2006) Complications and pitfalls of neuroendoscopic surgery in children. J Neurosurg 105(3 Suppl):187–193
68. Rezende MT, Spelle L, Piotin M, Mounayer C, Lucas Cde P, Abud DG, Moret J (2008) Selective endovascular treatment of a traumatic basilar aneurysm after endoscopic third ventriculostomy. Neuroradiology 50(5):443–446
69. Roux FE (2003) Death and third ventriculostomy. J Neurosurg 98(3):650; author reply 650–651
70. Schmidt RH (1999) Use of a microvascular Doppler probe to avoid basilar artery injury during endoscopic third ventriculostomy. Technical note. J Neurosurg 90(1):156–159
71. Schroeder HW, Niendorf WR, Gaab MR (2002) Complications of endoscopic third ventriculostomy. J Neurosurg 96(6):1032–1040
72. Vloeberghs M, Cartmill M (1999) Improved safety of neuroendoscopic third ventriculostomy by using an operative Doppler ultrasound probe. Technical note. Neurosurg Focus 6(4):e13
73. Beni-Adani L, Siomin V, Segev Y, Beni S, Constantini S (2000) Increasing chronic subdural hematoma after endoscopic III ventriculostomy. Childs Nerv Syst 16(7):402–405
74. Cinalli G, Spennato P, Ruggiero C, Aliberti F, Trischitta V, Buonocore MC, Cianciulli E, Maggi G (2007) Complications following endoscopic intracranial procedures in children. Childs Nerv Syst 23(6): 633–644
75. Depreitere B, Dasi N, Rutka J, Dirks P, Drake J (2007) Endoscopic biopsy for intraventricular tumors in children. J Neurosurg 106(5 Suppl):340–346
76. Di Rocco C, Massimi L, Tamburrini G (2006) Shunts vs endoscopic third ventriculostomy in infants: are there different types and/or rates of complications? A review. Childs Nerv Syst 22(12):1573–1589
77. El-Dawlatly AA, Murshid WR, Elshimy A, Magboul MA, Samarkandi A, Takrouri MS (2000) The incidence of bradycardia during endoscopic third ventriculostomy. Anesth Analg 91(5):1142–1144
78. Ersahin Y, Arslan D (2008) Complications of endoscopic third ventriculostomy. Childs Nerv Syst 24(8): 943–948
79. Hader WJ, Walker RL, Myles ST, Hamilton M (2008) Complications of endoscopic third ventriculostomy in previously shunted patients. Neurosurgery 63(1 Suppl 1):ONS168–ONS174; discussion ONS174–175
80. Husain M, Jha D, Vatsal DK, Thaman D, Gupta A, Husain N, Gupta RK (2003) Neuro-endoscopic surgery – experience and outcome analysis of 102 consecutive procedures in a busy neurosurgical centre of India. Acta Neurochir (Wien) 145(5):369–375; discussion 375–376
81. Massimi L, Di Rocco C, Tamburrini G, Caldarelli M, Iannelli A (2004) Endoscopic third ventriculostomy: complications and failures. Minerva Pediatr 56(2): 167–181
82. Navarro R, Gil-Parra R, Reitman AJ, Olavarria G, Grant JA, Tomita T (2006) Endoscopic third ventriculostomy in children: early and late complications and their avoidance. Childs Nerv Syst 22(5): 506–513
83. Constantini S, Siomin V (2005) Re: Death after late failure of endoscopic third ventriculostomy: a potential solution. Neurosurgery 56(3):E629
84. Constantini S, Siomin V (2005) Death after late failure of endoscopic third ventriculostomy: a potential solution. Neurosurgery 56(4):E873
85. Drake J, Chumas P, Kestle J, Pierre-Kahn A, Vinchon M, Brown J, Pollack IF, Arai H (2006) Late rapid deterioration after endoscopic third ventriculostomy: additional cases and review of the literature. J Neurosurg 105(2 Suppl):118–126
86. Fabiano AJ, Doyle K, Grand W (2010) Delayed stoma failure in adult communicating hydrocephalus after initial successful treatment by endoscopic third ventriculostomy: case report. Neurosurgery 66(6):E1210–E1211; discussion E1211
87. Hader WJ, Drake J, Cochrane D, Sparrow O, Johnson ES, Kestle J (2002) Death after late failure of third ventriculostomy in children. Report of three cases. J Neurosurg 97(1):211–215
88. Javadpour M, May P, Mallucci C (2003) Sudden death secondary to delayed closure of endoscopic third ventriculostomy. Br J Neurosurg 17(3):266–269
89. Lipina R, Palecek T, Reguli S, Kovarova M (2007) Death in consequence of late failure of endoscopic third ventriculostomy. Childs Nerv Syst 23(7): 815–819
90. Mobbs RJ, Vonau M, Davies MA (2003) Death after late failure of endoscopic third ventriculostomy: a potential solution. Neurosurgery 53(2):384–385; discussion 385–386
91. Mohanty A, Vasudev MK, Sampath S, Radhesh S, Sastry Kolluri VR (2002) Failed endoscopic third ventriculostomy in children: management options. Pediatr Neurosurg 37(6):304–309

92. Nigri F, Telles C, Acioly MA (2010) Late obstruction of an endoscopic third ventriculostomy stoma by metastatic seeding of a recurrent medulloblastoma. J Neurosurg Pediatr 5(6):641–644
93. Kulkarni AV, Shams I, Cochrane DD, McNeely PD (2010) Does treatment with endoscopic third ventriculostomy result in less concern among parents of children with hydrocephalus? Childs Nerv Syst 26(11):1529–1534
94. Bullivant KJ, Hader W, Hamilton M (2009) A pediatric experience with endoscopic third ventriculostomy for hydrocephalus. Can J Neurosci Nurs 31(2): 16–19
95. Cinalli G, Salazar C, Mallucci C, Yada JZ, Zerah M, Sainte-Rose C (1998) The role of endoscopic third ventriculostomy in the management of shunt malfunction. Neurosurgery 43(6):1323–1327; discussion 1327–1329
96. Cinalli G (1999) Alternatives to shunting. Childs Nerv Syst 15(11–12):718–731
97. Cinalli G, Sainte-Rose C, Chumas P, Zerah M, Brunelle F, Lot G, Pierre-Kahn A, Renier D (1999) Failure of third ventriculostomy in the treatment of aqueductal stenosis in children. Neurosurg Focus 6(4):e3
98. Di Rocco C, Cinalli G, Massimi L, Spennato P, Cianciulli E, Tamburrini G (2006) Endoscopic third ventriculostomy in the treatment of hydrocephalus in pediatric patients. Adv Tech Stand Neurosurg 31: 119–219
99. Drake JM (2007) Endoscopic third ventriculostomy in pediatric patients: the Canadian experience. Neurosurgery 60(5):881–886; discussion 881–886
100. Drake JM, Kulkarni AV, Kestle J (2009) Endoscopic third ventriculostomy versus ventriculoperitoneal shunt in pediatric patients: a decision analysis. Childs Nerv Syst 25(4):467–472
101. Elbabaa SK, Steinmetz M, Ross J, Moon D, Luciano MG (2001) Endoscopic third ventriculostomy for obstructive hydrocephalus in the pediatric population: evaluation of outcome. Eur J Pediatr Surg 11(Suppl 1):S52–S54
102. Fukuhara T, Vorster SJ, Luciano MG (2000) Risk factors for failure of endoscopic third ventriculostomy for obstructive hydrocephalus. Neurosurgery 46(5):1100–1109; discussion 1109–1111
103. Gangemi M, Donati P, Maiuri F, Longatti P, Godano U, Mascari C (1999) Endoscopic third ventriculostomy for hydrocephalus. Minim Invasive Neurosurg 42(3):128–132
104. Gangemi M, Mascari C, Maiuri F, Godano U, Donati P, Longatti PL (2007) Long-term outcome of endoscopic third ventriculostomy in obstructive hydrocephalus. Minim Invasive Neurosurg 50(5):265–269
105. Goumnerova LC, Frim DM (1997) Treatment of hydrocephalus with third ventriculocisternostomy: outcome and CSF flow patterns. Pediatr Neurosurg 27(3):149–152
106. Hopf NJ, Grunert P, Fries G, Resch KD, Perneczky A (1999) Endoscopic third ventriculostomy: outcome analysis of 100 consecutive procedures. Neurosurgery 44(4):795–804; discussion 804–806
107. Jones RF, Stening WA, Brydon M (1990) Endoscopic third ventriculostomy. Neurosurgery 26(1):86–91; discussion 91–92
108. Kadrian D, van Gelder J, Florida D, Jones R, Vonau M, Teo C, Stening W, Kwok B (2005) Long-term reliability of endoscopic third ventriculostomy. Neurosurgery 56(6):1271–1278; discussion 1278
109. Kulkarni AV, Drake JM, Kestle JR, Mallucci CL, Sgouros S, Constantini S (2010) Predicting who will benefit from endoscopic third ventriculostomy compared with shunt insertion in childhood hydrocephalus using the ETV Success Score. J Neurosurg Pediatr 6(4):310–315
110. Kulkarni AV, Drake JM, Kestle JR, Mallucci CL, Sgouros S, Constantini S (2010) Endoscopic third ventriculostomy vs cerebrospinal fluid shunt in the treatment of hydrocephalus in children: a propensity score-adjusted analysis. Neurosurgery 67(3): 588–593
111. Kulkarni AV, Hui S, Shams I, Donnelly R (2010) Quality of life in obstructive hydrocephalus: endoscopic third ventriculostomy compared to cerebrospinal fluid shunt. Childs Nerv Syst 26(1):75–79
112. Murshid WR (2000) Endoscopic third ventriculostomy: towards more indications for the treatment of non-communicating hydrocephalus. Minim Invasive Neurosurg 43(2):75–82
113. Singh D, Gupta V, Goyal A, Singh H, Sinha S, Singh AK, Kumar S (2003) Endoscopic third ventriculostomy in obstructed hydrocephalus. Neurol India 51(1):39–42
114. Siomin V, Weiner H, Wisoff J, Cinalli G, Pierre-Kahn A, Saint-Rose C, Abbott R, Elran H, Beni-Adani L, Ouaknine G, Constantini S (2001) Repeat endoscopic third ventriculostomy: is it worth trying? Childs Nerv Syst 17(9):551–555
115. Tisell M, Almstrom O, Stephensen H, Tullberg M, Wikkelso C (2000) How effective is endoscopic third ventriculostomy in treating adult hydrocephalus caused by primary aqueductal stenosis? Neurosurgery 46(1):104–110; discussion 101–110
116. Tuli S, Alshail E, Drake J (1999) Third ventriculostomy versus cerebrospinal fluid shunt as a first procedure in pediatric hydrocephalus. Pediatr Neurosurg 30(1):11–15
117. Warf BC, Mugamba J, Kulkarni AV (2010) Endoscopic third ventriculostomy in the treatment of childhood hydrocephalus in Uganda: report of a scoring system that predicts success. J Neurosurg Pediatr 5(2):143–148
118. Zong XY, Zhang YZ (2006) Endoscopic third ventriculostomy in treatment of obstructive hydrocephalus. Zhonghua Yi Xue Za Zhi 86(41):2905–2907
119. Klimo P Jr, Kestle JR (2005) Potentially useful outcome measures for clinical research in pediatric neurosurgery. J Neurosurg 103(3 Suppl):207–212
120. Dalrymple SJ, Kelly PJ (1992) Computer-assisted stereotactic third ventriculostomy in the man-

agement of noncommunicating hydrocephalus. Stereotact Funct Neurosurg 59(1–4):105–110
121. Hopf NJ, Perneczky A (1998) Endoscopic neurosurgery and endoscope-assisted microneurosurgery for the treatment of intracranial cysts. Neurosurgery 43(6):1330–1336; discussion 1336–1337
122. Cochrane DD, Kestle J (2002) Ventricular shunting for hydrocephalus in children: patients, procedures, surgeons and institutions in English Canada, 1989–2001. Eur J Pediatr Surg 12(Suppl 1):S6–S11
123. Cochrane DD, Kestle JR (2003) The influence of surgical operative experience on the duration of first ventriculoperitoneal shunt function and infection. Pediatr Neurosurg 38(6):295–301
124. Asai A, Hoffman HJ, Hendrick EB, Humphreys RP (1989) Dandy-Walker syndrome: experience at the Hospital for Sick Children, Toronto. Pediatr Neurosci 15(2):66–73
125. Beni-Adani L, Ben-Sira L, Constantini S (2010) Surgical treatment of post hemorrhagic hydrocephalus. In: Berger I, Schimmel MS (eds) Hot topics in neonatal neurology. Nova, New York, p Ch 9
126. Buxton N, Macarthur D, Mallucci C, Punt J, Vloeberghs M (1998) Neuroendoscopic third ventriculostomy in patients less than 1 year old. Pediatr Neurosurg 29(2):73–76
127. Buxton N, Jaspan T, Punt J (2002) Treatment of Chiari malformation, syringomyelia and hydrocephalus by neuroendoscopic third ventriculostomy. Minim Invasive Neurosurg 45(4):231–234
128. Chai WX (1995) Long-term results of fourth ventriculo-cisternostomy in complex versus simplex atresias of the fourth ventricle outlets. Acta Neurochir (Wien) 134(1–2):27–34
129. Cinalli G, Spennato P, Savarese L, Ruggiero C, Aliberti F, Cuomo L, Cianciulli E, Maggi G (2006) Endoscopic aqueductoplasty and placement of a stent in the cerebral aqueduct in the management of isolated fourth ventricle in children. J Neurosurg 104(1 Suppl):21–27
130. Decq P, Le Guerinel C, Sol JC, Brugieres P, Djindjian M, Nguyen JP (2001) Chiari I malformation: a rare cause of noncommunicating hydrocephalus treated by third ventriculostomy. J Neurosurg 95(5):783–790
131. Ersahin Y (2007) Endoscopic aqueductoplasty. Childs Nerv Syst 23(2):143–150
132. Faggin R, Bernardo A, Stieg P, Perilongo G, d'Avella D (2009) Hydrocephalus in infants less than six months of age: effectiveness of endoscopic third ventriculostomy. Eur J Pediatr Surg 19(4):216–219
133. Fritsch MJ, Kienke S, Manwaring KH, Mehdorn HM (2004) Endoscopic aqueductoplasty and interventriculostomy for the treatment of isolated fourth ventricle in children. Neurosurgery 55(2):372–377; discussion 377–379
134. Fritsch MJ, Kienke S, Ankermann T, Padoin M, Mehdorn HM (2005) Endoscopic third ventriculostomy in infants. J Neurosurg 103(1 Suppl):50–53
135. Fritsch MJ, Doerner L, Kienke S, Mehdorn HM (2005) Hydrocephalus in children with posterior fossa tumors: role of endoscopic third ventriculostomy. J Neurosurg 103(1 Suppl):40–42
136. Hamada H, Hayashi N, Endo S, Kurimoto M, Hirashima Y, Takaku A (1999) Endoscopic aqueductal plasty via the fourth ventricle through the cerebellar hemisphere under navigating system guidance–technical note. Neurol Med Chir (Tokyo) 39(13):950–952; discussion 952–954
137. Hayashi N, Hamada H, Hirashima Y, Kurimoto M, Takaku A, Endo S (2000) Clinical features in patients requiring reoperation after failed endoscopic procedures for hydrocephalus. Minim Invasive Neurosurg 43(4):181–186
138. Hayhurst C, Osman-Farah J, Das K, Mallucci C (2008) Initial management of hydrocephalus associated with Chiari malformation type I-syringomyelia complex via endoscopic third ventriculostomy: an outcome analysis. J Neurosurg 108(6):1211–1214
139. Hu ZQ, Zhu GT, Huang H, Dai B, Xiao ZY, Guan F, Zhang Y (2009) Endoscopic therapy for obstructive hydrocephalus caused by cysts in the pathway of CSF circulation. Zhonghua Yi Xue Za Zhi 89(17): 1179–1184
140. Inamura T, Morioka T, Nishio S, Ikezaki K, Nonaka H, Yoshiura T (2002) Diverticular enlargement of the foramina of Luschka and congenital hydrocephalus. Childs Nerv Syst 18(11):652–655
141. Jimenez-Leon JC, Jimenez CS, Betancourt YM (2007) Neuroendoscopy. Its usefulness in the hydrocephalus management of children in developing countries. Medicina (B Aires) 67(6 Pt 1):665–673
142. Kadri H, Mawla AA (2004) Variations of endoscopic ventricular anatomy in children suffering from hydrocephalus associated with myelomeningocele. Minim Invasive Neurosurg 47(6):339–341
143. Longatti P, Fiorindi A, Feletti A, Baratto V (2006) Endoscopic opening of the foramen of Magendie using transaqueductal navigation for membrane obstruction of the fourth ventricle outlets. Technical note. J Neurosurg 105(6):924–927
144. Macarthur DC, Buxton N, Vloeberghs M, Punt J (2001) The effectiveness of neuroendoscopic interventions in children with brain tumours. Childs Nerv Syst 17(10):589–594
145. Marlin AE (2004) Management of hydrocephalus in the patient with myelomeningocele: an argument against third ventriculostomy. Neurosurg Focus 16(2):E4
146. Mohanty A (2003) Endoscopic third ventriculostomy with cystoventricular stent placement in the management of dandy-walker malformation: technical case report of three patients. Neurosurgery 53(5):1223–1228; discussion 1228–1229
147. Mohanty A (2005) Endoscopic options in the management of isolated fourth ventricles. Case report. J Neurosurg 103(1 Suppl):73–78
148. Mohanty A, Biswas A, Satish S, Praharaj SS, Sastry KV (2006) Treatment options for Dandy-Walker malformation. J Neurosurg 105(5 Suppl):348–356

149. Mohanty A, Biswas A, Satish S, Vollmer DG (2008) Efficacy of endoscopic third ventriculostomy in fourth ventricular outlet obstruction. Neurosurgery 63(5):905–913; discussion 913–914
150. O'Brien DF, Seghedoni A, Collins DR, Hayhurst C, Mallucci CL (2006) Is there an indication for ETV in young infants in aetiologies other than isolated aqueduct stenosis? Childs Nerv Syst 22(12):1565–1572
151. O'Brien DF, Hayhurst C, Pizer B, Mallucci CL (2006) Outcomes in patients undergoing single-trajectory endoscopic third ventriculostomy and endoscopic biopsy for midline tumors presenting with obstructive hydrocephalus. J Neurosurg 105(3 Suppl):219–226
152. Oertel JM, Mondorf Y, Baldauf J, Schroeder HW, Gaab MR (2009) Endoscopic third ventriculostomy for obstructive hydrocephalus due to intracranial hemorrhage with intraventricular extension. J Neurosurg 111(6):1119–1126
153. Oertel JM, Mondorf Y, Schroeder HW, Gaab MR (2010) Endoscopic diagnosis and treatment of far distal obstructive hydrocephalus. Acta Neurochir (Wien) 152(2):229–240
154. Pavez A, Salazar C, Rivera R, Contreras J, Orellana A, Guzman C, Iribarren O, Hernandez H, Elzo J, Moraga D (2006) Description of endoscopic ventricular anatomy in myelomeningocele. Minim Invasive Neurosurg 49(3):161–167
155. Psarros TG, Coimbra C (2004) Endoscopic third ventriculostomy for patients with hydrocephalus and fourth ventricular cysticercosis: a review of five cases. Minim Invasive Neurosurg 47(6):346–349
156. Ray P, Jallo GI, Kim RY, Kim BS, Wilson S, Kothbauer K, Abbott R (2005) Endoscopic third ventriculostomy for tumor-related hydrocephalus in a pediatric population. Neurosurg Focus 19(6):E8
157. Ruggiero C, Cinalli G, Spennato P, Aliberti F, Cianciulli E, Trischitta V, Maggi G (2004) Endoscopic third ventriculostomy in the treatment of hydrocephalus in posterior fossa tumors in children. Childs Nerv Syst 20(11–12):828–833
158. Sainte-Rose C, Cinalli G, Roux FE, Maixner R, Chumas PD, Mansour M, Carpentier A, Bourgeois M, Zerah M, Pierre-Kahn A, Renier D (2001) Management of hydrocephalus in pediatric patients with posterior fossa tumors: the role of endoscopic third ventriculostomy. J Neurosurg 95(5):791–797
159. Schijman E, Peter JC, Rekate HL, Sgouros S, Wong TT (2004) Management of hydrocephalus in posterior fossa tumors: how, what, when? Childs Nerv Syst 20(3):192–194
160. Singh D, Sachdev V, Singh AK, Sinha S (2005) Endoscopic third ventriculostomy in post-tubercular meningitic hydrocephalus: a preliminary report. Minim Invasive Neurosurg 48(1):47–52
161. Siomin V, Cinalli G, Grotenhuis A, Golash A, Oi S, Kothbauer K, Weiner H, Roth J, Beni-Adani L, Pierre-Kahn A, Takahashi Y, Mallucci C, Abbott R, Wisoff J, Constantini S (2002) Endoscopic third ventriculostomy in patients with cerebrospinal fluid infection and/or hemorrhage. J Neurosurg 97(3):519–524
162. Tamburrini G, Pettorini BL, Massimi L, Caldarelli M, Di Rocco C (2008) Endoscopic third ventriculostomy: the best option in the treatment of persistent hydrocephalus after posterior cranial fossa tumour removal? Childs Nerv Syst 24(12):1405–1412
163. Teo C, Jones R (1996) Management of hydrocephalus by endoscopic third ventriculostomy in patients with myelomeningocele. Pediatr Neurosurg 25(2): 57–63; discussion 63
164. Villavicencio AT, Wellons JC 3rd, George TM (1998) Avoiding complicated shunt systems by open fenestration of symptomatic fourth ventricular cysts associated with hydrocephalus. Pediatr Neurosurg 29(6):314–319
165. Vindigni M, Tuniz F, Ius T, Cramaro A, Skrap M (2010) Endoscopic third ventriculostomy in patients with secondary triventricular hydrocephalus from a haemorrhage or ischaemia in the posterior cranial fossa. Minim Invasive Neurosurg 53(3):106–111
166. Warf BC (2005) Comparison of endoscopic third ventriculostomy alone and combined with choroid plexus cauterization in infants younger than 1 year of age: a prospective study in 550 African children. J Neurosurg 103(6 Suppl):475–481
167. Warf BC (2005) Hydrocephalus in Uganda: the predominance of infectious origin and primary management with endoscopic third ventriculostomy. J Neurosurg 102(1 Suppl):1–15
168. Warf BC, Campbell JW (2008) Combined endoscopic third ventriculostomy and choroid plexus cauterization as primary treatment of hydrocephalus for infants with myelomeningocele: long-term results of a prospective intent-to-treat study in 115 East African infants. J Neurosurg Pediatr 2(5):310–316
169. Warf B, Ondoma S, Kulkarni A, Donnelly R, Ampeire M, Akona J, Kabachelor CR, Mulondo R, Nsubuga BK (2009) Neurocognitive outcome and ventricular volume in children with myelomeningocele treated for hydrocephalus in Uganda. J Neurosurg Pediatr 4(6):564–570
170. Yamada H, Nakamura S, Tanaka Y, Tajima M, Kageyama N (1982) Ventriculography and cisternography with water-soluble contrast media in infants with myelomeningocele. Radiology 143(1):75–83
171. Yamini B, Refai D, Rubin CM, Frim DM (2004) Initial endoscopic management of pineal region tumors and associated hydrocephalus: clinical series and literature review. J Neurosurg 100(5 Suppl Pediatrics):437–441
172. Kulkarni AV, Shams I, Cochrane DD, McNeely PD (2010) Quality of life after endoscopic third ventriculostomy and cerebrospinal fluid shunting: an adjusted multivariable analysis in a large cohort. J Neurosurg Pediatr 6(1):11–16
173. Kulkarni AV, Warf BC, Drake JM, Mallucci CL, Sgouros S, Constantini S (2010) Surgery for hydrocephalus in sub-Saharan Africa versus developed

nations: a risk-adjusted comparison of outcome. Childs Nerv Syst 26(12):1711–1717
174. St George E, Natarajan K, Sgouros S (2004) Changes in ventricular volume in hydrocephalic children following successful endoscopic third ventriculostomy. Childs Nerv Syst 20(11–12):834–838
175. Hiraoka K, Yamasaki H, Takagi M, Saito M, Nishio Y, Iizuka O, Kanno S, Kikuchi H, Kondo T, Mori E (2010) Changes in the volumes of the brain and cerebrospinal fluid spaces after shunt surgery in idiopathic normal-pressure hydrocephalus. J Neurol Sci 296(1–2):7–12
176. Ammirati M, Raimondi AJ (1987) Cerebrospinal fluid shunt infections in children. A study on the relationship between the etiology of hydrocephalus, age at the time of shunt placement, and infection rate. Childs Nerv Syst 3(2):106–109
177. Bakar EE, Bakar B (2010) Neuropsychological assessment of adult patients with shunted hydrocephalus. J Korean Neurosurg Soc 47(3): 191–198
178. Kestle JR, Hoffman HJ, Soloniuk D, Humphreys RP, Drake JM, Hendrick EB (1993) A concerted effort to prevent shunt infection. Childs Nerv Syst 9(3):163–165
179. Kestle JR, Garton HJ, Whitehead WE, Drake JM, Kulkarni AV, Cochrane DD, Muszynski C, Walker ML (2006) Management of shunt infections: a multicenter pilot study. J Neurosurg 105(3 Suppl): 177–181
180. Lacy M, Oliveira M, Austria E, Frim MD (2009) Neurocognitive outcome after endoscopic third ventriculocisterostomy in patients with obstructive hydrocephalus. J Int Neuropsychol Soc 15(3):394–398
181. Lindquist B, Persson EK, Fernell E, Uvebrant P (2011) Very long-term follow-up of cognitive function in adults treated in infancy for hydrocephalus. Childs Nerv Syst 27(4):597–601
182. Pople IK, Bayston R, Hayward RD (1992) Infection of cerebrospinal fluid shunts in infants: a study of etiological factors. J Neurosurg 77(1):29–36
183. Renier D, Lacombe J, Pierre-Kahn A, Sainte-Rose C, Hirsch JF (1984) Factors causing acute shunt infection. Computer analysis of 1174 operations. J Neurosurg 61(6):1072–1078
184. Simon TD, Hall M, Riva-Cambrin J, Albert JE, Jeffries HE, Lafleur B, Dean JM, Kestle JR (2009) Infection rates following initial cerebrospinal fluid shunt placement across pediatric hospitals in the United States. Clinical article. J Neurosurg Pediatr 4(2):156–165
185. Takahashi Y (2006) Long-term outcome and neurologic development after endoscopic third ventriculostomy versus shunting during infancy. Childs Nerv Syst 22(12):1591–1602
186. Walters BC, Hoffman HJ, Hendrick EB, Humphreys RP (1984) Cerebrospinal fluid shunt infection. Influences on initial management and subsequent outcome. J Neurosurg 60(5):1014–1021
187. Buxton N, Macarthur D, Mallucci C, Punt J, Vloeberghs M (1998) Neuroendoscopy in the premature population. Childs Nerv Syst 14(11):649–652
188. Koch D, Wagner W (2004) Endoscopic third ventriculostomy in infants of less than 1 year of age: which factors influence the outcome? Childs Nerv Syst 20(6):405–411
189. Mori H, Nishiyama K, Tanaka R (2003) Endoscopic third ventriculostomy for pediatric hydrocephalic patients: discussion of the indication and strategy for shunt removal. Childs Nerv Syst 19:618
190. Wagner W, Koch D (2005) Mechanisms of failure after endoscopic third ventriculostomy in young infants. J Neurosurg 103(1 Suppl):43–49
191. Abdullah J, Ariff AR, Ghazaime G, Naing NN (2001) Stereotactic neuroendoscopic management of hydrocephalus: a three-year follow-up and analysis of Malaysian children with aqueduct stenosis. Stereotact Funct Neurosurg 76(3–4):175–180
192. Beems T, Grotenhuis JA (2002) Is the success rate of endoscopic third ventriculostomy age-dependent? An analysis of the results of endoscopic third ventriculostomy in young children. Childs Nerv Syst 18(11):605–608
193. Bilginer B, Oguz KK, Akalan N (2009) Endoscopic third ventriculostomy for malfunction in previously shunted infants. Childs Nerv Syst 25(6):683–688
194. Garg A, Suri A, Chandra PS, Kumar R, Sharma BS, Mahapatra AK (2009) Endoscopic third ventriculostomy: 5 years' experience at the All India Institute of Medical Sciences. Pediatr Neurosurg 45(1):1–5
195. Idowu O, Doherty A, Tiamiyu O (2008) Initial experience with endoscopic third ventriculostomy in Nigeria, West Africa. Childs Nerv Syst 24(2):253–255; discussion 257
196. Sufianov A, Sufianova G, Iakimov I (2008) Neuroendoscopic procedures in achievement of shunt independence: outcome analysis of 28 patients with shunt malfunction. Minim Invasive Neurosurg 51(3):158–164
197. Yadav YR, Jaiswal S, Adam N, Basoor A, Jain G (2006) Endoscopic third ventriculostomy in infants. Neurol India 54(2):161–163
198. Baldauf J, Oertel J, Gaab MR, Schroeder HW (2007) Endoscopic third ventriculostomy in children younger than 2 years of age. Childs Nerv Syst 23(6): 623–626
199. Helseth E, Due-Tonnessen B, Egge A, Eide PK, Meling T, Lundar T, Froslie KF (2002) Treatment of hydrocephalus with endoscopic third ventriculocisternostomy. Tidsskr Nor Laegeforen 122(10): 994–998
200. Kamikawa S, Inui A, Kobayashi N, Kuwamura K, Kasuga M, Yamadori T, Tamaki N (2001) Endoscopic treatment of hydrocephalus in children: a controlled study using newly developed Yamadori-type ventriculoscopes. Minim Invasive Neurosurg 44(1): 25–30

201. Koch-Wiewrodt D, Wagner W (2006) Success and failure of endoscopic third ventriculostomy in young infants: are there different age distributions? Childs Nerv Syst 22(12):1537–1541
202. Oertel JM, Baldauf J, Schroeder HW, Gaab MR (2009) Endoscopic options in children: experience with 134 procedures. J Neurosurg Pediatr 3(2): 81–89
203. Sacko O, Boetto S, Lauwers-Cances V, Dupuy M, Roux FE (2010) Endoscopic third ventriculostomy: outcome analysis in 368 procedures. J Neurosurg Pediatr 5(1):68–74
204. Lipina R, Reguli S, Dolezilova V, Kuncikova M, Podesvova H (2008) Endoscopic third ventriculostomy for obstructive hydrocephalus in children younger than 6 months of age: is it a first-choice method? Childs Nerv Syst 24(9):1021–1027
205. Algin O (2010) Role of complex hydrocephalus in unsuccessful endoscopic third ventriculostomy. Childs Nerv Syst 26(1):3–4; author reply 5–6
206. Balthasar AJ, Kort H, Cornips EM, Beuls EA, Weber JW, Vles JS (2007) Analysis of the success and failure of endoscopic third ventriculostomy in infants less than 1 year of age. Childs Nerv Syst 23(2):151–155
207. Burn SC, Saxena A, Tyagi A, Chumas PD (2003) Endoscopic third ventriculostomy in children during the first year of life. Childs Nerv Syst 19:618–619
208. Costa Val JA (2009) Minicraniotomy for endoscopic third ventriculostomy in babies: technical note with a 7-year-segment analysis. Childs Nerv Syst 25(3): 357–359
209. Cota Val JA, Lara A, Herval LM, Serrano P (2003) Endoscopic third ventriculostomy in children under 2 years old: experience of a neuropediatric service in Brazil. Childs Nerv Syst 19:688
210. de Ribaupierre S, Rilliet B, Vernet O, Regli L, Villemure JG (2007) Third ventriculostomy vs ventriculoperitoneal shunt in pediatric obstructive hydrocephalus: results from a Swiss series and literature review. Childs Nerv Syst 23(5):527–533
211. Egger D, Balmer B, Altermatt S, Meuli M (2010) Third ventriculostomy in a single pediatric surgical unit. Childs Nerv Syst 26(1):93–99
212. El-Ghandour NM (2011) Endoscopic third ventriculostomy versus ventriculoperitoneal shunt in the treatment of obstructive hydrocephalus due to posterior fossa tumors in children. Childs Nerv Syst 27(1):117–126
213. Elgamal EA (2010) Continuous monitoring of intracranial pressure after endoscopic third ventriculostomy in the management of CSF shunt failure. Minim Invasive Neurosurg 53(2):49–54
214. Elgamal EA, El-Dawlatly AA, Murshid WR, El-Watidy SM, Jamjoom ZA (2011) Endoscopic third ventriculostomy for hydrocephalus in children younger than 1 year of age. Childs Nerv Syst 27(1): 111–116
215. Etus V, Ceylan S (2005) Success of endoscopic third ventriculostomy in children less than 2 years of age. Neurosurg Rev 28(4):284–288
216. Fritsch MJ (2003) Indication and controversies for endoscopic third ventriculostomy in children. Childs Nerv Syst 19:706–707
217. Fritsch MJ, Mehdorn M (2002) Endoscopic intraventricular surgery for treatment of hydrocephalus and loculated CSF space in children less than one year of age. Pediatr Neurosurg 36(4):183–188
218. Galstian AG, Melikian AG, Korshunov AE, Arutoinov NV (2008) Endoscopic ventriculostomy of the third ventricle in infants of less than 2 years of age. Zh Vopr Neirokhir Im N N Burdenko 1:11–16; discussion 16–17
219. Gangemi M, Maiuri F, Colella G, Magro F, Seneca V, de Divitiis E (2007) Is endoscopic third ventriculostomy an internal shunt alone? Minim Invasive Neurosurg 50(1):47–50
220. Garg AK, Suri A, Sharma BS, Shamim SA, Bal CS (2009) Changes in cerebral perfusion hormone profile and cerebrospinal fluid flow across the third ventriculostomy after endoscopic third ventriculostomy in patients with aqueductal stenosis: a prospective study. Clinical article. J Neurosurg Pediatr 3(1): 29–36
221. Garton HJ, Kestle JR, Cochrane DD, Steinbok P (2002) A cost-effectiveness analysis of endoscopic third ventriculostomy. Neurosurgery 51(1):69–77; discussion 77–78
222. Gathura E, Poenaru D, Bransford R, Albright AL (2010) Outcomes of ventriculoperitoneal shunt insertion in Sub-Saharan Africa. J Neurosurg Pediatr 6(4):329–335
223. Genitori L, Peretta P, Mussa F, Giordano F (2003) Endoscopic third ventriculostomy in children: are age and etiology of hydrocephalus predictive factors influencing the outcome in primary and secondary treated patients? A series of 254 patients and 276 procedures. Childs Nerv Syst 19:619
224. Gorayeb RP, Cavalheiro S, Zymberg ST (2004) Endoscopic third ventriculostomy in children younger than 1 year of age. J Neurosurg 100(5 Suppl Pediatrics):427–429
225. Greenfield JP, Hoffman C, Kuo E, Christos PJ, Souweidane MM (2008) Intraoperative assessment of endoscopic third ventriculostomy success. J Neurosurg Pediatr 2(5):298–303
226. Javadpour M, Mallucci C, Brodbelt A, Golash A, May P (2001) The impact of endoscopic third ventriculostomy on the management of newly diagnosed hydrocephalus in infants. Pediatr Neurosurg 35(3):131–135
227. Jones RF, Kwok BC, Stening WA, Vonau M (1994) Neuroendoscopic third ventriculostomy. A practical alternative to extracranial shunts in noncommunicating hydrocephalus. Acta Neurochir Suppl 61:79–83
228. Kandasamy J, Dwan K, Hartley JC, Jenkinson MD, Hayhurst C, Gatscher S, Thompson D, Crimmins D, Mallucci C (2011) Antibiotic-impregnated ventriculoperitoneal shunts-a multi-centre British paediatric neurosurgery group (BPNG) study

using historical controls. Childs Nerv Syst 27(4): 575–581
229. Kim SK, Wang KC, Cho BK (2000) Surgical outcome of pediatric hydrocephalus treated by endoscopic III ventriculostomy: prognostic factors and interpretation of postoperative neuroimaging. Childs Nerv Syst 16(3):161–168; discussion 169
230. King JA, Auguste KI, Halliday W, Drake JM, Kulkarni AV (2010) Ventriculocystostomy and endoscopic third ventriculostomy/shunt placement in the management of hydrocephalus secondary to giant retrocerebellar cysts in infancy. J Neurosurg Pediatr 5(4):403–407
231. Koksal V, Oktem S (2010) Ventriculosubgaleal shunt procedure and its long-term outcomes in premature infants with post-hemorrhagic hydrocephalus. Childs Nerv Syst 26(11):1505–1515
232. Kombogiorgas D, Sgouros S (2006) Assessment of the influence of operative factors in the success of endoscopic third ventriculostomy in children. Childs Nerv Syst 22(10):1256–1262
233. Komolafe EO, Adeolu AA, Komolafe MA (2008) Treatment of cerebrospinal fluid shunting complications in a Nigerian neurosurgery programme. Case illustrations and review. Pediatr Neurosurg 44(1):36–42
234. Kulkarni AV (2010) Quality of life in childhood hydrocephalus: a review. Childs Nerv Syst 26(6):737–743
235. Lipina R, Reguli S, Novackova L, Podesvova H, Brichtova E (2010) Relation between TGF-beta 1 levels in cerebrospinal fluid and ETV outcome in premature newborns with posthemorrhagic hydrocephalus. Childs Nerv Syst 26(3):333–341
236. Marton E, Feletti A, Basaldella L, Longatti P (2010) Endoscopic third ventriculostomy in previously shunted children: a retrospective study. Childs Nerv Syst 26(7):937–943
237. Meling TR, Tiller C, Due-Tonnessen BJ, Egge A, Eide PK, Froslie KF, Lundar T, Helseth E (2007) Audits can improve neurosurgical practice–illustrated by endoscopic third ventriculostomy. Pediatr Neurosurg 43(6):482–487
238. Ogiwara H, Dipatri AJ Jr, Alden TD, Bowman RM, Tomita T (2010) Endoscopic third ventriculostomy for obstructive hydrocephalus in children younger than 6 months of age. Childs Nerv Syst 26(3): 343–347
239. Osman-Farah JJM, Buxton N, May P, Mallucci C (2003) Endoscopic ventricular fenestration and ETV for the treatment of multicompartmental neonatal hydrocephalus. Childs Nerv Syst 19:702–703
240. Peretta P, Cinalli G, Spennato P, Ragazzi P, Ruggiero C, Aliberti F, Carlino C, Cianciulli E (2009) Long-term results of a second endoscopic third ventriculostomy in children: retrospective analysis of 40 cases. Neurosurgery 65(3):539–547; discussion 547
241. Peretta P, Ragazzi P, Carlino CF, Gaglini P, Cinalli G (2007) The role of Ommaya reservoir and endoscopic third ventriculostomy in the management of post-hemorrhagic hydrocephalus of prematurity. Childs Nerv Syst 23(7):765–771
242. Rahme R, Rahme RJ, Hourani R, Moussa R, Nohra G, Okais N, Samaha E, Rizk T (2009) Endoscopic third ventriculostomy: the Lebanese experience. Pediatr Neurosurg 45(5):361–367
243. Ros-Lopez B, Jaramillo-Dallimonti AM, De Miguel-Pueyo LS, Rodriguez-Barcelo S, Dominguez-Paez M, Ibanez-Botella G, Marquez-Marquez B, Arraez-Sanchez MA (2009) Ventricular haemorrhage in preterm neonates and posthemorrhagic hydrocephalus. Proposal of a management protocol based on early ventriculo-peritoneal shunt. Neurocirugia (Astur) 20(1):15–24
244. Scarrow AM, Levy EI, Pascucci L, Albright AL (2000) Outcome analysis of endoscopic III ventriculostomy. Childs Nerv Syst 16(7):442–444; discussion 445
245. Scavarda D, Bednarek N, Litre F, Koch C, Lena G, Morville P, Rousseaux P (2003) Acquired aqueductal stenosis in preterm infants: an indication for neuroendoscopic third ventriculostomy. Childs Nerv Syst 19(10–11):756–759
246. Sharman A (2000) Endoscopic third ventriculocisternostomies in the infant: pre- & post-operative magnetic resonance imaging evaluation elective project. Clin Radiol 55(12):989
247. Shim KW, Kim DS, Choi JU (2008) Simultaneous endoscopic third ventriculostomy and ventriculoperitoneal shunt for infantile hydrocephalus. Childs Nerv Syst 24(4):443–451
248. Souweidane MM, Morgenstern PF, Kang S, Tsiouris AJ, Roth J (2010) Endoscopic third ventriculostomy in patients with a diminished prepontine interval. J Neurosurg Pediatr 5(3):250–254
249. Sufianov AA, Sufianova GZ, Iakimov IA (2010) Endoscopic third ventriculostomy in patients younger than 2 years: outcome analysis of 41 hydrocephalus cases. J Neurosurg Pediatr 5(4): 392–401
250. van Beijnum J, Hanlo PW, Fischer K, Majidpour MM, Kortekaas MF, Verdaasdonk RM, Vandertop WP (2008) Laser-assisted endoscopic third ventriculostomy: long-term results in a series of 202 patients. Neurosurgery 62(2):437–443; discussion 443–444
251. Wagner W (2006) Why a focus session on endoscopic third ventriculostomy in infants? Childs Nerv Syst 22(12):1527
252. Wagner W, Koch D (2003) Success or failure of endoscopic third ventriculostomy in young infants: is there a correlation with age in patients up to 12 months old? Childs Nerv Syst 19:618
253. Warf BC (2010) Pediatric hydrocephalus in East Africa: prevalence, causes, treatments, and strategies for the future. World Neurosurg 73(4):296–300
254. Warf BC, Kulkarni AV (2010) Intraoperative assessment of cerebral aqueduct patency and cisternal scarring: impact on success of endoscopic third ventriculostomy in 403 African children. J Neurosurg Pediatr 5(2):204–209

255. Warf BC (2007) Endoscopic third ventriculostomy and choroid plexus cauterization for pediatric hydrocephalus. Clin Neurosurg 54:78–82
256. Wiewrodt D, Schumacher R, Wagner W (2008) Hygromas after endoscopic third ventriculostomy in the first year of life: incidence, management and outcome in a series of 34 patients. Childs Nerv Syst 24(1):57–63
257. Sgouros S, Kulkharni AV, Constantini S (2006) The international infant hydrocephalus study: concept and rational. Childs Nerv Syst 22(4):338–345
258. Olschewski M, Schumacher M, Davis KB (1992) Analysis of randomized and nonrandomized patients in clinical trials using the comprehensive cohort follow-up study design. Control Clin Trials 13(3):226–239
259. Edwards RJ, Witchell C, Pople IK (2003) Chronic headaches in adults with spina bifida and associated hydrocephalus. Eur J Pediatr Surg 13(Suppl 1): S13–S17
260. Enchev Y, Oi S (2008) Historical trends of neuroendoscopic surgical techniques in the treatment of hydrocephalus. Neurosurg Rev 31(3): 249–262
261. Pople IK, Edwards RJ, Aquilina K (2001) Endoscopic methods of hydrocephalus treatment. Neurosurg Clin N Am 12(4):719–735, viii
262. Carmel PW, Antunes JL, Hilal SK, Gold AP (1977) Dandy-Walker syndrome: clinico-pathological features and re-evaluation of modes of treatment. Surg Neurol 8(2):132–138
263. Cinalli G, Vinikoff L, Zerah M, Renier D, Pierre-Kahn A (1997) Dandy-Walker malformation associated with syringomyelia. Case illustration. J Neurosurg 86(3):571
264. Hirsch JF, Pierre-Kahn A, Renier D, Sainte-Rose C, Hoppe-Hirsch E (1984) The Dandy-Walker malformation. A review of 40 cases. J Neurosurg 61(3):515–522
265. Klein O, Pierre-Kahn A (2006) Focus on Dandy-Walker malformation. Neurochirurgie 52(4):347–356
266. Klein O, Pierre-Kahn A, Boddaert N, Parisot D, Brunelle F (2003) Dandy-Walker malformation: prenatal diagnosis and prognosis. Childs Nerv Syst 19(7–8):484–489
267. Kumar R, Jain MK, Chhabra DK (2001) Dandy-Walker syndrome: different modalities of treatment and outcome in 42 cases. Childs Nerv Syst 17(6): 348–352
268. Sikorski CW, Curry DJ (2005) Endoscopic, single-catheter treatment of Dandy-Walker syndrome hydrocephalus: technical case report and review of treatment options. Pediatr Neurosurg 41(5): 264–268
269. Jones RF, Kwok BC, Stening WA, Vonau M (1996) Third ventriculostomy for hydrocephalus associated with spinal dysraphism: indications and contraindications. Eur J Pediatr Surg 6(Suppl 1):5–6

Controversies in the Endoscopic Management of the Various Forms of Hydrocephalus

4

Giuseppe Cinalli and Pietro Spennato

4.1 Introduction

Endoscopic third ventriculostomy (ETV) is nowadays considered the preferred treatment in case of obstructive hydrocephalus [1]. Indications to prefer ETV rather than a shunt operation increased in the last years. Initially prerequisite for ETV were [2, 3] acquired aqueductal stenosis, adequate size of third ventricle (at least 1 cm bicoronal diameter), extension of the floor of the third ventricle behind and below the dorsum sellae, and potential patency of subarachnoid spaces. Recently, there has been a tendency to include patients with myelomeningocele, Chiari malformation, congenital aqueductal stenosis, previous meningitis, age younger than 2 years, and prior ventriculoperitoneal shunt [4–8]. However, the success rate of ETV and the risk of complications vary according to the context in which ETV is performed, with some authors preferring alternative treatments. Controversies do surround not only the etiology of hydrocephalus but also other factors: the age of the patient, the role of ETV in case of posterior fossa tumors, the role of ETV in shunt malfunction, the role of ETV redo in case of obstruction of the stoma, and the influence on intellectual outcome of persistent ventricular dilatation following ETV.

4.2 ETV and Aqueductal Stenosis

Intrinsic aqueductal stenosis may be idiopathic or associated with other condition such as intracranial hemorrhage, bacterial or viral infections, and genetic diseases [9]. Hydrocephalus secondary to idiopathic aqueductal stenosis should be considered purely obstructive, without the influence of other factors on the mechanism of resorption of cerebrospinal fluid (CSF).

Despite the fact that the success rate of ETV in case of aqueductal stenosis does not approach 100 % in the series of the literature, there is unanimous consensus to propose ETV as first-line treatment in these cases. The reported success rate is quite homogeneous and stable, being above 60 % [10–12]; probably the high number of unsuccessful cases reflects the inclusion of patients with other factors, such as hemorrhages and infections.

Tumors arising within or around the aqueduct are responsible for the onset of secondary obstruction of the aqueduct. Usually tectal gliomas or hamartomas induce hydrocephalus when they are small, whereas pineal region tumors, inducing distortion of the whole mesencephalon from outside, are usually much larger by the time hydrocephalus is diagnosed. ETV has been

G. Cinalli, MD (✉)
Pediatric Neurosurgery, Santobono-Pausilipon Children's Hospital, Naples, Italy
e-mail: giuseppe.cinalli@gmail.com

P. Spennato, MD
Neurosurgery, Santobono-Pausilipon Children's Hospital, Naples, Italy

S. Sgouros (ed.), *Neuroendoscopy*,
DOI 10.1007/978-3-642-39085-2_4, © Springer-Verlag Berlin Heidelberg 2014

Table 4.1 Results of ETV in younger children, including only patients with idiopathic aqueductal stenosis

Author	No. of patients	Age	Successful ETV
Jones et al. [3]	15	<6 months	7 (47 %)
Buxton et al. [22]	4	<1 year	2 (50 %)
Cinalli et al. [10]	21	<6 months	Same outcome (measured using Kaplan–Meier survival analysis scoring) as did children older than 6 months
Beems and Grotenhuis [13]	16	<2 years	14 (87 %)
Gorayeb et al. [11]	11	<1 year	6 (55 %)
Fritsch et al. [16]	3	<1 year	3 (100 %)
Koch-Wiewrodt and Wagner [24]	13	<1 year	7 (54 %)
Baldauf et al. [18]	8	<2 years	4 (50 %)
Faggin et al. [15]	5	<6 months	4 (80 %)
Sufianov et al. [17]	2	<2 years	2 (100 %)
Ogiwara et al. [19]	11	<6 months	4 (36 %)
Elgamal et al. [14]	37	<1 year	28 (77, 4 %)

shown effective in treating this form of hydrocephalus in large series of patients.

4.3 ETV in Infants with Aqueductal Stenosis

The role of ETV in children younger than 1 year is very controversial in the literature. Many authors claim that ETV results in infants are as good as those in adults, ranging from 70 to 100 %, and do not consider age as a limiting factor in proposing ETV, even in newborns [10–17]. Other authors describe intermediate results, ranging from 47 to 52 % [18–21] and others have experienced very poor results (10–30 % success rate). These authors consider an age younger than 12 months as a contraindication to ETV [22–24]. These data should be considered with criticism; in fact, analyzing only patients with primary aqueductal stenosis, the success rate generally corresponds with an average of 50–70 %, with few exceptions (Table 4.1).

However, a trend in lower success rate in very young infant (under 6 months of age) is noticeable, probably correlated with a higher tendency to form new arachnoid membranes in younger patients [20] or an immature CSF absorption capacity [12, 25]. Considering that shunt surgery is burdened by higher rate of failures and complications in very young children [26], ETV should be preferred in well-selected cases of obstructive hydrocephalus also in this age group.

In conclusion, ETV should be proposed in infancy only in well-selected patients, in which preoperative diagnostic imaging confirms the obstructive nature of hydrocephalus and other factors that can impair the mechanisms of CSF absorption, in particular, infection, are excluded.

4.4 ETV in Infants with Myelomeningocele

The results of ETV in patients affected by myelomeningocele are not satisfactory in very young children [8], while they are good in older children and adolescents (>70 % success).

The presence of a neural tube defect with the consequent CSF leak before birth and its rapid closure immediately after birth may explain impaired development of the subarachnoid spaces and Pacchioni granulations. This could add the factor of poor resorption to the CSF pathways anatomic obstructions (aqueductal stenosis, Chiari II malformation). Later in life, subarachnoid spaces and Pacchioni granulations could develop and allow normal circulation and resorption, thus leaving only the anatomic, obstructive component of hydrocephalus and explaining the good results of ETV performed during shunt malfunction in older meningomyelocele patients.

4.5 ETV in Postinfectious and Posthemorrhagic Hydrocephalus

At the beginning of the experience with endoscopic surgery, patients who suffered CSF infection or intraventricular hemorrhage were considered poor candidates for ETV because of the fear for impairment of mechanisms of CSF absorption. Actually some forms of CNS infection, such as congenital toxoplasmosis, mumps meningoencephalitis, and tuberculous meningitis, can be complicated by obstructive hydrocephalus that can be successfully treated by ETV [1]. Also some cases of hydrocephalus secondary to intraventricular hemorrhage may be attributable to organization of the clot in the aqueduct with secondary aqueductal stenosis. Recent studies report that endoscopic third ventriculostomy is effective in approximately two-thirds of the patients who suffered meningitis, shunt infection, and subarachnoid and/or intraventricular hemorrhage [1, 27]. These data were first shown by the multicenter study of Siomin and colleagues that evaluated the safety, efficacy, and indications of ETV in patients with a history of subarachnoid hemorrhage or intraventricular hemorrhage and/or CSF infection [7]. These authors underlined the concept that patients with obstructive hydrocephalus with a history of either hemorrhage or infection may be good candidates for ETV, while patients who suffered both hemorrhage and infection should be poor candidates.

4.6 ETV in Hydrocephalus Secondary to Posterior Fossa Tumors

Hydrocephalus may complicate posterior fossa tumors during all phases of the disease. Most often hydrocephalus is already present at diagnosis, but it may also occur following surgical removal of the tumor, in case of tumor recurrence and in case of spreading of malignant tumors in the cerebrospinal fluid (CSF) [28].

Surgical options to manage this kind of hydrocephalus include steroids and early surgery, external ventricular drainage (EVD), placement of ventriculoperitoneal (VP) shunt, and ETV. Theoretically ETV offers the same advantage of implantation of ventriculoperitoneal shunting, such as rapid normalization of raised ICP, improvement of the patient's general condition, prevention of postoperative ICP elevation, and long-term control of hydrocephalus, without the shunt-related complications and the complication related to external ventricular drainage. At the beginning of the 2000s, since the publications of the group of Hôpital Necker-Enfants Malades of Paris [29], ETV obtained great popularity in this context, because it was considered able not only to control hydrocephalus in emergency but also to reduce incidence of postoperative hydrocephalus and to improve postoperative course following tumor removal reducing complications such as cerebellar swelling, pseudomeningocele, and CSF leak. However, subsequent studies reproduced only partially the initial good results of Sainte-Rose et al. [29], questioning, above all, the possibility of ETV to provide long-term control of hydrocephalus [30–32]. Moreover, some concern was raised about the systematic preoperative use of ETV in posterior fossa tumors, because a percentage of patients would be submitted to an unnecessary procedure [30, 31, 33], considering that ETV is not without risk [34] and that in most patients hydrocephalus can be resolved with surgical removal of posterior fossa tumor alone [35]. Therefore, the role of preoperative ETV still remains controversial [30, 31]. Moreover, it should be considered that preoperative ETV is at risk of secondary closure by blood products and tumor debris following operation for tumor removal. The risk of postoperative ETV failure might also depend on an impaired CSF absorption within the peripheral subarachnoid spaces because of inflammatory reactions secondary to the operation [34].

Recent orientation is to reserve preoperative ETV to those tumors with higher risk of postoperative hydrocephalus and only in cases where urgent management of hydrocephalus is required. Tumors of the midline, involving the fourth ventricle, especially if malignant and obstructing the foramina of Luschka and Magendie are at high risk of postoperative hydrocephalus and usually present with acute intracranial hypertension. The presence of papilledema at diagnosis is also considered to be significant in a recent study carried out to evaluate the risk of persisting hydrocephalus [36]. This study proposes a risk score where under the age two, the presence of cerebral metastases and the presence of initial hydrocephalus and its severity are confirmed to be the most important features to predict the persistence of postoperative hydrocephalus. The presumed histology of medulloblastoma, ependymoma, or dorsally exophytic brainstem glioma as well as the presence of papilledema seem also to have a role, even if less important.

In our center, patients with midline solid tumors and severe hydrocephalus are considered candidates for preoperative ETV, while patients with hemispheric cystic tumors undergo steroid therapy and early surgery. Urgent ETV is also important to obtain time to conclude the diagnostic workup and schedule tumor surgery in the first available surgical session, following improvement of signs and symptoms of intracranial hypertension.

This practice is in line with the more recent publication of the group of Hôpital Necker-Enfants Malades of Paris, in which it is underlined that correct indication for preresectional ETV concerns essentially tumors involving the fourth ventricle [34]. Preoperative ETV should also be avoided when CSF metastases are suggested by the neuroimaging investigations.

Recently, El-Ghandour [37] reported the first study specifically addressed to midline posterior fossa tumors (medulloblastomas and ependymomas) in pediatric patients with advanced hydrocephalus. He compared preresectional ETV vs. ventriculoperitoneal (VP) shunt. He concluded that the lower incidence of morbidity, the absence of mortality, the lower incidence of procedure failure of ETV as compared to VP shunt, and the significant advantage of not becoming shunt dependent render endoscopic third ventriculostomy the first choice in the treatment of pediatric patients with marked obstructive hydrocephalus due to midline posterior fossa tumors.

More agreement in the neurosurgical community is present in considering postoperative hydrocephalus obstructive in nature and to offer ETV as an alternative to shunt insertion to such patients [29–31].

Tamburrini et al. [38] recently have proposed a different strategy for management of hydrocephalus in posterior fossa tumors: perioperative external ventricular drainage positioned at time of tumor removal, postoperative ICP monitoring through the external ventricular drainage, ETV in case of persistent ventricular dilation and abnormally high ICP values, and VP shunt implantation in case of ETV failure.

In case of failure of ETV following posterior fossa tumor removal, a redo ETV can allow controlling the hydrocephalus when the failure is due to a closure of the stoma; conversely, in case of permeable ETV, the hydrocephalus must be treated with an extrathecal shunt [34].

4.7 ETV in Shunt Malfunction

At the beginning of the experience with ETV, patients previously shunted were considered as poor candidates. The shunt, diverting CSF away from the site of CSF absorption (Pacchioni granulations), was believed to impair the mechanism of CSF absorption. This belief led to the assumption: "once a shunt, always a shunt." More recent observations did not confirm this; on the contrary, it is now believed that a shunt, diverting CSF away from the ventricular system, may allow the CSF spaces around the brain to re-expand, increasing the likelihood of CSF resorption following an ETV [39]. Moreover, it was shown that the anatomy of initially communicating hydrocephalus may change over time following shunt insertion, increasing the likelihood of success of an ETV after a shunt malfunction [4, 6, 40]. Following shunting of originally communicating hydrocephalus, an acquired aqueductal stenosis may develop: the continuous CSF diversion from the lateral ventricle may create a pressure gradient between the supratentorial and infratentorial compartment, causing an anterior rotation of the upper vermis, with subsequent aqueductal stenosis. The results of Siomin in 2002 [7] and O'Brien [6] in 2005 support this hypothesis: Siomin reported an increase in ETV efficacy in posthemorrhagic hydrocephalus from 60.9 to 100 % in primary and secondary ETV, and O'Brien reported an increase of success rate from 27 to 71 % in posthemorrhagic hydrocephalus and from 0 to 75 % in post-meningitic hydrocephalus. Also, in patients with myelomeningocele, a better outcome after secondary ETV has been reported by Teo (84 % vs. 24 %) [8].

In summary, candidates for ETV as alternative to shunt revision are those patients who present an obstructive hydrocephalus at the time of shunt malfunction, regardless of the original cause and radiological appearance of the hydrocephalus. Etiologies of hydrocephalus in which secondary ETV may be considered include aqueductal stenosis, meningomyelocele, obstruction caused by tumor, and posthemorrhagic or post-meningitic hydrocephalus with secondary aqueductal stenosis. We do not agree with those authors who perform ETV whatever radiological appearance of hydrocephalus at time of shunt malfunction.

Preoperative evaluation by magnetic resonance imaging is mandatory to assess anatomical suitability and the patency of the aqueduct and fourth ventricle outlets. MRI T2 sagittal images, with CISS or DRIVE sequences (which are particularly useful in defining structures with two CSF interfaces), should be carefully checked in order to verify the patency and morphology of the prepontine cisterns and, above all, the anatomical features of the third ventricle floor, to be sure that there is enough space to perform the perforation of the floor.

Overall, successful ETV in selected patients who had previously undergone shunt placement has been reported in 42–100 % of patients in different studies [4, 6, 40–44]. In most series the results of secondary ETV are not different from those of primary ETV. It should be remembered that a higher number of complications and abandoned procedures are reported [27, 44–46]. Performing ETV for malfunctioning or infected shunts, in fact, is more difficult than in primary cases because presentation is usually acute, with less severe ventricular dilatation and a third ventricular floor thicker than those seen in chronic hydrocephalus. Moreover, other anatomical abnormalities can be found [39, 47]. The CSF, in case of infection, may be not clear, affecting the surgeon's view through the optic device. Considering these factors, ETV in shunt malfunction should be performed by expert neuro-endoscopists.

4.8 ETV in Shunt Infection

The usual management of shunt infection consists of shunt removal, external ventricular drainage placement, and antibiotics administration, until CSF sterilization. ETV may be performed as alternative to shunt reinsertion in case of compatible anatomy. In case of distal shunt infection (i.e., abdominal pseudocyst or ascites) without ventriculitis (normal CSF sampling), ETV may be performed at the time of shunt removal. There are few reports in the literature specifically addressing the role of ETV in shunt infection. However, preliminary results are encouraging [4, 48–50]. Recently, Shimizu et al. retrospectively reviewed children with shunted hydrocephalus extracting data on CSF shunt infection. They observed a 30 % risk of CSF reinfection in the patients treated with shunt reinsertion and a 11 % risk in the patients in which ETV was performed as alternative to shunt reinsertion. There were no significant differences between the longevity of the reinserted shunt and of ETV. ETV allowed to completely remove the shunt in only a minority of cases (<20 %). The authors conclude that even if a high number of ETV finally fail, the reinserted VP shunt has significantly better longevity than a VP shunt reinserted without using ETV [51].

In conclusion, shunt infection should not be considered a contraindication to ETV, in case of compatible anatomy. ETV may help in managing those difficult cases of chronic bacterial shunt colonization, avoiding reimplantation of foreign material [4].

4.9 ETV in Communicating and Normal Pressure Hydrocephalus

ETV is the treatment of choice of obstructive hydrocephalus, with limited role in case of communicating hydrocephalus. However, reports attesting its efficacy also in case of communicating hydrocephalus have been published, with a successful rate of 45–70 % [52, 53].

The rationale of efficacy of ETV in case of communicating hydrocephalus is more difficult to understand. Differently from obstructive hydrocephalus, where the treatment is aimed to bypass the obstruction, the primary goal in chronic communicating hydrocephalus is to restore intracranial compliance: after opening the ventricle into the basal subarachnoid space, there is an increased expulsion of ventricular CSF during systole, thus reducing the intraventricular pulse pressure, the transmantle pulsatile stress, and the ventricular size. As a consequence, the subarachnoid spaces and their contents expand including the cortical veins, thus restoring intracranial compliance, cerebral blood flow, and perfusion pressure. ETV decreases the transmantle pulsatile stress, thereby reducing the resistance to CSF reabsorption [53, 54]. However, these results should be considered with caution, because in these series a number of patients with shunt malfunction or blockage at the level of the fourth ventricle outlet or basal cistern may be included.

In series of ETV performed in case of normal pressure hydrocephalus (NPH), the success rate is surprisingly high, usually exceeding 65 % [53, 55]. This can be explained with the same physiopathologic considerations as for communicating hydrocephalus. In patients with NPH, the brain elasticity is lost due to multiple factors, including an insufficient transcortical subarachnoid space, fibrosis meningitis, and, above all, periventricular ischemic lesions that weaken the cerebral ventricles. Fenestration of the floor of the third ventricle results in a decrease in the intraventricular pressure, consequently increasing cerebral blood flow and perfusion pressure. However, these cases should also be considered with skepticism, because some cases classified as NPH actually are secondary to a condition known as LOVA (long-standing overt ventriculomegaly in adults) [56]. This is a form of chronic obstructive hydrocephalus with its roots in childhood but that manifests in middle-aged adults: the patients had severe triventriculomegaly and macrocephalus and become symptomatic during adulthood, mimicking a normal pressure hydrocephalus syndrome (dementia, gait disturbances, and urinary incontinence). In these cases, ETV usually restores CSF dynamics.

4.10 ETV Redo in Obstruction of the Stoma

ETV may fail if the stoma becomes blocked by clot, debris, or development of new membranes [57]. A repeat ETV can be proposed in alternative to shunt insertion in well-selected cases: in patients that had experienced excellent clinical response to the first ETV and have favorable radiological presentation (disappearance of the flow artifact on sagittal T2-weighted MRI sequences and presence of typical anatomic deformation of the third ventricle) [58]. In these cases reopening or enlargement of the stoma carries the same success rate as the primary treatment (>65 %) [57–59]. The presence, at surgery, of membranes and arachnoid adhesions in the subarachnoid cisterns and age younger of 2 years at first ETV are important predictors of failure of the second ETV [58].

4.11 ETV in Faciocraniosynostosis

Various forms of syndromic faciocraniosynostosis are associated with hypertensive ventricular dilation in about 20 % of cases. Traditionally this form of hydrocephalus is treated by shunting. The nature of the hydrocephalus is not completely understood, with multiple factors implicated.

Hypoplastic subarachnoid spaces over the cerebral convexities and venous hypertension caused by jugular foramina stenosis may affect CSF absorption mechanisms. Recently, Di Rocco et al. [60] stressed the importance of obstructive cofactors in pathogenesis of hydrocephalus. In particular, the sylvian aqueduct may be restricted or distorted because of the abnormal anatomy within the posterior cranial fossa. The posterior fossa cisterns may be reduced in volume or be completely obliterated. A caudal dislocation of the cerebellar tonsils may affect the CSF flow at the level of the craniocervical junction and/or cisterna magna. In singular cases, the contribution of obstructive and non-obstructive factors may be variable in pathogenesis of hydrocephalus.

Di Rocco et al. [60] reported their preliminary and encouraging results on a group of selected patients treated with ETV. On 46 patients with craniosynostosis and hypertensive hydrocephalus, they selected 11 patients in which, on the basis of MRI findings, an obstructive nature of hydrocephalus was assumed. These findings included not only aqueductal stenosis (that was present in three cases) but also a small and "crowded" posterior fossa, with absence of the cisterna magna and small fourth ventricle and/or cerebellar tonsils herniation, especially when they were associated with downward displacement of the floor of the third ventricle. A long-term success rate of 60 % was obtained. This can be considered a good result, because it was achieved in a group of patients difficult to treat, mostly younger than 1 year of age and more prone to shunt complications.

4.12 Combined ETV and Choroid Plexus Cauterization (CPC)

Endoscopic cauterization of the choroid plexus (CPC) can be combined with ETV in order to reduce the CSF production and increase the success rate of ETV. The most important experience is that of the group of Warf in Uganda, who, since the beginning of 2000s, has adopted the policy to treat hydrocephalus endoscopically whenever possible, regardless of the patient's age or the cause of hydrocephalus. Most of their cases were postinfection hydrocephalus and hydrocephalus associated with myelomeningocele. This choice was determined by the high risk of shunt dependence in the context of rural Africa, because of the inability to obtain timely treatment in case of shunt malfunction. The overall success of combined ETV/CPC in those younger than 1 year of age was significantly better than that for ETV alone, (reaching 66 %) except in those with postinfectious aqueduct obstruction, for whom there was no significant advantage. There was also no significant effect of adding CPC to ETV in children older than 1 year of age, in which the success rate was 80 %. For hydrocephalus associated with myelomeningocele, the effect of adding CPC to ETV was particularly evident (35 % success for ETV alone and 76 % success for combined ETV/CPC) [21, 61]. There was no increased morbidity or mortality over ETV alone. The neurocognitive outcome of children treated by ETV/CPC was as good as those whose hydrocephalus had been shunted [62].

Combined ETV/CPC may be effective in avoiding shunt dependence in the majority of infants presenting with hydrocephalus in the context of a developing country. However, other studies are necessary in order to assess this efficacy also in other geographic contexts.

4.13 ETV Versus Shunt

The main advantages of shunting are that it can be used for all types of hydrocephalus whatever the etiology, it is technically straightforward, and the intraoperative mortality is very low. The benefits of ETV are that the mechanical problems of shunt such as disconnection, occlusion, overdrainage, and valve dysfunction can be avoided. Also, the risk of infection is significantly lower.

The most important difference between ETV and shunt is the effect on the volume of the cerebral ventricles as demonstrated by neuroimaging. The ventricular size usually decreases rapidly and significantly following the shunt implantation, while it decreases much slower and smaller after ETV [63, 64]. This is cause for concern regarding neuropsychological outcome. Hirsch et al. [65] observed a similar postoperative IQ in patients affected by aqueductal stenosis treated with ETV and shunting. Also, Sainte-Rose and Tuli [26, 66] did not find statistical difference between the two groups.

De Ribaupierre et al. [67] observed less revisions and larger revision-free time in children treated with ETV. At 5 years of follow-up, the failure rate of ETV was 26 % and that of VP shunt 42 %.

The group of Kulkarni et al. studied the effect of ETV on quality of life. They observed [68, 69] that the relative risk of ETV failure is initially higher than that for shunt, but after about 3 months following surgery, the relative risk becomes progressively lower for ETV. Furthermore, patients treated with ETV had less frequently repeat surgery, had larger ventricle size at last follow-up, spent fewer days in hospital for CSF obstruction, and spent fewer days per year in hospital for any hydrocephalus-related complications. The outcome measures of quality of life and IQ scores were slightly lower in the ETV group, but these data were not statistically significant.

References

1. Cinalli G (2004) Endoscopic third ventriculostomy. In: Cinalli G, Maixner WJ, Saint-Rose C (eds) Pediatric hydrocephalus. Springer, Milan, pp 361–388
2. Høffman HJ, Harwood-Nash D, Gilday DL (1980) Percutaneous third ventriculostomy in the management of non-communicating hydrocephalus. Neurosurgery 7:313–321
3. Jones RFC, Stening WA, Brydon M (1990) Endoscopic third ventriculostomy. Neurosurgery 26: 86–92
4. Cinalli G, Salazar C, Mallucci C, Yada JZ, Zerah M, Sainte-Rose C (1998) The role of third ventriculostomy in the management of shunt malfunction. Neurosurgery 43:1323–1329
5. Jones RF, Kwok BC, Stening WA, Vonau M (1996) Third ventriculostomy in patients with spinal dysraphism. Indications and contraindications. Eur J Pediatr Surg 6(Suppl):5–6
6. O'Brien DF, Javadpour M, Collins DR, Spennato P, Mallucci CL (2005) Endoscopic third ventriculostomy: an outcome analysis of primary cases and procedures performed after ventriculoperitoneal shunt malfunction. J Neurosurg 103(5 Suppl Pediatrics):393–400
7. Siomin V, Cinalli G, Grotenhuis A, Golash A, Oi S, Kothbauer K, Weiner H, Roth J, Beni-Adani L, Pierre-Kahn A, Takahashi Y, Mallucci C, Abbott R, Wisoff J, Constantini S (2002) Endoscopic third ventriculostomy in patients with cerebrospinal fluid infection and/or hemorrhage. J Neurosurg 97: 519–524
8. Teo C, Jones R (1996) Management of hydrocephalus by endoscopic third ventriculostomy in patients with myelomeningocele. Pediatr Neurosurg 25:57–63
9. Cinalli G, Spennato P, Nastro A, Aliberti F, Trischitta V, Ruggiero C, Mirone G, Cianciulli E (2011) Hydrocephalus in aqueductal stenosis. Childs Nerv Syst 27:1621–1642
10. Cinalli G, Sainte-Rose C, Chumas P, Zerah M, Brunelle F, Lot G, Pierre-Kahn A, Renier D (1999) Failure of third ventriculostomy in the treatment of aqueductal stenosis in children. J Neurosurg 90: 448–454
11. Gorayeb RP, Cavalheiro S, Zymberg SY (2004) Endoscopic third ventriculostomy in children younger than 1 year of age. J Neurosurg 100:427–429
12. Javadpour M, Mallucci C, Brodbelt A, Golash A, May P (2001) The impact of endoscopic third ventriculostomy on the management of newly diagnosed hydrocephalus in infants. Pediatr Neurosurg 35:131–135
13. Beems T, Grotenhuis A (2002) Is the success rate of third ventriculostomy age dependent? An analysis of the results of endoscopic third ventriculostomy in young children. Childs Nerv Syst 18:605–608
14. Elgamal EA, El-Dawlatly AA, Murshid WR, El-Watidy SM, Jamjoom ZA (2011) Endoscopic third ventriculostomy for hydrocephalus in children younger than 1 year of age. Childs Nerv Syst 27: 111–116
15. Faggin R, Bernardo A, Stieg P, Perilongo G, d'Avella D (2009) Hydrocephalus in infants less than six months of age: effectiveness of endoscopic third ventriculostomy. Eur J Pediatr Surg 19:216–219
16. Fritsch MJ, Kienke S, Ankermann T, Padoin M, Mehdorn HM (2005) Endoscopic third ventriculostomy in infants. J Neurosurg 103(1 Suppl):50–53
17. Sufianov AA, Sufianova GZ, Iakimov IA (2010) Endoscopic third ventriculostomy in patients younger than 2 years: outcome analysis of 41 hydrocephalus cases. J Neurosurg Pediatr 5:392–401
18. Baldauf J, Oertel J, Gaab MR, Schroeder HW (2007) Endoscopic third ventriculostomy in children younger than 2 years of age. Childs Nerv Syst 23: 623–626
19. Ogiwara H, Dipatri AJ Jr, Alden TD, Bowman RM, Tomita T (2010) Endoscopic third ventriculostomy for obstructive hydrocephalus in children younger than 6 months of age. Childs Nerv Syst 26:343–347
20. Wagner W, Koch D (2005) Mechanisms of failure after endoscopic third ventriculostomy in young infants. J Neurosurg 103:43–49

21. Warf BC (2005) Comparison of endoscopic third ventriculostomy alone and combined with choroid plexus cauterization in infants younger than 1 year of age: a prospective study in 550 African children. J Neurosurg 103(6 Suppl Pediatrics):475–481
22. Buxton N, Macarthur D, Mallucci C, Punt J, Vloeberghs M (1998) Neuroendoscopic third ventriculostomy in patients less than 1 year old. Pediatr Neurosurg 29:73–76
23. Kadrian D, van Gelder J, Florida D, Jones R, Vonau M, Teo C, Stening W, Kwok B (2005) Long-term reliability of endoscopic third ventriculostomy. Neurosurgery 56:1272–1278
24. Koch-Wiewrodt D, Wagner W (2006) Success and failure of endoscopic third ventriculostomy in young infants: are there different age distributions? Childs Nerv Syst 22:1537–1541
25. Oi S, Di Rocco C (2006) Proposal of "evolution theory in cerebrospinal fluid dynamics" and minor pathway hydrocephalus in developing immature brain. Childs Nerv Syst 22:662–669
26. Tuli S, Alshail E, Drake JM (1999) Third ventriculostomy versus cerebrospinal fluid shunt as a first procedure in pediatric hydrocephalus. Pediatr Neurosurg 30:11–15
27. Hopf NJ, Grunert P, Fries G, Resch KD, Perneczky A (1999) Endoscopic third ventriculostomy: outcome analysis of 100 consecutive procedures. Neurosurgery 44:795–804
28. Di Rocco C, Cinalli G, Massimi L, Spennato P, Cianciulli E, Tamburini G (2006) Endoscopic third ventriculostomy in the treatment of hydrocephalus in pediatric patients. Adv Tech Stand Neurosurg 31:119–219
29. Sainte-Rose C, Cinalli G, Roux FE, Maixner R, Chumas PD, Mansour M, Carpentier A, Bourgeois M, Zerah M, Pierre-Kahn A, Renier D (2001) Management of hydrocephalus in pediatric patients with posterior fossa tumors: the role of endoscopic third ventriculostomy. J Neurosurg 95:791–797
30. Fritsch MJ, Doerner L, Kienke S, Mehdorn HM (2005) Hydrocephalus in children with posterior fossa tumors: role of endoscopic third ventriculostomy. J Neurosurg 103(1 Suppl):40–42
31. Morelli D, Pirotte B, Lubansu A, Detemmerman D, Aeby A, Fricx C, Berre J, David P, Brotchi J (2005) Persistent hydrocephalus after early surgical management of posterior fossa tumors in children: is routine preoperative endoscopic third ventriculostomy justified? J Neurosurg 103(3 Suppl):247–252
32. Ruggiero C, Cinalli G, Spennato P, Aliberti F, Cianciulli E, Trischitta V, Maggi G (2004) Endoscopic third ventriculostomy in the treatment of hydrocephalus in posterior fossa tumors in children. Childs Nerv Syst 20:828–833
33. Ray P, Jallo GI, Kim RYH, Kim BS, Wilson S, Kothbauer K, Abbott R (2005) Endoscopic third ventriculostomy for tumor-related hydrocephalus in a pediatric population. Neurosurg Focus 19(6):E8
34. Di Rocco F, Jucá CE, Zerah M, Sainte-Rose C (2012) Endoscopic third ventriculostomy and posterior fossa tumors. World Neurosurg. doi:10.1016/j.wneu.2012.02.018
35. Due-Tonnessen BJ, Helseth E (2007) Management of hydrocephalus in children with posterior fossa tumors: role of tumor surgery. Pediatr Neurosurg 43:92–96
36. Riva-Cambrin J, Detsky AS, Lamberti-Pasculli M, Sargent MA, Armstrong D, Moineddin R, Cochrane DD, Drake JM (2009) Predicting postresection hydrocephalus in pediatric patients with posterior fossa tumors. J Neurosurg Pediatr 3:378–385
37. El-Ghandour NM (2011) Endoscopic third ventriculostomy versus ventriculoperitoneal shunt in the treatment of obstructive hydrocephalus due to posterior fossa tumors in children. Childs Nerv Syst 27: 117–126
38. Tamburrini G, Pettorini BL, Massimi L, Caldarelli M, Di Rocco C (2008) Endoscopic third ventriculostomy: the best option in the treatment of persistent hydrocephalus after posterior cranial fossa tumor removal? Childs Nerv Syst 24:1405–1412
39. Spennato P, Ruggiero C, Aliberti F, Nastro A, Mirone G, Cinalli G (2013) Third ventriculostomy in shunt malfunction. World Neurosurg 79:S22.e21–S22.e26
40. Marton E, Feletti A, Basaldella L, Longatti P (2010) Endoscopic third ventriculostomy in previously shunted children: a retrospective study. Childs Nerv Syst 26:937–943
41. Bilginer B, Oguz KK, Akalan N (2009) Endoscopic third ventriculostomy for malfunction in previously shunted infants. Childs Nerv Syst 25:683–688
42. Boschert J, Hellwig D, Krauss JK (2003) Endoscopic third ventriculostomy for shunt dysfunction in occlusive hydrocephalus: long term follow up and review. J Neurosurg 98:1032–1039
43. Buxton N, Macarthur D, Robertson I, Punt J (2003) Neuroendoscopic third ventriculostomy for failed shunts. Surg Neurol 60:201–204
44. Hader WJ, Walker RL, Myles ST, Hamilton M (2008) Complications of endoscopic third ventriculostomy in previously shunted patients. Neurosurgery 63(Suppl 1):ONS168–ONS174
45. Brockmeyer D, Abtin K, Carey L, Walker ML (1998) Endoscopic third ventriculostomy: an outcome analysis. Pediatr Neurosurg 28:236–240
46. Jones RF, Kwok BC, Stening WA, Vonau M (1994) The current status of endoscopic third ventriculostomy in the management of noncommunicating hydrocephalus. Minim Invasive Neurosurg 37: 28–36
47. Punt J (2004) Third ventriculostomy in shunt malfunction. In: Cinalli G, Maixner WJ, Sainte-Rose C (eds) Pediatric hydrocephalus. Springer, Milan, pp 389–396
48. Jones RFC, Stening WA, Kwok BCT, Sands TM (1993) Third ventriculostomy for shunt infections in children (technique and application). Neurosurgery 32:855–860

49. Fukuhara T, Vorster SJ, Luciano MG (2000) Risk factors for failure of endoscopic third ventriculostomy for obstructive hydrocephalus. Neurosurgery 46: 1100–1111
50. Punt J, Vloeberghs M (1998) Endoscopy in neurosurgery. Minim Invasive Ther Allied Technol 7:159–170
51. Shimizu T, Luciano MG, Fukuhara T (2012) Role of endoscopic third ventriculostomy at infected cerebrospinal fluid shunt removal. J Neurosurg Pediatr 9: 320–326
52. Hailong F, Guangfu H, Haibin T, Hong P, Yong C, Weidong L, Dongdong Z (2008) Endoscopic third ventriculostomy in the management of communicating hydrocephalus: a preliminary study. J Neurosurg 109:923–930
53. Rangel-Castilla L, Barber S, Zhang YJ (2012) The role of endoscopic third ventriculostomy in the treatment of communicating hydrocephalus. World Neurosurg 77:555–560
54. Greitz D (2004) Radiological assessment of hydrocephalus: new theories and implications for therapy. Neurosurg Rev 27:145–165; discussion 166–167
55. Gangemi M, Maiuri F, Buonamassa S, Colella G, de Divitiis E (2004) Endoscopic third ventriculostomy in idiopathic normal pressure hydrocephalus. Neurosurgery 55:129–134
56. Oi S, Shimoda M, Shibata M, Honda Y, Togo K, Shinoda M, Tsugane R, Sato O (2000) Pathophysiology of long-standing overt ventriculomegaly in adults. J Neurosurg 92:933–940
57. Fukuhara T, Luciano M, Kowalski RJ (2002) Clinical features of third ventriculostomy failures classified by fenestration patency. Surg Neurol 58:102–110
58. Peretta P, Cinalli G, Spennato P, Ragazzi P, Ruggiero C, Aliberti F, Carlino C, Cianciulli E (2009) Long-term results of a second endoscopic third ventriculostomy in children: retrospective analysis of 40 cases. Neurosurgery 65:539–547
59. Surash S, Chumas P, Bhargava D, Crimmins D, Straiton J, Tyagi A (2010) A retrospective analysis of revision endoscopic third ventriculostomy. Childs Nerv Syst 26:1693–1698
60. Di Rocco F, Jucá CE, Arnaud E, Renier D, Sainte-Rose C (2010) The role of endoscopic third ventriculostomy in the treatment of hydrocephalus associated with faciocraniosynostosis. J Neurosurg Pediatr 6:17–22
61. Warf BC, Campbell JW (2008) Combined endoscopic third ventriculostomy and choroid plexus cauterization (ETV/CPC) as primary treatment of hydrocephalus for infants with myelomeningocele: long-term results of a prospective intention to treat study in 115 African infants. J Neurosurg Pediatr 2:310–316
62. Warf BC, Ondoma S, Kulkarni A, Donnelly R, Ampeire M, Akona J, Kabachelor C, Mulondo R, Nsubuga B (2009) Neurocognitive outcome and ventricular volume in myelomeningocele children treated for hydrocephalus in Uganda. J Neurosurg Pediatr 4:564–570
63. Xenos C, Sgouros S, Natarajan K, Walsh AR, Hockley AD (2003) Influence of shunt type on ventricular volume changes in children with hydrocephalus. J Neurosurg 98:277–283
64. St George E, Natarajan K, Sgouros S (2004) Changes in ventricular volume in hydrocephalic children following successful endoscopic third ventriculostomy. Childs Nerv Syst 20:834–838
65. Hirsch JF (1982) Percutaneous ventriculocisternostomies in non-communicating hydrocephalus. Monogr Neural Sci 8:170–178
66. Sainte-Rose C (1992) Third ventriculostomy. In: Manwaring KH, Crone KR (eds) Neuroendoscopy. Mary Ann Liebert, New York, pp 47–62
67. de Ribaupierre S, Rilliet B, Vernet O, Regli L, Villemure J-G (2007) Third ventriculostomy vs ventriculoperitoneal shunt in pediatric obstructive hydrocephalus: results from a Swiss series and literature review. Childs Nerv Syst 23:527–533
68. Kulkarni AV, Drake JM, Kestle JR, Mallucci CL, Sgouros S, Constantini S (2010) Endoscopic third ventriculostomy vs cerebrospinal fluid shunt in the treatment of hydrocephalus in children: a propensity score-adjusted analysis. Neurosurgery 67: 588–593
69. Kulkarni AV, Hui S, Shams I, Donnelly R (2010) Quality of life in obstructive hydrocephalus: endoscopic third ventriculostomy compared to cerebrospinal fluid shunt. Childs Nerv Syst 26:75–79

Current Status and Future Developments of Neuroendoscopic Management of Pituitary Tumours and Craniopharyngiomas

5

Paolo Cappabianca, Luigi Maria Cavallo, Isabella Esposito, and Felice Esposito

5.1 Introduction

Pituitary tumours and craniopharyngiomas are benign midline skull base lesions, which frequently involve adjacent structures such as the pituitary stalk, optic apparatus, major blood vessels and hypothalamus. Following the evolution of the concept of "minimally invasive surgery", the endoscopic endonasal technique has been applied for pituitary adenomas and craniopharyngiomas in both endoscope-assisted and endoscope-controlled modality with encouraging results [3, 7, 11, 16, 19, 24, 25, 29, 30, 34, 45, 49]. During the last decade, the use of the endoscope through the nose underwent a progressive optimization, driven not only by the development of superior optic systems but also by the contemporary improvement of image-guided surgery techniques, dedicated instruments, haemostatic materials and dural and bone substitutes. Technological advancement of the endoscopic endonasal technique allowed progressive extension of the endonasal route to lesions which have been regularly treated transcranially [1, 19, 20, 23, 26, 29, 37]. In order to maximize such technique, the main preconditions are thorough anatomic knowledge, endoscopic surgical skill, familiarity with haemostasis techniques and reconstruction strategies.

P. Cappabianca, MD (✉) • L.M. Cavallo, MD
I. Esposito, MD • F. Esposito, MD
Department of Neurosciences and Reproductive and Odontostomatological Sciences,
Division of Neurosurgery,
Università degli Studi di Napoli Federico II,
Naples, Italy
e-mail: cappabia@unina.it

5.2 Management of Pituitary Tumours

The endoscope has become part of the standard equipment in most neurosurgical operating theatres; several studies demonstrated that the endoscopic endonasal transphenoidal technique to treat pituitary adenomas is superior or at least equal to the microsurgical approach in terms of vision of the relevant surgical targets, exposure of the tumour-brain/gland interface, complication rate and results [4–7, 21, 27, 32, 50]. It has to be underlined that in the management of pituitary adenomas the indications for surgery by means of the endoscopic transphenoidal technique are the same used since the 1960s, as with the microscopic transphenoidal route [31].

Surgical excision of hormonally inactive adenomas has a low morbidity and leads to an improvement of visual symptoms in the majority of cases; in patients with macroadenomas and preoperative normal pituitary function, the endoscopic close-up view may increase the chance to identify and preserve residual pituitary gland. Patients with hormonally active prolactinomas are referred for surgery for cystic lesions, after failure of medical treatment or for complications related to it (CSF leak, pituitary apoplexy) or when they

S. Sgouros (ed.), *Neuroendoscopy*,
DOI 10.1007/978-3-642-39085-2_5, © Springer-Verlag Berlin Heidelberg 2014

refuse long-term medical therapy. Furthermore, possible deleterious effects of cabergoline on heart valve abnormalities have been recently investigated [18], and endocrinologists are referring PRL adenoma patients to experienced pituitary surgeons in a greater number than in the previous recent years. In patients with acromegaly, despite advances in pharmacological suppression of GH levels by means of somatostatin analogues or GH-receptor antagonists [2, 17, 47], transphenoidal surgery remains the first-line therapy [32]. In experienced hands, surgery has the advantage of immediate lowering of the growth hormone excess, with endocrine remission rates of 70 % for microadenomas and 50 % for macroadenomas [40]. In recurrences of GH-secreting pituitary adenomas, 48 % of cases can achieve remission with repeated transphenoidal surgery [41], and the endoscopic technique has proved to be safe and effective for such purpose [3]. In ACTH-secreting pituitary adenomas, surgery is offered as a primary therapy. Management of recurrences is still controversial [22, 42, 46]; we favour repeat surgery and, in case of failure, radiosurgery, with reported encouraging results [33]. Medical therapy with cabergoline has been proposed as an adjuvant therapy in selected patients [44].

5.2.1 Operative Technique

The patient's nasal anatomy, the characteristics of the lesion and the surgeon's preference determine the side of approach. For microadenomas that are off the midline, and for those macroadenomas extending into the medial cavernous sinus, the contralateral nasal cavity allows a better exposure. More recently, a binostril approach with a partial posterior septectomy has been favoured since it allows for more than one instrument to be inserted in addition to the endoscope, which is used freehand during the whole procedure ("two nostrils-four hands technique") [12, 14, 35]. The surgical corridor between the nasal septum and the middle turbinate is enlarged by pushing laterally the middle turbinate. The appropriate trajectory toward the sphenoid sinus is maintained running the endoscope parallel to the nasal floor, toward the choana, and then angling it up along the sphenoethmoid recess. Failure to adhere to this principle may result in misdirection superiorly, into the ethmoid sinus and/or the anterior cranial fossa. After anterior sphenoidotomy, careful identification of the anatomic landmarks over the posterior wall of the sphenoid sinus guides the opening of the sellar floor.

After meticulous haemostasis of the endonasal corridor, dural opening and tumour removal are tailored to the lesion extension.

In case of microadenoma, the endoscope can highlight its pseudocapsule and enable a radical en bloc resection. When a surgical plane cannot be developed, adenomatous tissue, yellowish and softer than normal pituitary gland, is easily aspirated and/or piecemeal removed. When decompressed, pituitary tissue appears yellowish-orange, thanks to its microvasculature. In case of intra- and suprasellar macroadenoma, during tumour removal the diaphragma may descend rapidly while pockets of tumour are left behind; to avoid such side effect, a gradual emptying technique should be used: tumour debulking should start from the bottom of the sella, then from the lateral tumour extension and finally from the suprasellar component (Fig. 5.1). When the suprasellar cistern is thinned and infiltrated, a capsule remnant may be left in place to avoid CSF leakage. After tumour removal, the suprasellar cistern should be explored all around to check for eventual retained tumour and/or CSF leakage.

Intra- and suprasellar fibrous adenoma and giant adenomas with a prevalent suprasellar extension can be unlocked through an extended endoscopic approach to the planum, by expanding the bone window upon the tuberculum sellae and planum sphenoidale. After internal debulking, the tumour is gently pulled downward and removed through an extracapsular dissection. The endoscopic multiangled close-up view allows precise and effective dissection of tumour capsule from the arachnoid covering the optic pathway and anterior cerebral artery-anterior communicating artery complex.

The endoscopic approach offers the possibility to manage even wide parasellar adenomatous

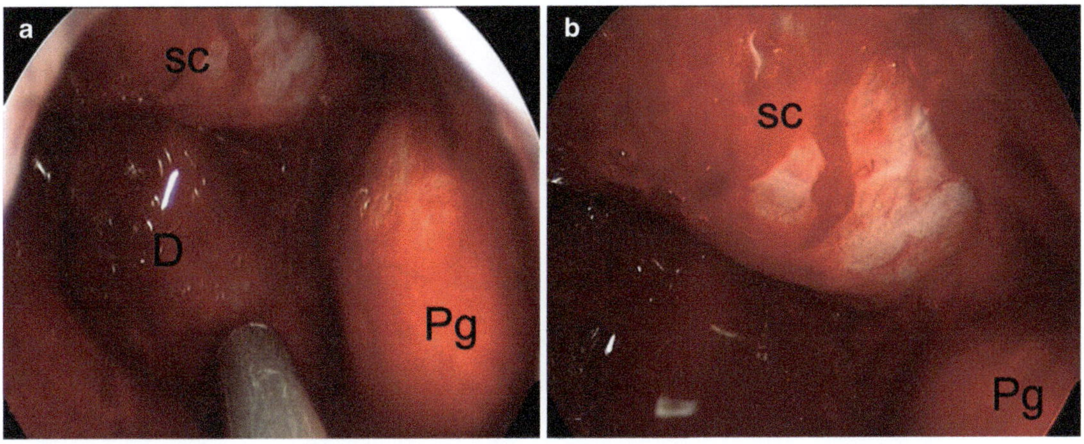

Fig. 5.1 Endoscopic view of the surgical field after the removal of a large pituitary adenoma. Note the residual gland pushed toward the left wall of the sella (**a**). Endoscopic close-up view of the suprasellar cistern (**b**). *D* dorsum sellae, *Sc* suprasellar cistern, *Pg* pituitary gland

extension; in such cases, the medial wall of the cavernous sinus has been already fenestrated by the tumour, mainly at level of its superior aspect, which is thinner, thus representing a "natural gate" toward the medial compartment of the cavernous sinus [48]. The venous bleeding indicates the completeness of tumour removal and is easily controlled with warm saline irrigation, cottonoid compression and, if brisky, with thrombin-gelatine matrix (Floseal, Baxter BioSurgery, Vienna, Austria) [10].

When the pituitary adenoma extends to the lateral compartment of the cavernous sinus, it can be delivered through an ipsilateral transethmoid transpterygoid route [13, 25, 36]. The endonasal corridor is widened along the coronal plane by removing the posterior ethmoid and drilling the root of the medial pterygoid process; the lateral recess of the sphenoid sinus is exposed, and the lateral compartment of the cavernous sinus is entered through a quadrangular safety area, bordered superiorly by V2, inferiorly by the vidian nerve and posteriorly by the parasellar and paraclival carotid artery [13, 39].

After tumour removal, the sellar reconstruction is required mainly when an intraoperative CSF leak has occurred. Autologous or heterologous materials, either resorbable or not, are used, if necessary, to achieve a safe and effective sellar reconstruction. The aim of the repair is to provide a watertight closure, reduce the dead space and prevent the descent of the chiasm into the sellar cavity. Overpacking and subsequent damage to the optic chiasm should be avoided. In addition to accurately packing the sellar cavity, it is necessary to close the sellar floor. Different techniques are used (intra- and/or extradural closure of the sella and packing of the sella with or without packing of the sphenoid sinus), depending on the size of osteodural defect and of the dead space inside the sella [9, 15].

5.3 Craniopharyngiomas

The current management of craniopharyngioma aims for complete resection, which remains the gold standard, although recurrence is a common event [8, 16, 19, 26, 28, 29]. The multitude of operative approaches to these midline deep-seated lesions reflects their challenging nature. Several factors can guide a case-specific choice of the approach:

- Patient's characteristics: age, pituitary function and ophthalmologic status, degree of hypothalamic dysfunction, primary or recurrent pathology and in the latter, history of previous surgery and/or radiosurgery
- Lesion's configuration: consistency, presence of cysts and calcification, dimension, growth

direction, lateral extension, relationship with the ICA and with the third ventricle, pial invasion
- Surgeon's personal experience

Systematic review of these factors has a critical role when designing the appropriate surgical approach.

A pure intrasellar lesion with enlargement of the sella turcica is a well-established indication for the standard transphenoidal approach.

In case of intra-suprasellar infradiaphragmatic lesion, the sella turcica is enlarged, and the diaphragma sellae is pushed upward. In the majority of cases, a standard transphenoidal approach allows the removal of the lesion since the suprasellar part usually collapses down into the sella after the removal of the intrasellar compartment of the lesion. In case of suprasellar craniopharyngiomas, some selected cases can be treated using the transtuberculum-transplanum approach. The main steps of the procedure are:

- Creation of a wide endonasal corridor with middle turbinectomy (uni- or bilateral), posterior septectomy and a wide anterior sphenoidotomy [35].
- Drilling of the sellar floor and of the tuberculum sellae, with bone removal extended between the medial opto-carotid recesses (Fig. 5.2). We routinely use some additional tools (neuronavigator, dedicated instruments, micro-Doppler probe) that improve safety and effectiveness of the procedure.

Among supradiaphragmatic lesions, Kassam has recently proposed an approach-based classification useful when removing the craniopharyngioma from the endonasal route; he brings out four main types: pre-, trans- and retroinfundibular and lesions isolated to the third ventricle [37].

In suprasellar prechiasmatic preinfundibular lesions, the transtuberculum-transplanum sphenoidale approach provides a direct midline exposure of the tumour, which is seen immediately after dural opening. The optic nerves and chiasm are usually stretched superiorly by the tumour, and the endoscopic view from below highlights in a safe way the distal branches of the superior hypophyseal arteries, which supply the inferior surface of the optic chiasm and the pars tuberalis

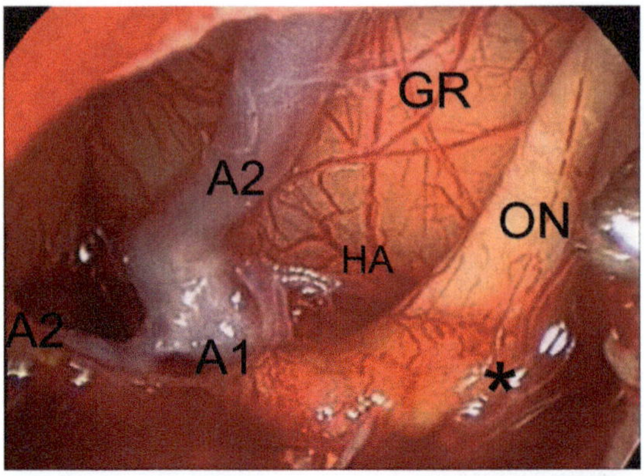

Fig. 5.2 Intra-op image shows suprasellar neurovascular structures after the removal of a suprasellar prechiasmatic craniopharyngioma. *A1* precommunicating segment of the anterior cerebral artery, *A2* postcommunicating segment of the anterior cerebral artery, *HA* Heubner's artery, *GR* gyrus rectus, *ON* optic nerve, *asterisk* thickened arachnoid

of the pituitary; their preservation is critical for the visual and endocrine outcome. As for transcranial techniques, tolerance of the optic system to surgical manipulation depends on its preoperative status: an optic nerve or chiasm already stretched and distorted by adjacent tumour is extremely sensitive to any type of manipulation; however, the endoscopic endonasal technique offers the opportunity to early decompress the nerves and to dissect the tumour from the nerve and not vice versa as usually occurs during transcranial procedures, thus minimizing the surgical manipulation over the optic pathways (Fig. 5.2).

Concerning retrochiasmatic retroinfundibular craniopharyngiomas, the number of surgical classifications and cranial approaches (subfrontal, pterional, transcallosal, transpetrosal) proposed for such lesions over the years reflects the difficulty in exposing them widely through a single approach. The endoscopic endonasal route provides a coaxial route to the lesion extension. The starting gate is the pituitary stalk [37]; depending on the pattern of growth of the lesion, intra- and/or para-pituitary stalk routes can be followed toward the retrosellar and even intraventricular area (Fig. 5.3).

When dealing with retroinfundibular lesions, the pituitary stalk can be preserved by running

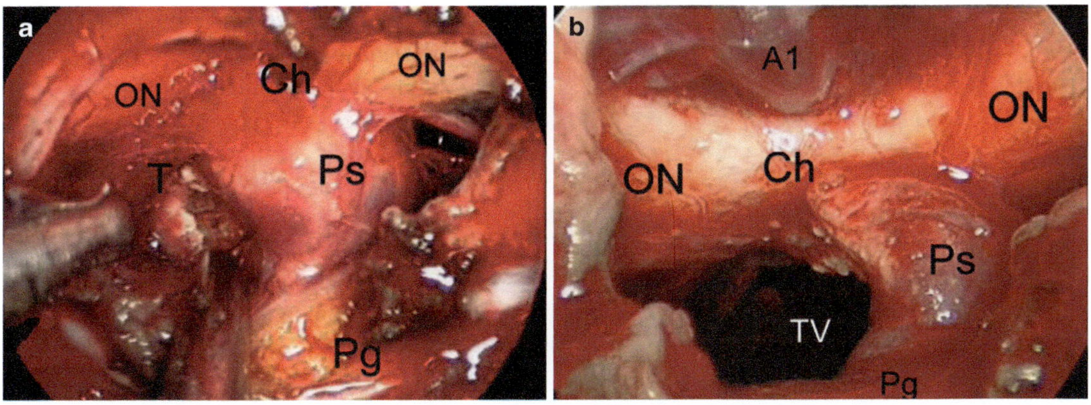

Fig. 5.3 Intra-op image during the removal of a suprasellar retroinfundibular craniopharyngioma before (**a**) and after (**b**) tumour removal. *ON* optic nerve, *Ch* chiasm, *Ps* pituitary stalk, *T* tumour, *Pg* pituitary gland, *A1* precommunicating segment of the anterior cerebral artery, *TV* third ventricle

the endoscope and instruments along the para-pituitary stalk corridors and/or by mobilizing the gland upward as proposed by Kassam et al. [38]. However, such procedure requires extensive experience in endonasal skull base surgery. Furthermore, depending on downward extension in the posterior cranial fossa, retroinfundibular lesions can also require drilling of the dorsum sellae and removal of the posterior clinoids [37].

When the lesion grows into the infundibulum, the pituitary stalk is usually enlarged by the tumour, which creates a corridor to enter the ventricular chamber; since it may be hard to understand how the third ventricle can be unlocked through the nose, some considerations supporting such strategy have to be clarified. When dealing with a lesion inside the third ventricle, the possibility to apply the endoscopic endonasal technique depends on two main factors:

- The position of the floor of the third ventricle
- The size and position of the infundibulum and of the pituitary stalk

A craniopharyngioma which displaces the floor of the third ventricle inferiorly and enlarges the infundibulum, pushing it over the sella, creates the surgical space needed to face the lesion just after the dural opening over the suprasellar area.

Some points have to be considered when approaching such intraventricular lesions:

1. The dura should be opened carefully in the suprasellar area since the chiasm may lie just behind the dura in a prefixed position, pushed anteriorly by the intraventricular lesion; preoperative MRI is of value to highlight the distance between the tuberculum sellae and the chiasm.
2. When dissecting the tumour from the floor of the third ventricle, the latter should never be violated at the level of the mammillary bodies or even more posteriorly to avoid the risk of brain stem injury.
3. Invasive fingerlike tumoural infiltration and/or gliotic tissue adherent to the hypothalamus represents a contraindication to further dissection.

5.4 Reconstruction in Extended Approaches

After tumour removal and careful haemostasis, the reconstruction of the osteodural defect is tailored in order to avoid CSF leakage. The latter is related to the degree of subarachnoid dissection and/or opening of the third ventricle.

In standard transphenoidal surgery, the integrity of the subarachnoid space is usually preserved, whereas in extended transplanum approaches wide arachnoidal opening is a prerequisite to a successful surgery. In the

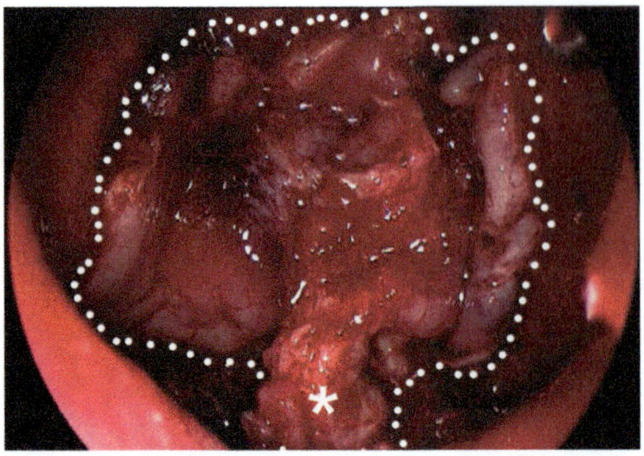

Fig. 5.4 Intra-op image showing a vascularized nasoseptal flap. *Dotted line* borders of the flap, *asterisk* vascular pedicle containing the septal branches of the sphenopalatine artery

transtuberculum-transplanum approach, the bone window has an irregular shape and is bordered by neurovascular structures such as the optic nerve and the internal carotid artery. The reconstruction technique comprises the following main steps:

1. Arachnoid sealing. A thin layer of fibrin glue (Tisseel, Baxter, Vienna, Austria) is injected intradurally to create a first barrier to CSF leakage.
2. The osteodural defect is reconstructed extradurally with a foil of collagen-derived dural substitute which exceeds the bone defect, held in place with a fragment of bone substitute (Lactosorb®, Walter Lorenz Surgical, INC., Florida, USA) which fits the bone opening.
3. The whole skull base defect is then covered with a vascularized nasoseptal flap, which is designed preoperatively, depending on the size of the craniectomy; due to its shrinkage, it should be about 30 % larger than the defect (Fig. 5.4) [43].

5.5 Future Perspectives

Despite significant improvements in medical therapy, surgery still has an important role in the management of pituitary adenomas and craniopharyngiomas. Further development of the endoscopic techniques will be driven by several technological advances such as high-definition intraoperative digital imaging, three-dimensional endoscopy and dedicated instruments [47, 51]. Another important determinant in improving the global outcomes of such techniques is the advancement in the anatomic research, which is of utmost importance to define the advantages and limits of skull base surgery with the endoscopic endonasal technique. At the same time, the evolution of reconstruction materials and of reconstruction techniques will greatly affect this still critical step of the procedure.

Among the sophisticated features of modern integrated operating rooms, the availability of advanced capabilities in telemedicine and live telesurgery allows surgeons to view any procedure live all over the world. This possibility will further speed the widespreading of the endoscopic techniques: Distance education courses can be organized and more experienced neurosurgeons can be called for consulting during surgery.

References

1. Akutsu H, Kreutzer J, Fahlbusch R, Buchfelder M (2009) Transsphenoidal decompression of the sellar floor for cavernous sinus meningiomas: experience with 21 patients. Neurosurgery 65:54–62; discussion 62
2. Bollerslev J, Fougner SL, Berg JP (2009) New directions in pharmacological treatment of acromegaly. Expert Opin Investig Drugs 18:13–22
3. Cappabianca P, Alfieri A, Colao A, Cavallo LM, Fusco M, Peca C, Lombardi G, de Divitiis E (2000) Endoscopic endonasal transsphenoidal surgery in recurrent and residual pituitary adenomas: technical note. Minim Invasive Neurosurg 43:38–43
4. Cappabianca P, Alfieri A, de Divitiis E (1998) Endoscopic endonasal transsphenoidal approach to the sella: towards functional endoscopic pituitary surgery (FEPS). Minim Invasive Neurosurg 41:66–73
5. Cappabianca P, Cavallo LM, Colao A, de Divitiis E (2002) Surgical complications associated with the endoscopic endonasal transsphenoidal approach for pituitary adenomas. J Neurosurg 97:293–298
6. Cappabianca P, Cavallo LM, Colao A, Del Basso De Caro M, Esposito F, Cirillo S, Lombardi G, de Divitiis E (2002) Endoscopic endonasal transsphenoidal approach: outcome analysis of 100 consecutive procedures. Minim Invasive Neurosurg 45:193–200
7. Cappabianca P, Cavallo LM, de Divitiis E (2004) Endoscopic endonasal transsphenoidal surgery. Neurosurgery 55:933–940; discussion 940–941

8. Cappabianca P, Cavallo LM, Esposito F, De Divitiis E (2008) Craniopharyngiomas. J Neurosurg 109:1–3; reply 3–5
9. Cappabianca P, Cavallo LM, Valente V, Romano I, D'Enza AI, Esposito F, de Divitiis E (2004) Sellar repair with fibrin sealant and collagen fleece after endoscopic endonasal transsphenoidal surgery. Surg Neurol 62:227–233; discussion 233
10. Cappabianca P, Esposito F, Esposito I, Cavallo LM, Leone CA (2009) Use of a thrombin-gelatin haemostatic matrix in endoscopic endonasal extended approaches: technical note. Acta Neurochir (Wien) 151:69–77; discussion 77
11. Carrau RL, Kassam AB, Snyderman CH (2001) Pituitary surgery. Otolaryngol Clin North Am 34: 1143–1155, ix
12. Castelnuovo P, Pistochini A, Locatelli D (2006) Different surgical approaches to the sellar region: focusing on the "two nostrils four hands technique". Rhinology 44:2–7
13. Cavallo LM, Cappabianca P, Galzio R, Iaconetta G, de Divitiis E, Tschabitscher M (2005) Endoscopic transnasal approach to the cavernous sinus versus transcranial route: anatomic study. Neurosurgery 56:379–389; discussion 379–389
14. Cavallo LM, Dal Fabbro M, Jalalod'din H, Messina A, Esposito I, Esposito F, de Divitiis E, Cappabianca P (2007) Endoscopic endonasal transsphenoidal surgery. Before scrubbing in: tips and tricks. Surg Neurol 67:342–347
15. Cavallo LM, Messina A, Esposito F, de Divitiis O, Dal Fabbro M, de Divitiis E, Cappabianca P (2007) Skull base reconstruction in the extended endoscopic transsphenoidal approach for suprasellar lesions. J Neurosurg 107:713–720
16. Cavallo LM, Prevedello DM, Solari D, Gardner PA, Esposito F, Snyderman CH, Carrau RL, Kassam AB, Cappabianca P (2009) Extended endoscopic endonasal transsphenoidal approach for residual or recurrent craniopharyngiomas. J Neurosurg 111:578–589
17. Colao A, Auriemma RS, Galdiero M, Lombardi G, Pivonello R (2009) Effects of initial therapy for five years with somatostatin analogs for acromegaly on growth hormone and insulin-like growth factor-I levels, tumor shrinkage, and cardiovascular disease: a prospective study. J Clin Endocrinol Metab 94: 3746–3756
18. Colao A, Galderisi M, Di Sarno A, Pardo M, Gaccione M, D'Andrea M, Guerra E, Pivonello R, Lerro G, Lombardi G (2008) Increased prevalence of tricuspid regurgitation in patients with prolactinomas chronically treated with cabergoline. J Clin Endocrinol Metab 93:3777–3784
19. de Divitiis E, Cappabianca P, Cavallo LM, Esposito F, de Divitiis O, Messina A (2007) Extended endoscopic transsphenoidal approach for extrasellar craniopharyngiomas. Neurosurgery 61:219–227; discussion 228
20. de Divitiis E, Esposito F, Cappabianca P, Cavallo LM, de Divitiis O, Esposito I (2008) Endoscopic transnasal resection of anterior cranial fossa meningiomas. Neurosurg Focus 25:E8
21. Dehdashti AR, Gentili F (2007) Current state of the art in the diagnosis and surgical treatment of Cushing disease: early experience with a purely endoscopic endonasal technique. Neurosurg Focus 23:E9
22. Dickerman RD, Oldfield EH (2002) Basis of persistent and recurrent Cushing disease: an analysis of findings at repeated pituitary surgery. J Neurosurg 97: 1343–1349
23. Fatemi N, Dusick JR, de Paiva Neto MA, Malkasian D, Kelly DF (2009) Endonasal versus supraorbital keyhole removal of craniopharyngiomas and tuberculum sellae meningiomas. Neurosurgery 64:269–284; discussion 284–286
24. Fatemi N, Dusick JR, Mattozo C, McArthur DL, Cohan P, Boscardin J, Wang C, Swerdloff RS, Kelly DF (2008) Pituitary hormonal loss and recovery after transsphenoidal adenoma removal. Neurosurgery 63:709–718; discussion 718–719
25. Frank G, Pasquini E (2002) Endoscopic endonasal approaches to the cavernous sinus: surgical approaches. Neurosurgery 50:675
26. Frank G, Pasquini E, Doglietto F, Mazzatenta D, Sciarretta V, Farneti G, Calbucci F (2006) The endoscopic extended transsphenoidal approach for craniopharyngiomas. Neurosurgery 59:ONS75–ONS83; discussion ONS75–83
27. Frank G, Pasquini E, Farneti G, Mazzatenta D, Sciarretta V, Grasso V, Faustini Fustini M (2006) The endoscopic versus the traditional approach in pituitary surgery. Neuroendocrinology 83:240–248
28. Gardner PA, Kassam AB, Snyderman CH, Carrau RL, Mintz AH, Grahovac S, Stefko S (2008) Outcomes following endoscopic, expanded endonasal resection of suprasellar craniopharyngiomas: a case series. J Neurosurg 109:6–16
29. Gardner PA, Prevedello DM, Kassam AB, Snyderman CH, Carrau RL, Mintz AH (2008) The evolution of the endonasal approach for craniopharyngiomas. J Neurosurg 108:1043–1047
30. Grosvenor AE, Laws ER (2008) The evolution of extracranial approaches to the pituitary and anterior skull base. Pituitary 11:337–345
31. Guiot G (1973) Transsphenoidal approach in surgical treatment of pituitary adenomas: general principles and indications in non-functioning adenomas. In: Kohler PO, Rossi GT (eds) Diagnosis and treatment of pituitary adenomas. Excerpta Medica, Amsterdam, pp 159–178
32. Jagannathan J, Laws E, Jane JA Jr (2009) Evaluation and management of sellar tumors. In: Hanna EY, DeMonte F (eds) Comprehensive management of skull base tumors. Informa Heathcare, New York/London, pp 355–365
33. Jagannathan J, Yen CP, Pouratian N, Laws ER, Sheehan JP (2009) Stereotactic radiosurgery for pituitary adenomas: a comprehensive review of indications, techniques and long-term results using the Gamma Knife. J Neurooncol 92:345–356

34. Kaptain GJ, Vincent DA, Sheehan JP, Laws ER Jr (2001) Transsphenoidal approaches for the extracapsular resection of midline suprasellar and anterior cranial base lesions. Neurosurgery 49:94–100; discussion 100–101
35. Kassam A, Snyderman CH, Mintz A, Gardner P, Carrau RL (2005) Expanded endonasal approach: the rostrocaudal axis. Part I. Crista galli to the sella turcica. Neurosurg Focus 19:E3
36. Kassam AB, Gardner P, Snyderman C, Mintz A, Carrau R (2005) Expanded endonasal approach: fully endoscopic, completely transnasal approach to the middle third of the clivus, petrous bone, middle cranial fossa, and infratemporal fossa. Neurosurg Focus 19:E6
37. Kassam AB, Gardner PA, Snyderman CH, Carrau RL, Mintz AH, Prevedello DM (2008) Expanded endonasal approach, a fully endoscopic transnasal approach for the resection of midline suprasellar craniopharyngiomas: a new classification based on the infundibulum. J Neurosurg 108:715–728
38. Kassam AB, Prevedello DM, Thomas A, Gardner P, Mintz A, Snyderman C, Carrau R (2008) Endoscopic endonasal pituitary transposition for a transdorsum sellae approach to the interpeduncular cistern. Neurosurgery 62:57–72; discussion 72–74
39. Kassam AB, Vescan AD, Carrau RL, Prevedello DM, Gardner P, Mintz AH, Snyderman CH, Rhoton AL (2008) Expanded endonasal approach: vidian canal as a landmark to the petrous internal carotid artery. J Neurosurg 108:177–183
40. Laws ER (2008) Surgery for acromegaly: evolution of the techniques and outcomes. Rev Endocr Metab Disord 9:67–70
41. Melmed S, Colao A, Barkan A, Molitch M, Grossman AB, Kleinberg D, Clemmons D, Chanson P, Laws E, Schlechte J, Vance ML, Ho K, Giustina A (2009) Guidelines for acromegaly management: an update. J Clin Endocrinol Metab 94:1509–1517
42. Patil CG, Veeravagu A, Prevedello DM, Katznelson L, Vance ML, Laws ER Jr (2008) Outcomes after repeat transsphenoidal surgery for recurrent Cushing's disease. Neurosurgery 63:266–270; discussion 270–271
43. Pinheiro-Neto CD, Prevedello DM, Carrau RL, Snyderman CH, Mintz A, Gardner P, Kassam A (2007) Improving the design of the pedicled nasoseptal flap for skull base reconstruction: a radioanatomic study. Laryngoscope 117:1560–1569
44. Pivonello R, De Martino MC, Cappabianca P, De Leo M, Faggiano A, Lombardi G, Hofland LJ, Lamberts SW, Colao A (2009) The medical treatment of Cushing's disease: effectiveness of chronic treatment with the dopamine agonist cabergoline in patients unsuccessfully treated by surgery. J Clin Endocrinol Metab 94:223–230
45. Powell M (2009) Microscope and endoscopic pituitary surgery. Acta Neurochir (Wien) 151:723–728
46. Prevedello DM, Pouratian N, Sherman J, Jane JA Jr, Vance ML, Lopes MB, Laws ER Jr (2008) Management of Cushing's disease: outcome in patients with microadenoma detected on pituitary magnetic resonance imaging. J Neurosurg 109: 751–759
47. Roelfsema F, Biermasz NR, Pereira AM, Romijn J (2006) Nanomedicines in the treatment of acromegaly: focus on pegvisomant. Int J Nanomedicine 1: 385–398
48. Songtao Q, Yuntao L, Jun P, Chuanping H, Xiaofeng S (2009) Membranous layers of the pituitary gland: histological anatomic study and related clinical issues. Neurosurgery 64:1–9; discussion 9–10
49. Tabaee A, Anand VK, Barron Y, Hiltzik DH, Brown SM, Kacker A, Mazumdar M, Schwartz TH (2009) Endoscopic pituitary surgery: a systematic review and meta-analysis. J Neurosurg 111:545–554
50. Tabaee A, Anand VK, Barron Y, Hiltzik DH, Brown SM, Kacker A, Mazumdar M, Schwartz TH (2009) Predictors of short-term outcomes following endoscopic pituitary surgery. Clin Neurol Neurosurg 111: 119–122
51. Tabaee A, Anand VK, Fraser JF, Brown SM, Singh A, Schwartz TH (2009) Three-dimensional endoscopic pituitary surgery. Neurosurgery 64:288–293; discussion 294–295

Current Status and Future Developments of Neuroendoscopically Assisted Neurosurgery

6

Henry W.S. Schroeder

6.1 Introduction

The use of the operating microscope in neurosurgery has been well established since more than 30 years. A major improvement in surgical results has been obtained by using microsurgical techniques. Especially in complex skull base and vascular surgery, the microscope is a prerequisite to achieve excellent outcomes for the patients. The microscope provides a superb stereoscopic view. However, in deep and narrow surgical corridors, there is a considerable loss of light at the entry site (Fig. 6.1a). Furthermore, the surgeon is working within the light beam which further decreases the light intensity in the surgical field. With the microscope, only structures which are visible in a straight line can be explored.

6.2 Rationale of Endoscope-Assisted Microsurgery

Compared with the operating microscope, the endoscope provides a completely different view. "State-of-the-art" endoscopes containing a Hopkins II® rod lens have a wide angle viewing field resulting in a panoramic view (Fig. 6.1b). Therefore, even lesions which are not located in front of the endoscope tip can be recognized early. This is a major advantage in narrow and deep surgical approaches. Using endoscopes with angulated optics gives the ability to look around a corner or behind neurovascular structures which is very useful in skull base surgery (Fig. 6.1c). With the use of the endoscope, the surgeon brings the eye close to the target area with perfect illumination even in the depth. Another important advantage of the endoscope compared with the microscope is the excellent depth of field. Refocusing which is frequently required with the microscope particularly with high magnification is rarely necessary.

Of course, the endoscope has also limitations. The major drawback of the endoscope is the lack of true 3D viewing. However, because of the fish-eye effect, the endoscopic image is distorted and provides a pseudo 3D impression. Furthermore, motion parallax which means closer objects move more than distal objects contributes to the pseudo 3D impression of an endoscopic image. Therefore, the lack of stereopsis is usually compensated for with some training. Another disadvantage of the endoscope is the lower resolution compared to the microscope. Because of the smaller lens diameter of the endoscopes used in neuroendoscopy, the operating microscope has still better resolution than the endoscope. Furthermore, when using the operating microscope, the surgeon has a very good resolution because he is looking directly through the lens system. The sensor is the retina which is much better then CCD chips in the mini video cameras which are attached to the endoscope. Although recently introduced high-definition cameras gen-

H.W.S. Schroeder, MD, PhD
Department of Neurosurgery,
University Medicine Greifswald,
Greifswald, Germany

S. Sgouros (ed.), *Neuroendoscopy*,
DOI 10.1007/978-3-642-39085-2_6, © Springer-Verlag Berlin Heidelberg 2014

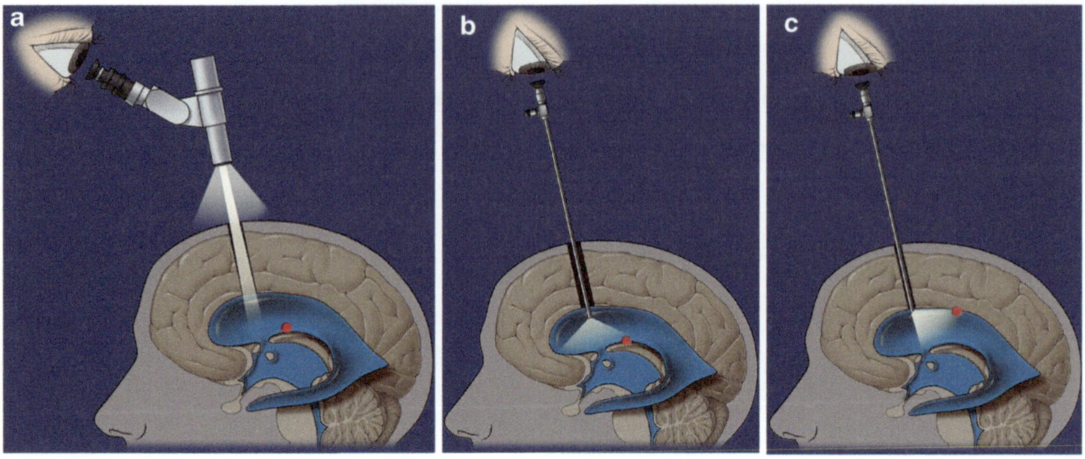

Fig. 6.1 Schematic drawing of microscopic and endoscopic visualization. (**a**) Microscopic visualization. (**b**) Endoscopic 0° visualization. (**c**) Endoscopic 45° visualization

Fig. 6.2 Endoscopes with angulated eyepiece with 0°, 30°, and 70° of view

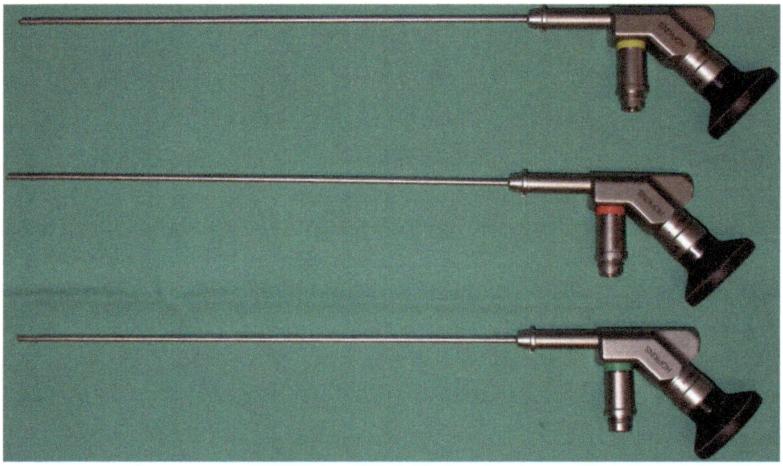

erate images with 1080 lines and over two million pixels, the image quality is still inferior when comparing with the direct look of the human eye through the microscope.

In conclusion, microscope as well as endoscope has advantages and disadvantages. Therefore, it sounds reasonable to combine the advantages of both optical instruments during neurosurgery.

6.3 Endoscopic Equipment

For endoscope-assisted procedures endoscopes with angulated eye pieces are preferred to bring the video camera away from the surgical field and avoid interference with the surgical instruments (Fig. 6.2). Various angles of view (0°, 30°, 45°, and 70°) are available to be able to inspect any corner. The endoscope outer diameter should not exceed 4 mm. For the cerebellopontine angle 2.7 mm scopes are recommended because of the narrow spaces between the cranial nerves in this area. Angulated instruments are required for removing tumor tissue around a corner (Fig. 6.3). Xenon light sources provide the best illumination, since the color temperature of xenon light resembles that of sunlight (6,000 K) which improves the color fidelity. High-definition (HD) video cameras should be used whenever possible as the image quality is

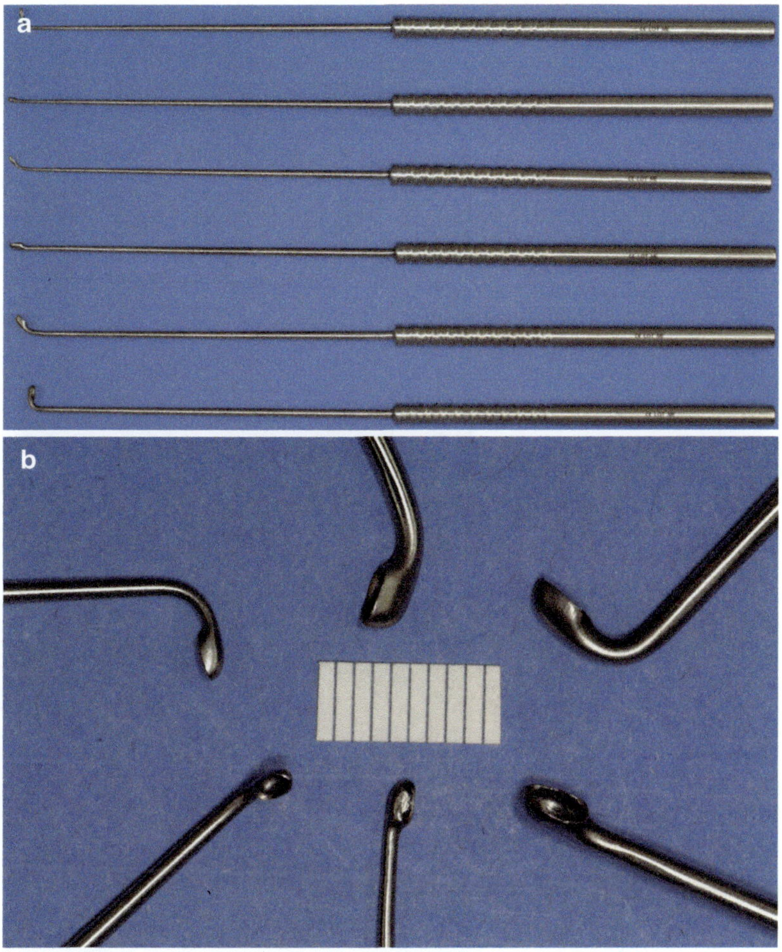

Fig. 6.3 Instruments for endoscope-assisted surgery with angulated tips. (**a**) Curettes of various sizes. (**b**) Close-up view of the tips

much better compared with the standard cameras [12].

6.4 Surgical Technique

In endoscope-assisted microsurgery, usually the major part of the procedure is performed under microscopic view because of the better image quality and the 3D view. However, certain steps of the surgery are carried out under endoscopic view. The endoscope is mostly used to look around bony or dural corners as well as neurovascular structures to avoid extensive skull base drilling and retraction. Furthermore, the endoscope is applied in deep and narrow surgical corridors to improve illumination and viewing field.

Frequently, the endoscope is used freehand simply for inspection (Fig. 6.4a). However, when bimanual dissection is required, the endoscope is fixed to a self-retaining holding device, and the surgeon has both hands free for manipulation (Fig. 6.4b, c). The monitor is placed straight in front of the surgeon for ergonomic purposes (Fig. 6.4d).

Care has to be taken when moving the endoscope and inserting or removing the instruments from the surgical field to avoid damage to neurovascular structures which are behind the tip of the endoscope and therefore not under endoscopic view. It is important to keep in mind that the tip of the endoscopes may become really hot which may damage neurovascular structures especially during prolonged dissections under endoscopic view. Therefore, frequent irrigation is recommended.

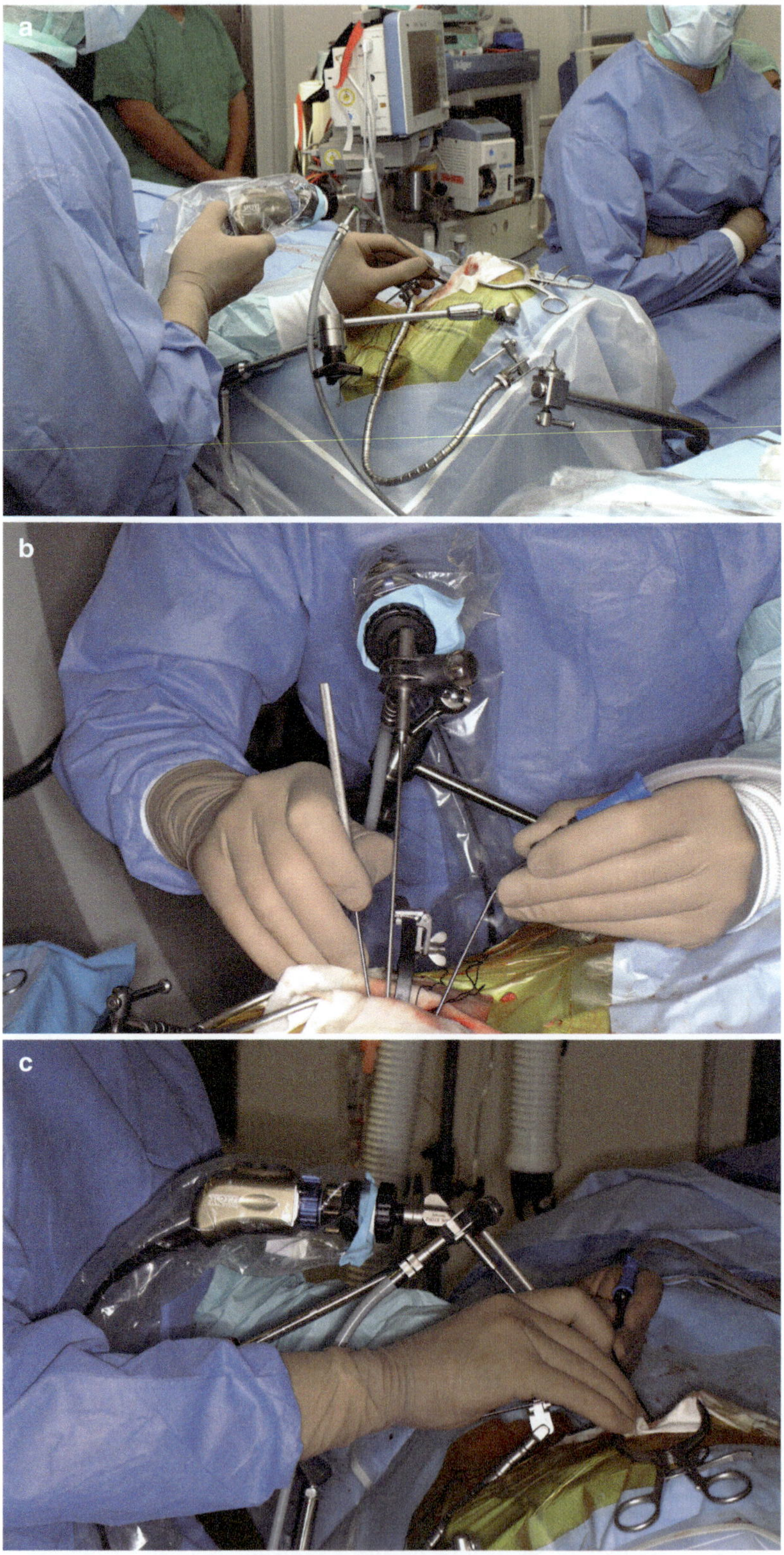

Fig. 6.4 Use of endoscopes in endoscope-assisted procedures. (**a**) Freehand endoscopic inspection. (**b**, **c**) Bimanual endoscopic dissection. Endoscope with self-retaining holding arm. (**d**) Ergonomic positioning of the screen in straight line in front of the surgeon

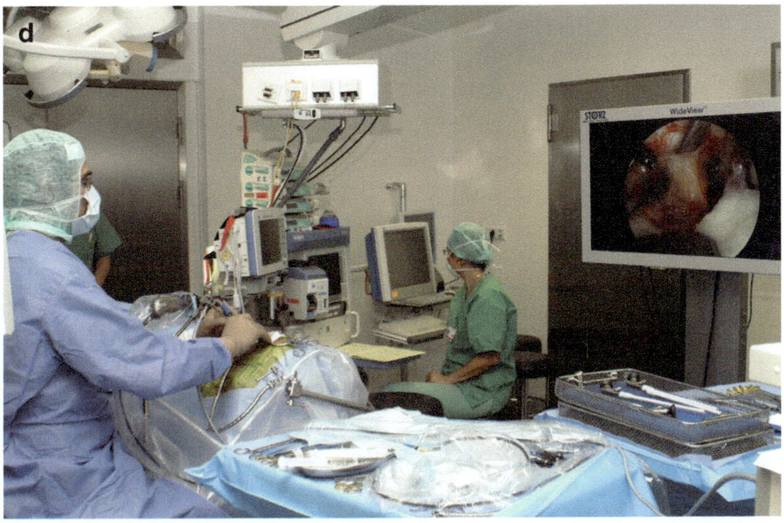

Fig. 6.4 (continued)

6.5 Indications

The endoscope-assisted technique has turned out to be particularly useful in skull base tumor surgery, aneurysm clipping, and microvascular decompression [1–11, 13, 14].

6.5.1 Vestibular Schwannomas

Vestibular schwannomas with tumor extension deeply into the internal auditory canal are good indications for an endoscope-assisted retrosigmoid approach (Fig. 6.5). When hearing preservation is demanded, the extent of drilling of the posterior wall of the internal auditory canal is limited by the vestibule and the posterior semicircular canal. The angle of viewing does not allow the direct inspection of the fundus of the internal auditory canal with the aid of the microscope even after extensive drilling of the posterior wall of the internal auditory canal (Fig. 6.5f). Therefore, very often a blind dissection of the distal tumor pole is performed with the aid of a hook dissector. Using a 30°, 45°, and 70° endoscope enables a perfect visualization of the fundus (Fig. 6.5e). The endoscope can be used freehand for inspection after tumor removal to make sure that the tumor is totally removed or for dissection of the tumor in the fundus. After tumor removal, the drilled area of the internal auditory canal is inspected to find open air cells which might cause CSF leak (Fig. 6.5d).

6.5.2 Epidermoids

Epidermoids spread along the subarachnoid CSF spaces and have very often a considerable extension. Frequently, two or more compartments are involved, e.g., posterior and middle cranial fossa. The endoscope is useful in removing tumor parts which are hidden behind dural (e.g., tentorium) or bony corners (Meckel's cave) as well as neurovascular structures (Fig. 6.6). Epidermoids involving two compartments can be removed via a single craniotomy in one of the compartments.

6.5.3 Skull Base Meningiomas

In skull base meningiomas, the endoscope-assisted technique is mostly applied in tumors of the posterior cranial fossa to remove tumor parts hidden behind bony corners (e.g., jugular tubercle, Meckel's cave, or internal auditory canal) in order to reduce the amount of drilling. In frontal skull base meningiomas, the endoscope is usually not required because standard frontolateral or pterional approaches give enough space to inspect the entire frontal skull base with the microscope. However, when keyhole supraorbital approaches are used, the endoscope is mandatory to achieve a radical resection (Fig. 6.7). Because of the limited viewing angle and the prominent orbital roof, the entire skull base cannot be visualized in a

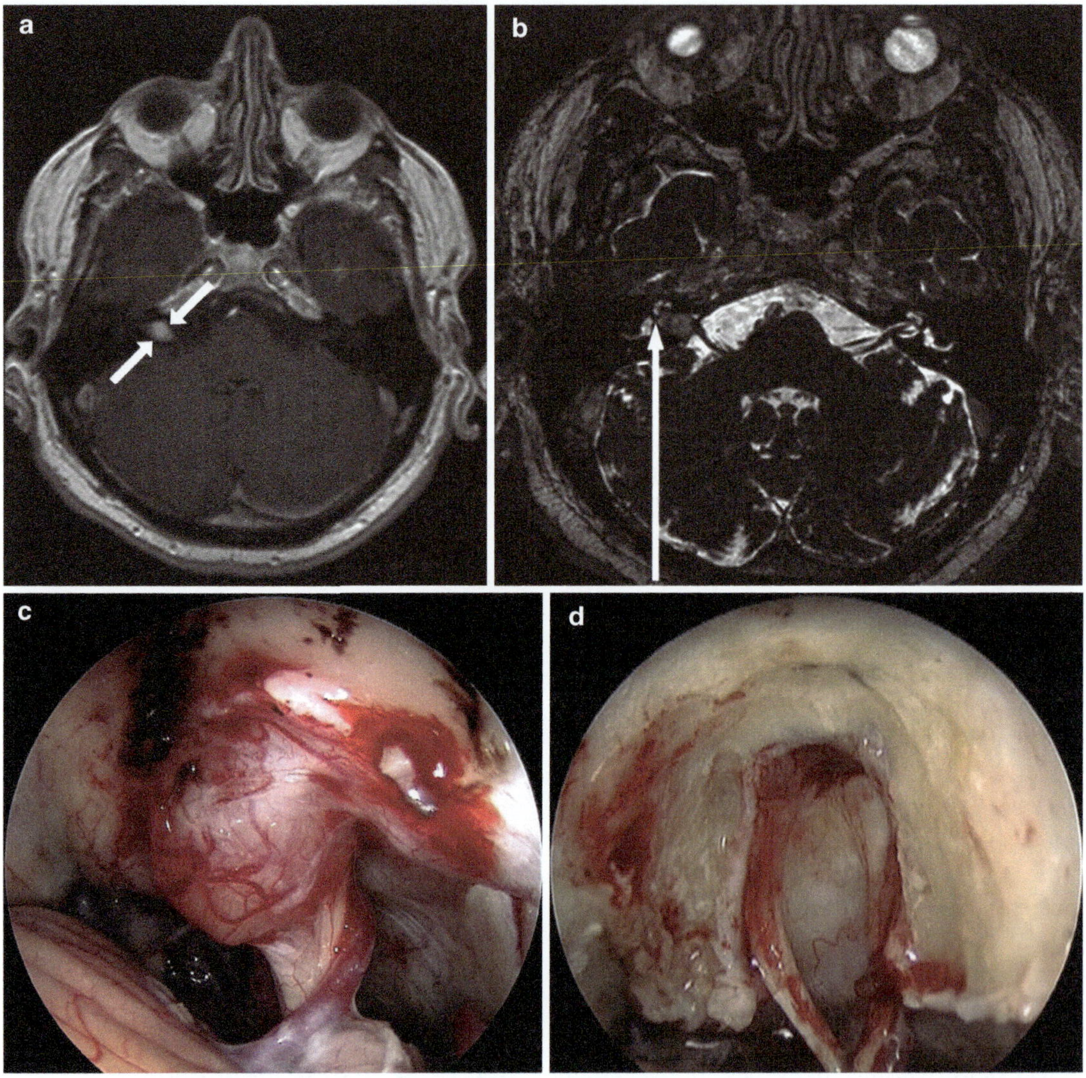

Fig. 6.5 Intra-extrameatal vestibular schwannoma in a 58-year-old male presenting with hearing loss. (**a**) T1-weighted axial MR image showing a contrast-enhancing lesion (*arrows*) within the cerebellopontine angle. (**b**) Axial CISS MR image showing the accurate extension of the lesion with the internal auditory canal (*arrow*). (**c**) Endoscopic image of the tumor. (**d**) Endoscopic inspection of the internal auditory canal after tumor removal showing preserved facial and cochlear nerve. (**e**) Endoscopic inspection of the fundus proving gross total tumor resection. (**f**) Axial bony CT scan obtained after surgery showing the extent of drilling of the posterior wall of the internal auditory canal with preservation of vestibule and posterior semicircular canal and the trajectory of the microscopic view (*arrow*). The fundus cannot be inspected with the microscope. (**g, h**) Axial T1-weighted contrast-enhanced (**g**) and axial CISS (**h**) MR image obtained 4 years after surgery showing no recurrence

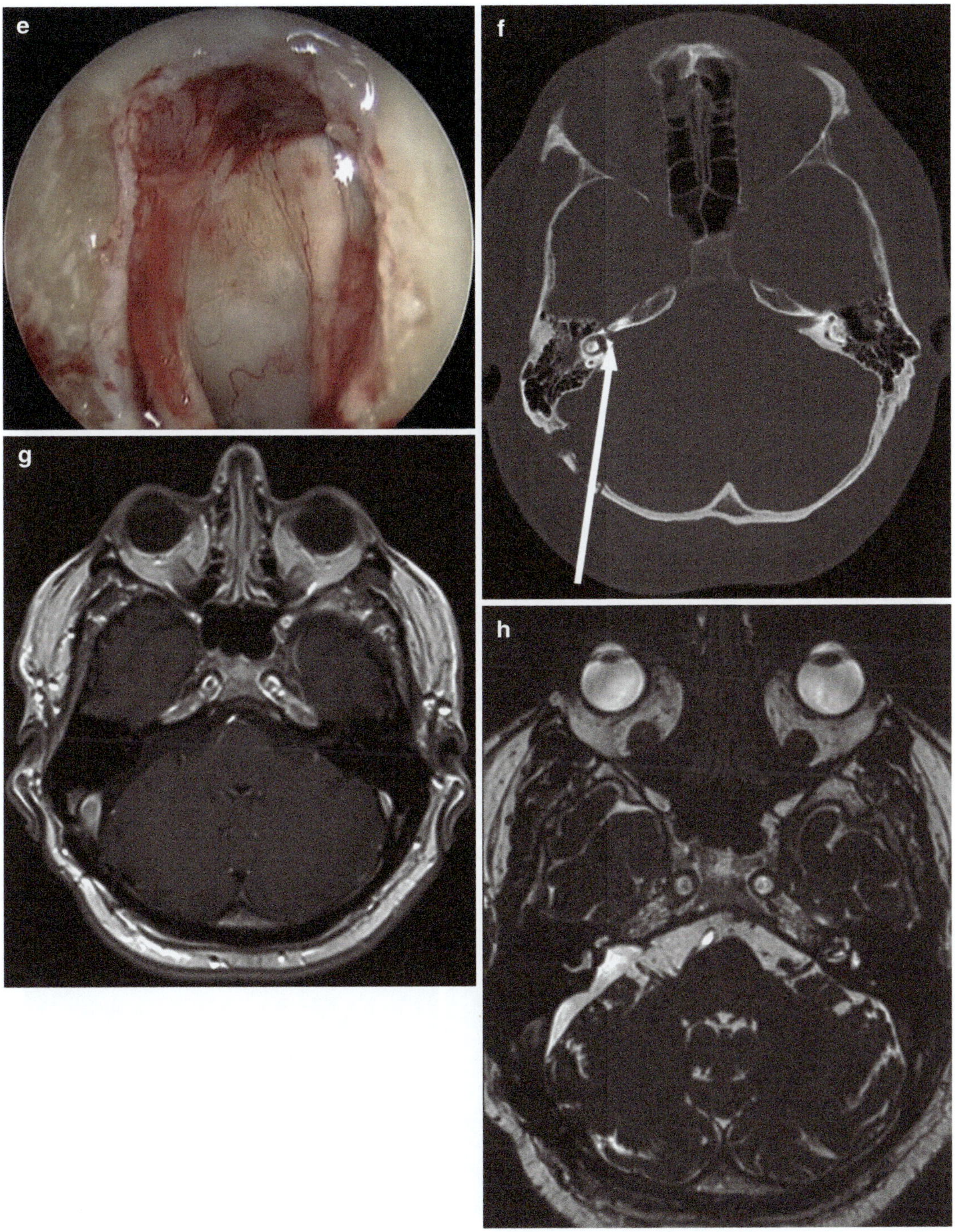

Fig. 6.5 (continued)

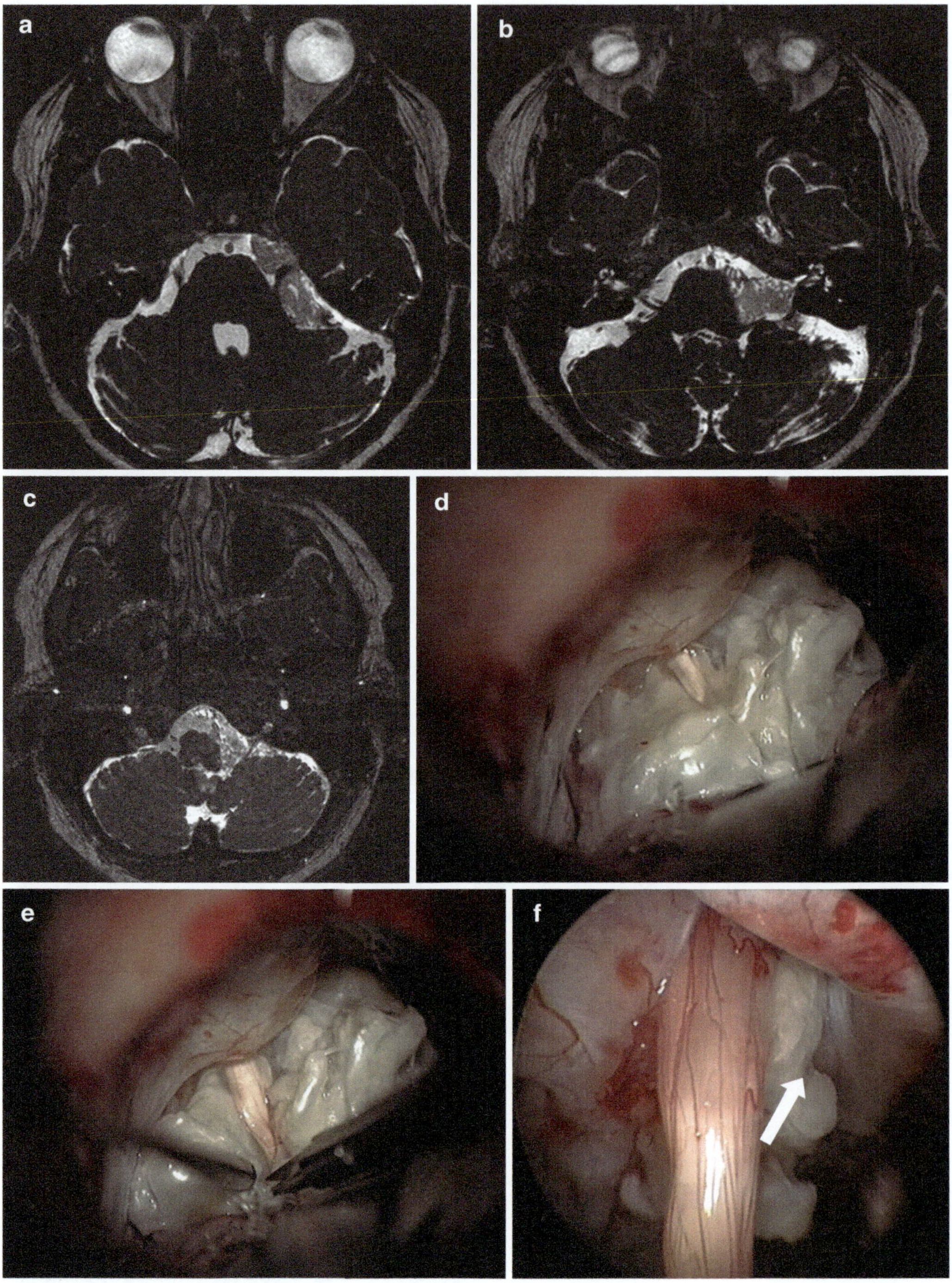

Fig. 6.6 Epidermoid of the cerebellopontine angle in a 45-year-old female presenting with trigeminal neuralgia and hearing loss. (**a–c**) Axial CISS MR images showing a large space-occupying lesion within the cerebellopontine angle. (**d**) Microscopic view of the pearly tumor. (**e**) Bimanual microsurgical dissection. (**f**) Endoscopic inspection of the entrance of the internal auditory canal with tumor behind the nerves (*arrow*). (**g**) Endoscopic inspection after microsurgical resection showing a tumor remnant behind the tentorium (*arrow*). (**h**) Endoscopic tumor removal. (**i**) Microscopic view after gross total tumor resection. (**j–l**) Axial CISS MR images obtained 2 years after surgery showing the total tumor resection

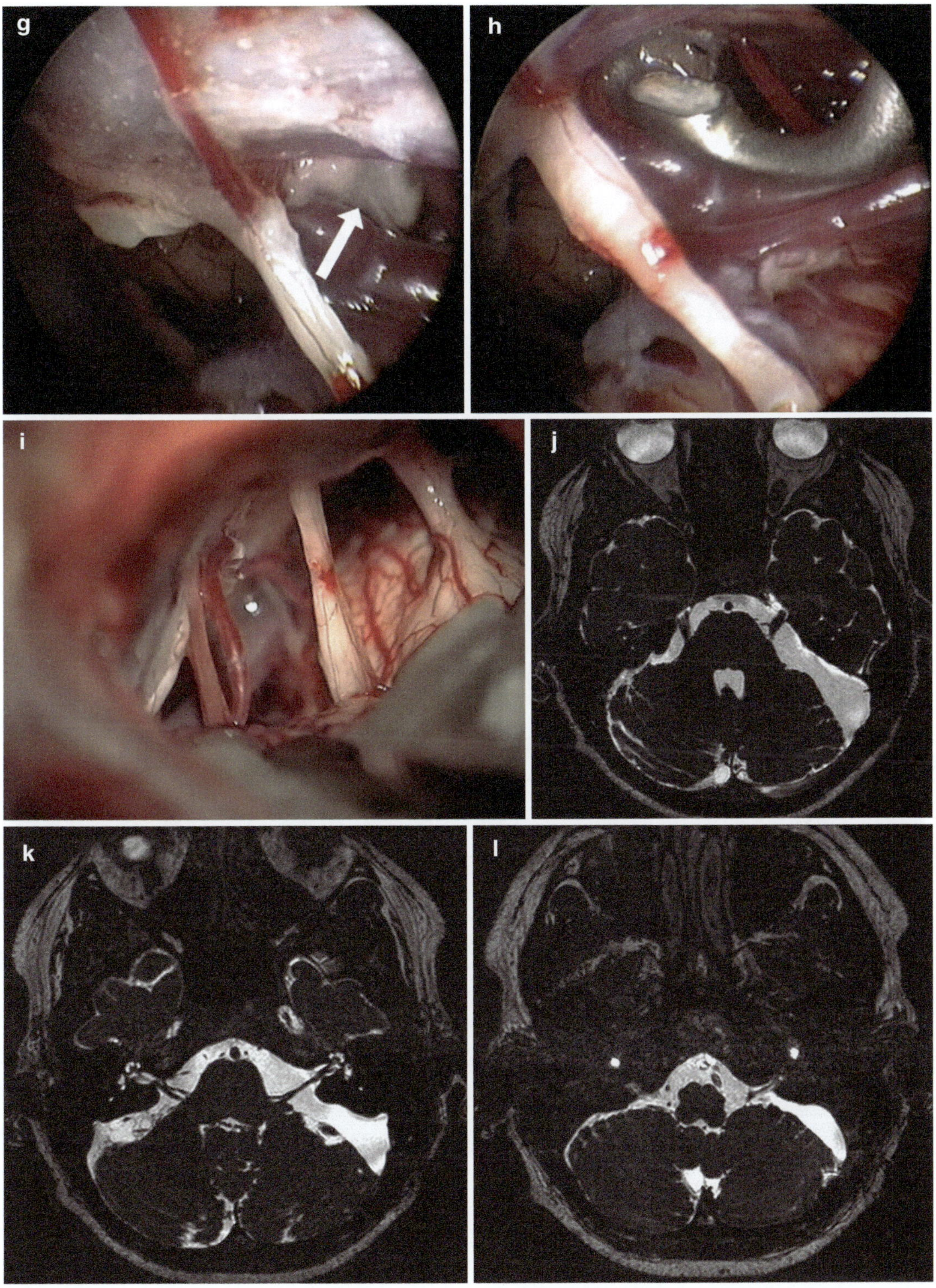

Fig. 6.6 (continued)

straight line with the microscope; 30° and 45° endoscopes are required to visualize the sellar diaphragm, the depth of the olfactory grove, and the space behind the ipsilateral carotid artery.

6.5.4 Aneurysms

In aneurysm surgery, the endoscope is helpful when the aneurysm neck with parent and efferent arteries or perforators cannot be visualized with

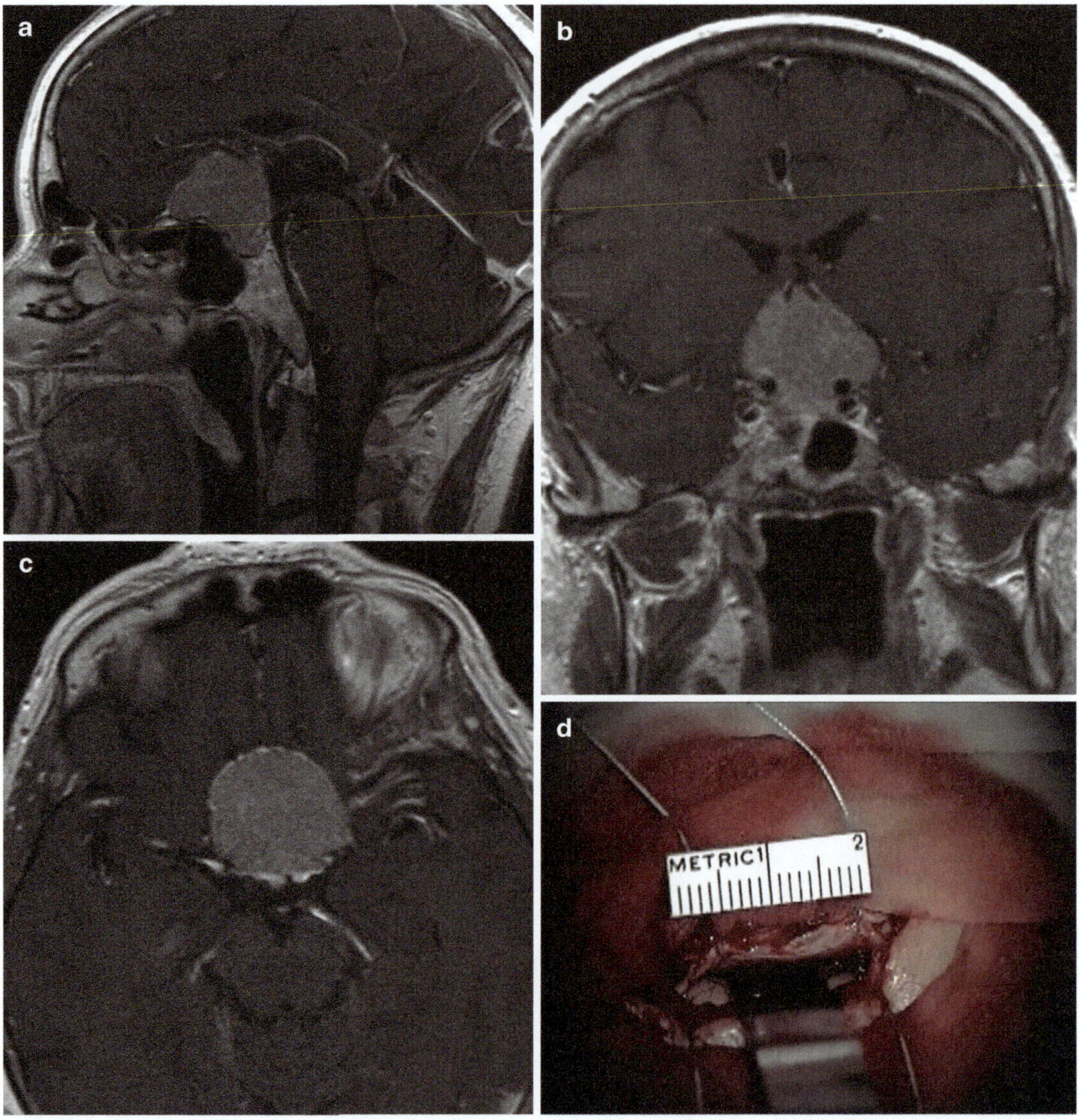

Fig. 6.7 Tuberculum sellae meningioma in a 61-year-old female presenting with visual loss and visual field deficits. (**a–c**) Sagittal, coronal, and axial T1-weighted MR images showing a contrast-enhancing lesion arising from the tuberculum sellae. (**d**) Microsurgical approach via eyebrow incision and supraorbital craniotomy. (**e**) Microsurgical exposure of the right optic nerve (*arrows*) and tumor (*T*). (**f**) Endoscopic dissection of tumor remnants (*T*) at the sellar diaphragm close to the ipsilateral carotid artery (*right arrow*), pituitary stalk (*middle arrow*), and contralateral carotid artery (*left arrow*). (**g**) Axial bony CT scan obtained after surgery showing the size of the craniotomy (*arrows*). (**h, i**) Sagittal and coronal T1-weighted MR images obtained 5 years after surgery showing total tumor resection and no recurrence. (**j**) Excellent cosmetic result after 1 year

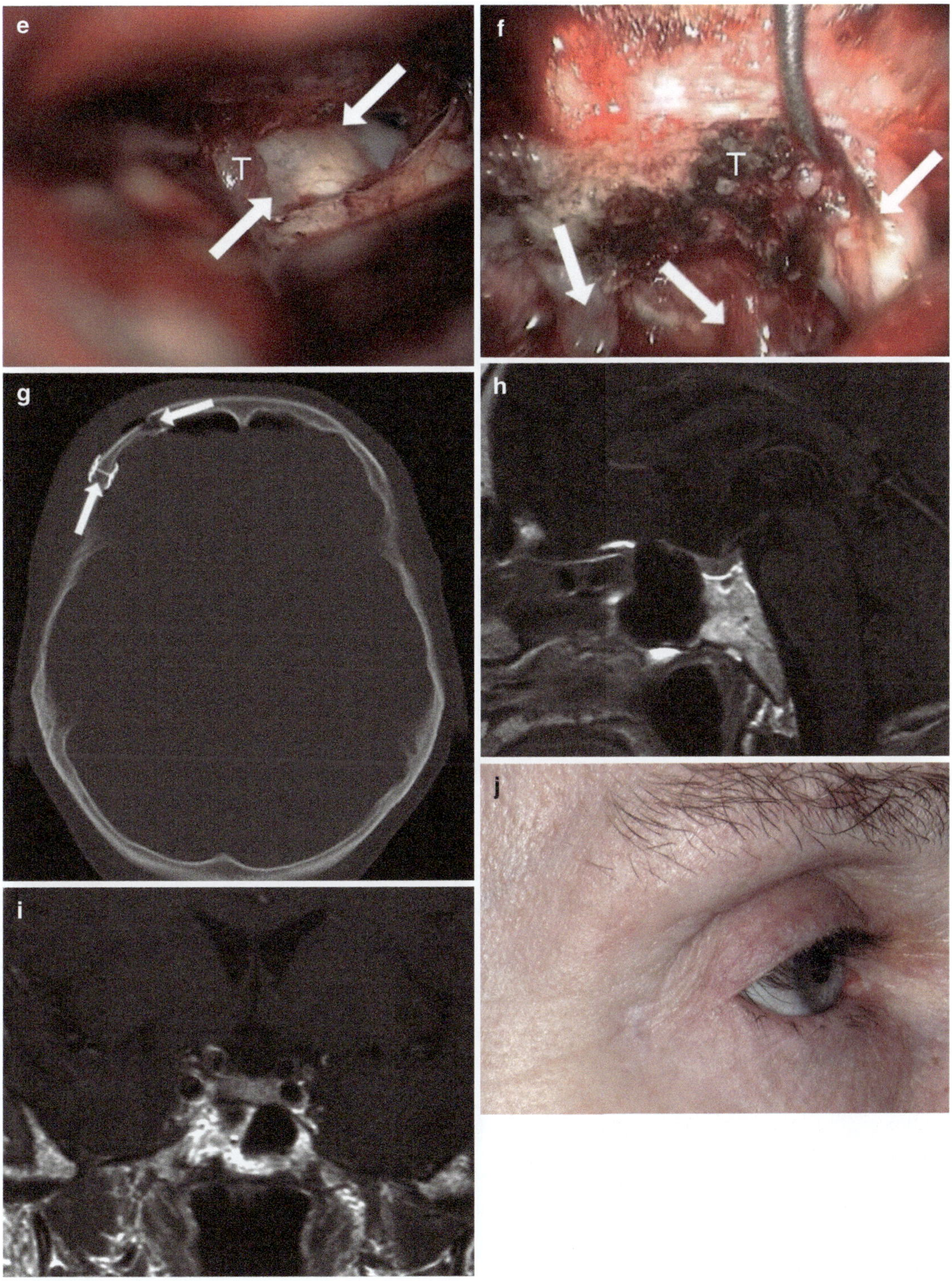

Fig. 6.7 (continued)

the microscope (Fig. 6.8). In keyhole approaches with nearly coaxial vision, the endoscope is often mandatory to make sure that a proper clip position has been achieved. Using standard pterional approaches in aneurysms of the anterior circulation, the application of endoscopes is rarely

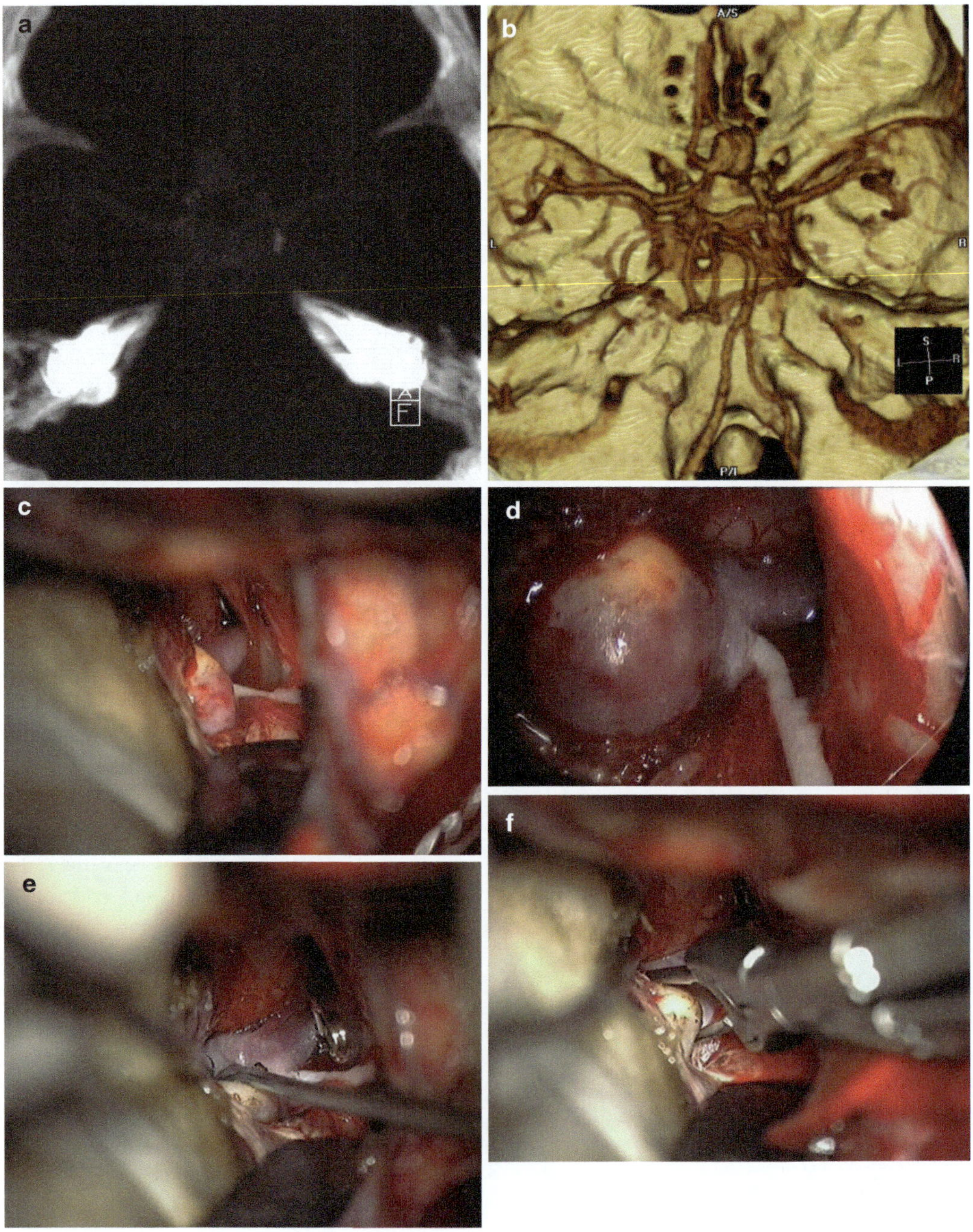

Fig. 6.8 Unruptured anterior communicating artery aneurysm in a 57-year-old male. The aneurysm was an incidental finding. (**a**, **b**) CT angiography and 3D reconstruction showing an anterior communicating artery aneurysm. (**c**) Microsurgical exposure of the aneurysm via a pterional approach. The neck cannot be visualized. (**d**) Endoscopic inspection of the neck. (**e**) Microsurgical aneurysm dissection. (**f**) Microsurgical clipping of the aneurysm. (**g**) Clipped aneurysm. (**h**) Endoscopic inspection of the clip position. (**i**) Indocyanine-green angiography showing complete occlusion of the aneurysm and patency of all vessels. (**j**) DSA obtained 5 days after surgery showing the complete obliteration of the aneurysm

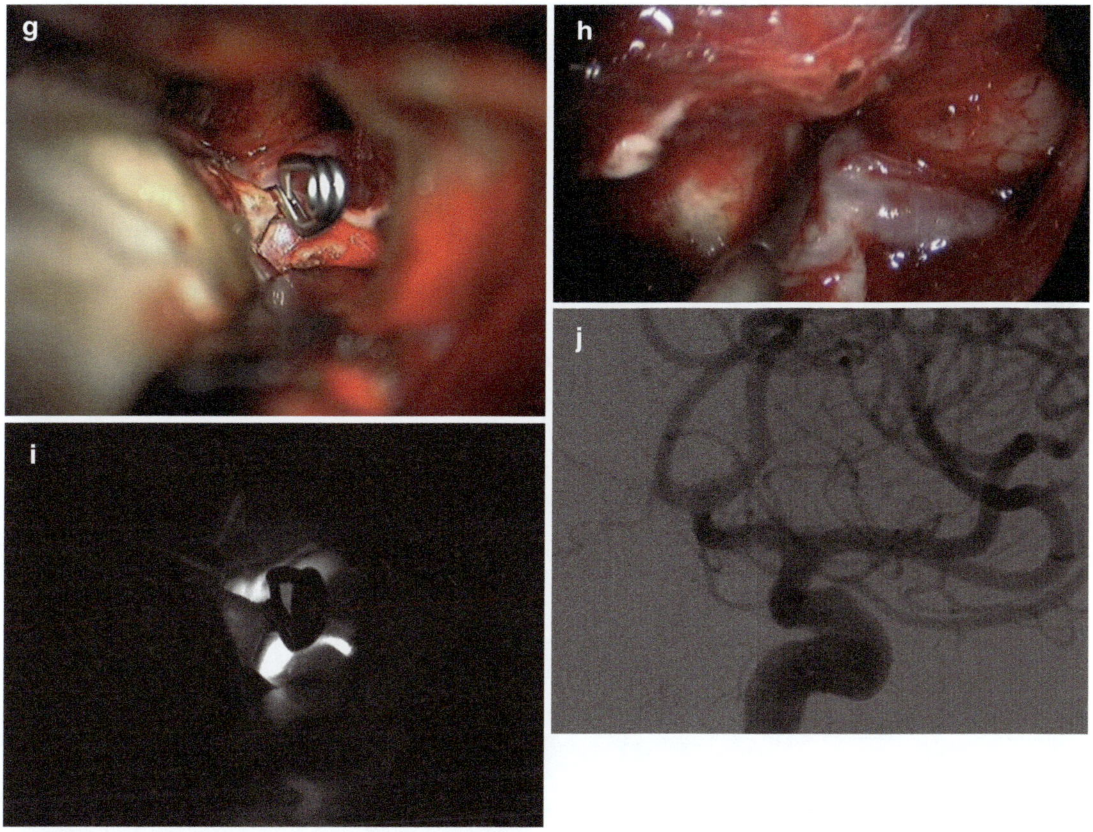

Fig. 6.8 (continued)

required. However, for aneurysms of the posterior circulation at the basilar tip, the endoscope is very beneficial to get an overview of the anatomy before applying the clip and to check the clip position. I use the endoscope in aneurysm surgery nearly always only for inspection before and after clipping. In my attempts of using the endoscope for visualization during the aneurysm clipping, the endoscope mostly interfered with my suction and clip applicator.

6.5.5 Trigeminal Neuralgia and Hemifacial Spasm

The application of the endoscope in microvascular decompression for trigeminal neuralgia and hemifacial spasm is another good example of endoscope-assisted microsurgery (Fig. 6.9). After microsurgical exposure of the nerves and vessels, the endoscope is used to inspect the trigeminal nerve at the entrance into Meckel's cave. Small veins which can compress the trigeminal nerve are frequently found at the entry point into Meckel's cave. When a prominent suprameatal tubercle is present, a direct microscopic view to this area cannot be obtained. Using an endoscope, drilling of the suprameatal tubercle can be avoided. In hemifacial spasm, the compression site is often very medially located and direct microscopic visualization requires considerable retraction of the cerebellum. With the endoscope the compression site can be inspected avoiding any retraction.

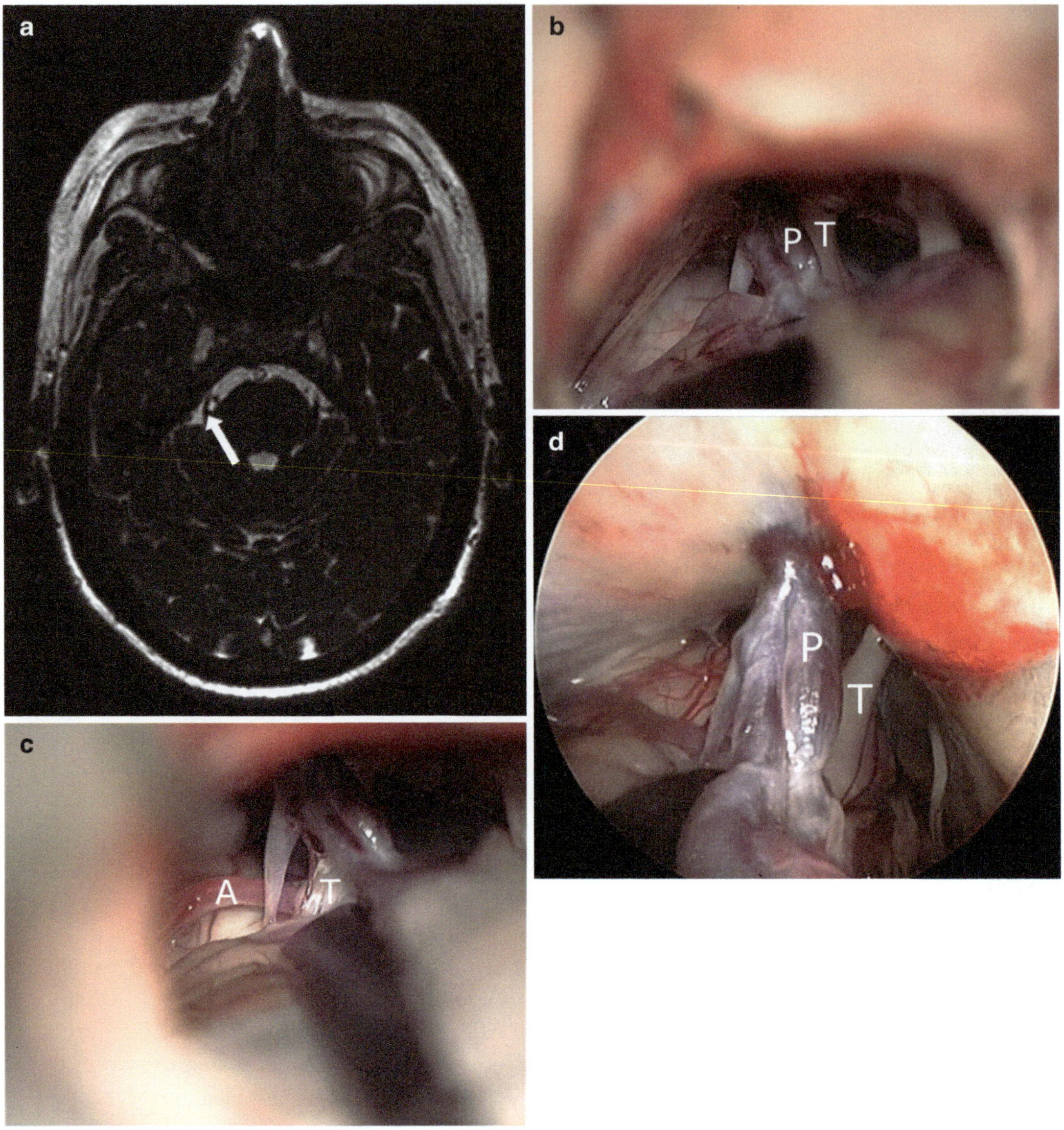

Fig. 6.9 A 63-year-old female presenting with typical trigeminal neuralgia on the right side. (**a**) Axial CISS MR image showing the juxtapontine compression of the right trigeminal nerve at the root entry zone by a loop of the superior cerebellar artery (*arrow*). (**b**) Microsurgical approach via a superior retrosigmoid craniotomy showing the superior petrosal vein (*P*) and the trigeminal nerve (*T*). (**c**) Microsurgical exposure of the offending branch of the superior cerebellar artery (*A*) at the root of the trigeminal nerve (*T*). (**d**) Endoscopic inspection with 0° endoscope showing initially a similar image like the microscope with superior petrosal vein (*P*) and trigeminal nerve (*T*). (**e**) However, after passing the petrosal vein with the endoscope tip, the compression of the trigeminal nerve (*T*) by the branch of the superior cerebellar artery (*A*) is clearly visible. (**f**) Endoscopic inspection with 30° optic showing nicely the compression of the trigeminal nerve root (*T*). (**g, h**) Endoscopic dissection of the loop. (**i**) Decompression with the aid of Teflon wool

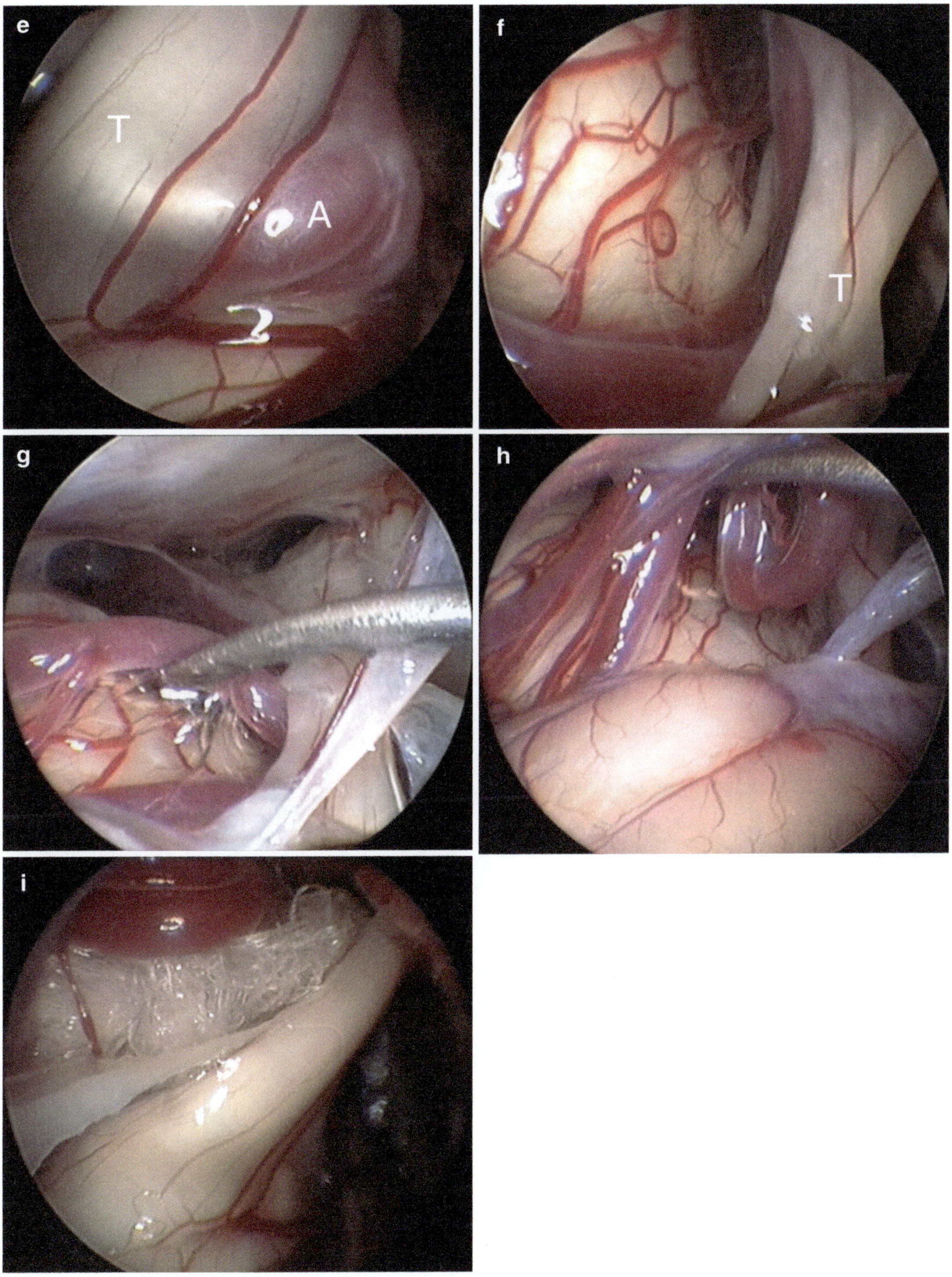

Fig. 6.9 (continued)

6.6 Future Developments

It is expected that high-resolution 3D video camera systems will replace the surgical microscope in the future. Video cameras with resolution much beyond the resolution of the HD system we currently use will be developed. Chip technology will advance more and more, and the resolution will be even superior to the human eye. These 3D cameras will be adapted to the endoscopes too. The surgeon will look at only one screen where all information including navigation data and preoperative MR images will be displayed. Nowadays, however, the surgical microscope remains the most frequently used optical tool in neurosurgery which can be assisted by the endoscope in certain procedures.

Conclusion

Endoscope-assisted microsurgery combines the advantages of the microscope with those of the endoscope. For dissection of structures which are visible in a straight line, the microscope with high resolution, excellent color fidelity, as well as stereoscopic vision is used. For working "around a corner," the endoscope is applied to reduce the amount of retraction and skull base drilling.

References

1. Baldauf J, Junghans D, Schroeder HW (2005) Endoscope-assisted microsurgical resection of an intraneural ganglion cyst of the hypoglossal nerve. J Neurosurg 103:920–922
2. Fries G, Perneczky A (1998) Endoscope-assisted brain surgery: part 2 – analysis of 380 procedures. Neurosurgery 42:226–232
3. Fries G, Perneczky A (2000) Endoscope-assisted keyhole surgery for aneurysms of the anterior circulation and the basilar apex. Oper Tech Neurosurg 3: 216–230
4. Grotenhuis JA (1996) Endoscope-assisted craniotomy. Tech Neurosurg 1:201–212
5. Kalavakonda C, Sekhar LN, Ramachandran P, Hechl P (2002) Endoscope-assisted microsurgery for intracranial aneurysms. Neurosurgery 51:1119–1126
6. Menovsky T, Grotenhuis JA, de Vries J, Bartels RH (1999) Endoscope-assisted supraorbital craniotomy for lesions of the interpeduncular fossa. Neurosurgery 44:106–110
7. Perneczky A, Boecher-Schwarz HG (1998) Endoscope-assisted microsurgery for cerebral aneurysms. Neurol Med Chir (Tokyo) 38(Suppl):33–34
8. Perneczky A, Fries G (1998) Endoscope-assisted brain surgery: part 1 – evolution, basic concept, and current technique. Neurosurgery 42:219–225
9. Rak R, Sekhar LN, Stimac D, Hechl P (2004) Endoscope-assisted microsurgery for microvascular compression syndromes. Neurosurgery 54:876–881
10. Reisch R, Perneczky A (2005) Ten-year experience with the supraorbital subfrontal approach through an eyebrow skin incision. Neurosurgery 57:242–255
11. Reisch R, Perneczky A, Filippi R (2003) Surgical technique of the supraorbital key-hole craniotomy. Surg Neurol 59:223–227
12. Schroeder HW, Nehlsen M (2009) Value of high-definition imaging in neuroendoscopy. Neurosurg Rev 32:303–308
13. Schroeder HW, Oertel J, Gaab MR (2004) Endoscope-assisted microsurgical resection of epidermoid tumors of the cerebellopontine angle. J Neurosurg 101:227–232
14. Tatagiba M, Matthies C, Samii M (1996) Microendoscopy of the internal auditory canal in vestibular schwannoma surgery. Neurosurgery 38: 737–740

Neuroendoscopic Instruments and Surgical Technique

7

André Grotenhuis

7.1 Introduction

Neuroendoscopic surgery has evolved from an initially diagnostic modality over a treatment modality for obstructive hydrocephalus to a widespread neurosurgical technique. It reflects the tendency of modern neurosurgery to aim towards minimum invasiveness, that is, access and visualization through the narrowest practical surgical approach with, at the same time, maximum effectiveness. Transventricular neuroendoscopic approaches allow the treatment of several pathologies inside the ventricular system, such as obstructive hydrocephalus and intra- and paraventricular tumors and cysts.

However, an endoscope may be used to assist microneurosurgery in virtually any kind of neurosurgical procedures, particularly in aneurysm and tumor surgery. This endoscope-assisted microneurosurgery allows precise clipping of aneurysms and visual control to avoid inadvertent clipping of perforators and parent arteries and allows to "look around the corner" in tumor surgery to identify vital structures that are hidden behind the tumor itself or bony protrusions. Endoscope-controlled microneurosurgery is the replacement of the operating microscope by a larger lenscope. It is best illustrated by the rapidly evolving technique of endoscopic endonasal transphenoidal surgery that allows the treatment of pathologies of the sellar and parasellar region and frontal skull base such as pituitary adenomas, craniopharyngiomas, meningiomas, and clival chordomas, with the advantage of a wide vision of the surgical field.

This evolution occurred in response to the reported benefits of endoscopic surgery compared to conventional surgical procedures for patients. The use of neuroendoscopic surgery has increased exponentially during the past 10 years. Previously lengthy and difficult procedures now are being performed endoscopically. Advances in instrumentation, dissection and hemostasis techniques, and improved camera technologies have simplified these procedures and expanded the application of the minimally invasive neurosurgical approach.

The earliest reported endoscopic neurosurgery was performed in 1910 when two children were treated for hydrocephalus by endoscopic fulguration of the choroid plexus. By 1960, technological advances in flexible and rigid lens endoscopes allowed for additional endoscopic procedures, but it was not rapidly adopted by neurosurgeons. In the 1970s it was Fukushima (Japan) who used fiber optics to inspect the ventricular system. Vries and Jones used it for the treatment of hydrocephalus and Prott and Oppel for the inspection of the subarachnoid space.

Further use of neuroendoscopy was hampered by the lack of dedicated endoscopes and dedicated instruments for the specific needs inside the ventricular system and subarachnoid space.

A. Grotenhuis, MD, PhD
Department of Neurosurgery, Radboud University Nijmegen Medical Center, Nijmegen, The Netherlands

S. Sgouros (ed.), *Neuroendoscopy*,
DOI 10.1007/978-3-642-39085-2_7, © Springer-Verlag Berlin Heidelberg 2014

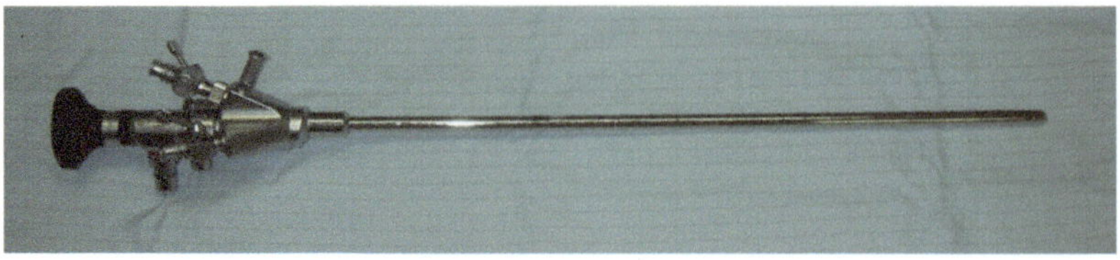

Fig. 7.1 Wolf rigid neuroendoscope, with 6-mm outer diameter, three working channels, and sheath of 25 cm, long enough to be used in conjunction with the Leksell stereotactic frame, designed by Prof J. Caemaert, originally introduced in 1986, and still in production in an updated form (Richard Wolf GmbH, Knittlingen, Germany) (Photograph courtesy of Dr S. Sgouros)

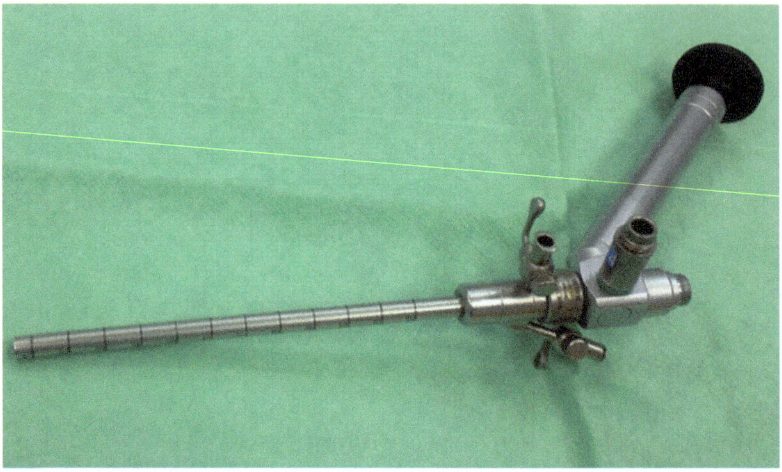

Fig. 7.2 Endoscope system Storz Gaab (Karl Storz GmbH & Co KG, Tuttlingen, Germany) (Photograph courtesy of Dr S. Sgouros)

When I started to use neuroendoscopy I used pediatric cystoscopes and flexible bronchoscopes and makeshift instruments to perform fenestrations and biopsies. But soon the development of such suitable and specially designed neuroendoscopic equipment started.

7.2 Neuroendoscopes and Endoscopic Equipment

Requirements for modern endoscopes suitable for neurosurgery are brilliant visualization and illumination, high-quality equipment for intricate surgical manipulations, small outer diameter of the endoscope, and an ergonomic and convenient way of handling the endoscope and the instruments in order to compete with minimally invasive microneurosurgery.

In 1986 Jacques Caemaert, from the Department of Neurosurgery of the University Hospital of Ghent, Belgium, designed the first prototype of a new multipurpose neuroendoscope. The requirements for this instrument were a maximum outer diameter of 6 mm, round in cross section to permit rotation around its own axis, a long rigid sheath suitable for freehand introduction with any stereotactic frame, simultaneous visual control and operating possibilities, and continuous irrigation via separate inlet and outlet channels which are themselves wide enough to take small auxiliary operating instruments. He developed this endoscope together with the company Richard Wolf, Germany, and is still in production in an updated form (Fig. 7.1).

Professor Michael Gaab, an endoscopic pioneer from Germany, developed an endoscopic system for intraventricular use in the early 1990s together with company Storz. It consists of a 6.5-mm rigid shaft, which is equipped with three channels for instruments, suction, and irrigation (Fig. 7.2). There are the so-called diagnostic optics that are larger than the therapeutic optics. When the latter is used, it fills up less space inside

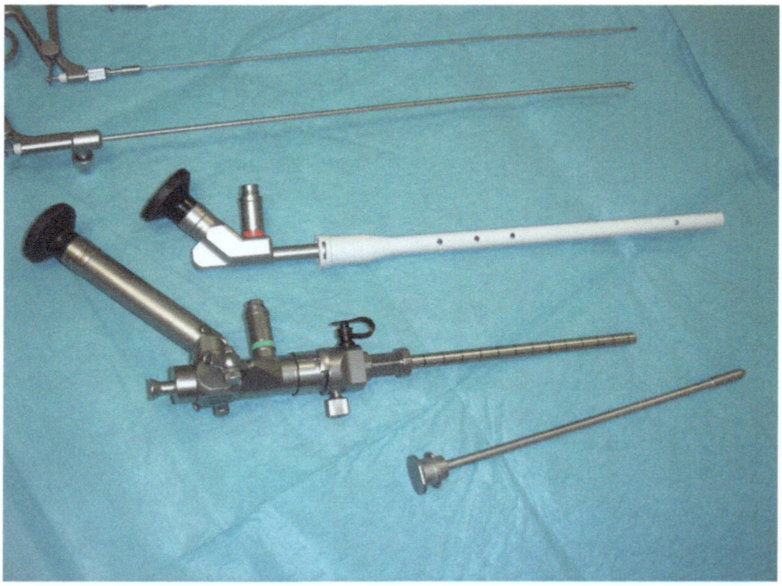

Fig. 7.3 Endoscope system Storz Schroeder LOTTA, with main endoscope shaft, obturator, and optical rod lens. Some instruments (grabbing forceps and scissors) are shown as well (Karl Storz GmbH & Co KG, Tuttlingen, Germany) (Photograph courtesy of Dr S. Sgouros)

the shaft and leaves more room for instruments. The same company offers a variety of specific neuroendoscopic systems, e.g., the LOTTA neuroendoscope for intraventricular use designed by Professor Henry Schroeder (Fig. 7.3), the universal endoscopy set designed by Professor Philippe Decq, the Oi HandyPro system designed by Professor Shizuo Oi for pediatric patients (Fig. 7.4), and the endonasal transphenoidal endoscope set with Thumfart suction and irrigation system designed by Professor Martin Bettag and Peter Schäfer (Fig. 7.5). Each of these endoscope systems comes with a complete set of optics of different viewing angles (0° and 30°) and a multitude of purpose-designed instruments.

Another important company in this field, also from Germany, B. Braun/Aesculap, has developed in close cooperation with Professor Axel Perneczky from the University Hospital in Mainz, Germany, until his untimely death in 2009, several specialized endoscopic instruments and endoscopes. This led to the development of a modular system for all applications of endoscopic neurosurgery, called the MINOP® Modular Neuroendoscopy System.

The MINOP® system is a multifunctional and modular neuroendoscopy system for intraventricular indications and endoscope-assisted neurosurgery. It consists of three trocars, with outer diameters 3.2 mm/4.6 mm/6 mm, for diagnostic and therapeutic purposes; several instruments; electrodes; accessories; and especially two FULL HD compatible endoscopes, outer diameter 2.7 mm, viewing direction 0° and 30°. Its angled design makes the MINOP® system easy to handle and universal in use (Fig. 7.6). It has blunt distal tip of trocar and depth marking for atraumatic insertion and straight working channel for rigid instruments which increases control and precision. Its rigid instruments have steering wheel, which allows rotation of their tip without turning your holding hand and offers the possibility to work bi-instrumental with both hands. It has lateral connection of cables for unhindered view along the trocar shaft.

A disposable introducer set (also known as "peel away sheath," manufactured by several companies) facilitates the process of introducing the endoscope through the brain parenchyma.

Although the neuroendoscopes can be held freehand, there are mechanical and pneumatic holder systems available. For short and straightforward procedures, like an endoscopic third ventriculostomy, they are not necessary, but they can help to facilitate dissection in procedures like intra- and paraventricular tumor removal, when bimanual instrumentation is indicated. Such a holding arm is the Aesculap

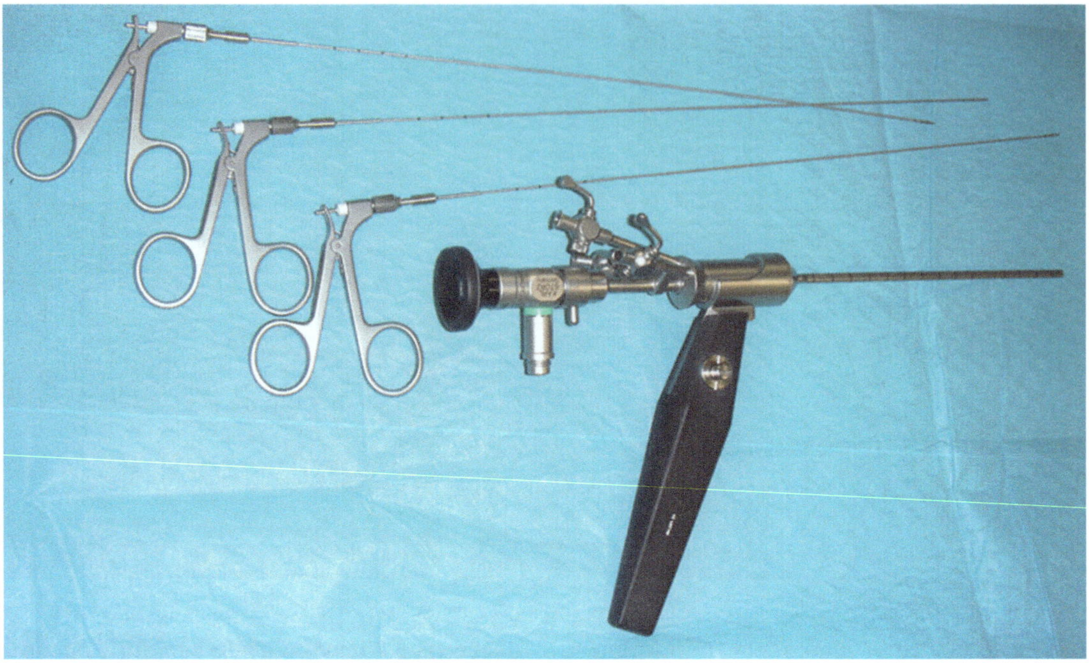

Fig. 7.4 Endoscope system Storz Oi Handy Pro, designed mainly for pediatric work, shown with its instrument set (grabbing forceps and scissors) (Karl Storz GmbH & Co KG, Tuttlingen, Germany) (Photograph courtesy of Dr S. Sgouros)

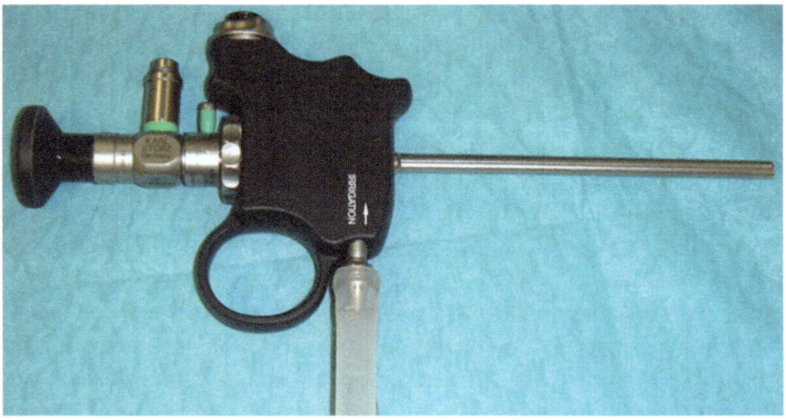

Fig. 7.5 Endoscope system Storz Bettag Schäfer with the Thumfart suction-irrigation system, specifically designed for transnasal skull base work (Karl Storz GmbH & Co KG, Tuttlingen, Germany) (Photograph courtesy of Dr S. Sgouros)

M-TRAC, which gives both a stable performance (especially for FULL HD cameras) and excellent flexibility and maneuverability for the neuroendoscope. It has an easy mechanical fixation by clamping handle with small, flexible joints for fine positioning and can be used for any surgical intervention when holding of, e.g., optical systems, cameras, instruments, and trocars is needed. Other companies make similar holding arms for their endoscopes.

Other more sophisticated pneumatic systems are also available to hold the endoscope secure during operation. Such a system is the Aesculap UNITRAC®, which is an aid for exact positioning of instruments and video endoscopic systems and for holding retractors in a stable manner over a long period. It is a pneumatic supported system with easy connection to the air supply in the OR with integrated safety systems that prevent collapse of the holding arm if OR compressed air

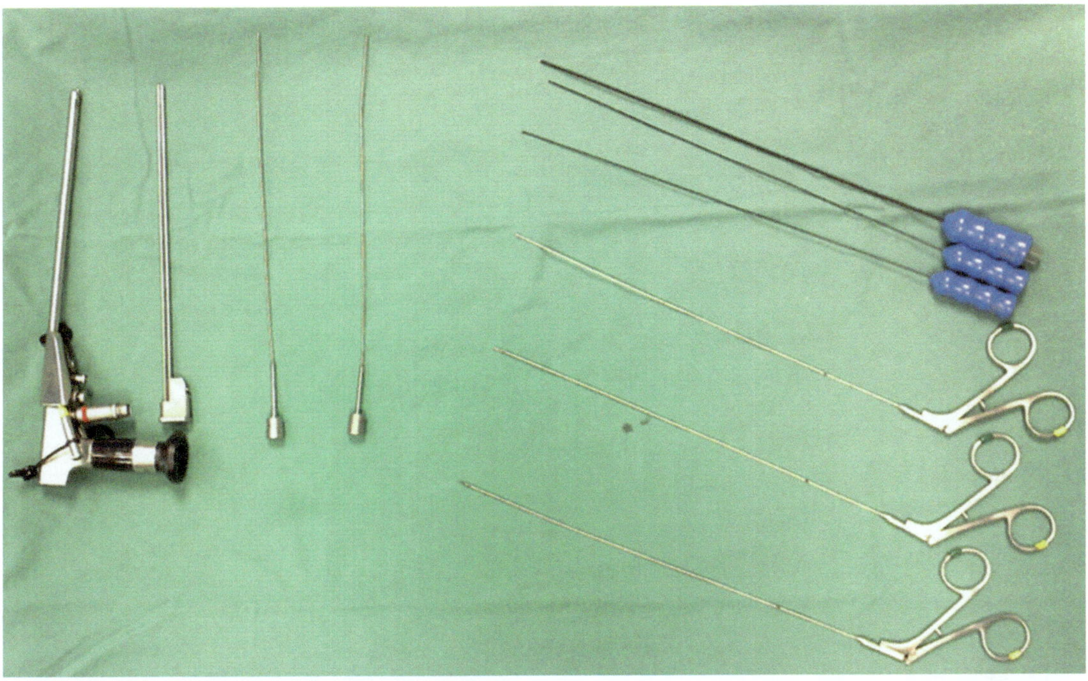

Fig. 7.6 Endoscope system Aesculap MINOP®, shown with its complete instrument set, including obturator, diathermies, biopsy forceps, and scissors (Aesculap AG, Tuttlingen, Germany) (Photograph courtesy of Dr S. Sgouros)

supply is interrupted. It is single-handed in use just by pressing the release button. Other companies make similar pneumatic holding arms for their endoscopes.

The Aesculap NeuroPilot® is a unique steering mechanism for neuroendoscopes offering precise steering of the neuroendoscope by the use of three screws in three dimensions allowing submillimeter maneuvering. After positioning of the neuroendoscope in situ finest corrections or adjustments are often necessary to receive the optimal endoscopic image. With traditional holding devices only a rough positioning is possible; a precise and fine steering of the neuroendoscope is difficult or even not possible.

Altogether, these components allow safe bimanual endoscopic surgery through the endoscope.

For endoscope-controlled procedures like the endoscopic endonasal transphenoidal procedures, dedicated systems have been developed such as the Storz Bettag-Schäfer system with the Thumfart suction-irrigation device (Fig. 7.5) or the Aesculap MINOP® TREND (Fig. 7.7). The MINOP® TREND (TRansnasal ENDoscopy) has a bright 4-mm optic in 0° and 30°. These systems not only are a good to start with transnasal endoscopy but also inspire advanced users to go further and perform extended approaches of the pituitary region and areas of the skull base.

Most surgeons are using a particular system and acquire over the years significant expertise over it. My personal experience with the MINOP® TREND system allows me to say that it is a well-balanced endoscope system offering high ergonomics, a brilliant picture, as well as specially developed instruments. It has an ergonomic handle design and optimum weight distribution, suction, and irrigation that prevents the optic from misting; a revolvable endoscope shaft with angled optics permitting direct visualization of hidden corners of the operating field; and a slim handle for unimpeded panendoscopic manipulation (Fig. 7.8). It can be easily secured to a holding arm.

One very important component of the whole endoscopic equipment is the camera. Compared to the one-chip cameras used in the 1990s, the present-day's full high-definition three-chip

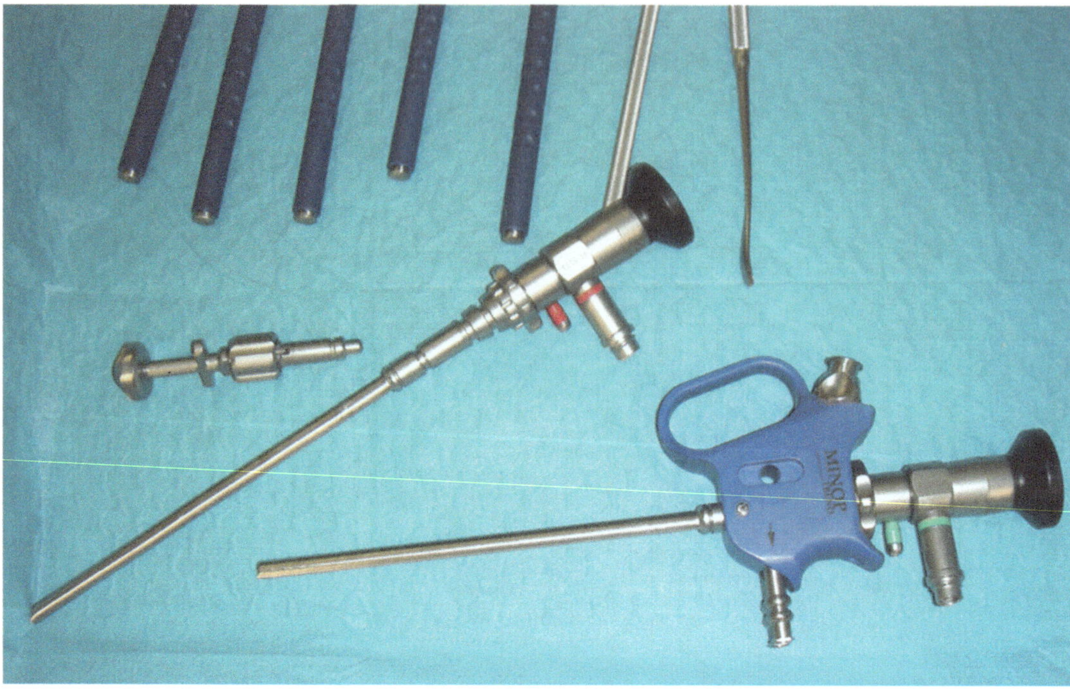

Fig. 7.7 Endoscope system Aesculap MINOP Trend, designed for skull base work (Aesculap AG, Tuttlingen, Germany) (Photograph courtesy of Dr S. Sgouros)

Fig. 7.8 Bimanual two-hand transnasal endoscopic work, using the Aesculap MINOP Trend system, and a bone drill, during a transnasal transphenoidal operation

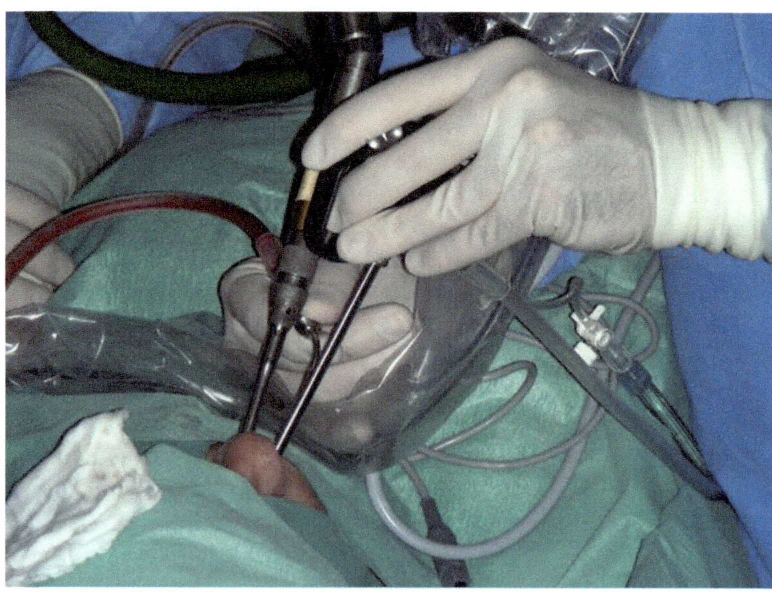

cameras give excellent views that are indeed comparable to what can be seen through the operating microscope. The full HD camera has a six times higher resolution than conventional standard cameras and delivers crystal clear images of the highest quality (1920×1080 pixels). The three-chip technology provides impressive color depth and brilliant red differentiation. The latest Full HD technology delivers lag-free images, even with rapid camera movements. The world's first 5× zoom in an endoscopy camera shows even the tiniest details in perfect HD quality.

The light source should be a xenon light. Xenon technology achieves a higher efficiency than halogen light sources. It gives extremely high light intensity and excellent color reproduction due to an absolute natural light with a color temperature of 6,000 K (daylight). Special integrated UV filters reduce the highest amount of heat in the visible light.

Apart from the companies mentioned above (Wolf, Storz, Aesculap), other companies are making similar neuroendoscopic equipment systems, e.g., Rudolf, but obviously it is difficult to give full account of all systems that are currently commercially available.

7.3 Neuroendoscopic Instruments

The MINOP® Modular Neuroendoscopy System comes with dedicated rigid tube shaft instruments with an outer diameter 2.0 mm, with a rotation knob for easy rotation of the jaw part for more precise action of the instrument tip and flexible instruments for bi-instrumental working with an outer diameter 1.0 mm. Sharp and blunt scissors, biopsy forceps, dissecting forceps, surgical micro-forceps, and several bipolar and monopolar electrodes are available.

All the neuroendoscope systems manufactured by Storz company offer also a complete set of instruments, dissectors, scissors, and bipolar and monopolar diathermy electrodes.

Next to these instruments, balloon catheters can be used for widening of a small fenestration or for localized pressure on a bleeding point (Fig. 7.9).

Other instruments have been developed for specific use in certain situations, like the Grotenhuis endoscopic fenestration system with a special perforator and dilator (Synergetics, Inc.) for third ventriculostomy and cyst fenestration.

There are also specialized instruments (tube shaft instruments) that are ideal for use through small approach, e.g., supraorbital keyhole craniotomy or subtemporal and retromastoid keyhole craniotomies. They need less space than the conventional micro-instruments. In endoscopic endonasal surgery, straight instruments are preferable over the bayonet-shaped instruments used in the microscopic procedure. But otherwise, the same array of instruments is available.

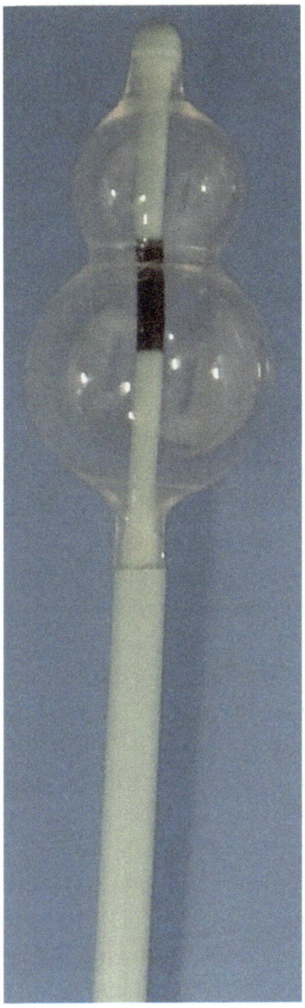

Fig. 7.9 Integra NeuroBalloon, utilized to enlarge the stoma on the floor of the third ventricle and any other stoma created with the endoscope (Integra, Plainsboro, NY, USA) (Photograph courtesy of Dr F. Di Rocco)

7.4 Surgical Technique

Whether a neuroendoscope should be rigid or flexible is an irrelevant question. The famous quote from Professor Jacques Caemaert is: "The endoscope should be rigid, the neurosurgeon should be flexible." The real problem is to know when to use a rigid instrument and when a flexible one is preferable. In the vast majority of cases a rigid endoscope is perfectly suitable to reach all targets and to perform a wide variety of actions. The action radius is mostly wide enough because of the 100° field of view, the eventual use of an angled lens at the tip of the rigid telescope, the possibility of rotating the endoscope around its own axis, and the use of instruments with curved tips. In cases where a flexible endoscope is necessary, it is preferable to use a small flexible and movable endoscope through the working channel of the rigid endoscope in what is called the "mother-and-baby" principle.

This permits visual control of the movements of the flexible instrument. The problem when using a flexible endoscope alone is that "you see what you see but you don't see what you do." The fornix might, for example, be damaged after entering the third ventricle through the foramen of Monro. Obviously two video cameras and two light cables are necessary. Direct visual control by the naked eye through the flexible endoscope is not advisable for sterility reasons.

The neuroendoscope can be introduced stereotactically, either frame-based or frameless or freehand [28, 38, 42]. In many cases guidance is used to reach the target after which procedure is then continued freehand. The angle of approach and the trajectory are of the utmost importance to be able to perform the planned operation.

The use of the different instruments will depend on the specific indications. Today's challenge is to expand the range of working instruments available and to extend the operative possibilities both safely but also as simply as possible.

Endoscopy has revolutionized neurosurgical treatment modalities in many ways [1, 6, 8, 10, 12, 13, 18]. Today, many cases of hydrocephalus, cystic lesions, and other intraventricular pathologies are approached endoscopically. Endoscopy has also revolutionized our approach to sellar lesions, skull base tumors, aneurysm surgery, and microvascular decompression.

7.4.1 Hydrocephalus

The most frequently performed endoscopic procedure is endoscopic third ventriculostomy in patients with obstructive hydrocephalus [9, 16, 20, 21, 26, 27, 37, 40]. Here, a communication between the third ventricle and the prepontine cistern through the floor of the third ventricle reestablishes physiological CSF pressure dynamics and enables a shunt-free life for the patient. An additional indication for endoscopic surgery is asymmetric hydrocephalus, caused by unilateral obstruction of the foramen of Monro. A fenestration of the septum pellucidum, the so-called endoscopic pellucidotomy, restores a communication between both lateral ventricles and avoids shunting or, in case of impaired CSF reabsorption, avoids a second shunt system. Furthermore, endoscopic shunt placement and endoscopic removal of adherent intracranial shunt catheters facilitate shunting procedures to a great degree and improve long-term function of the shunt system [30].

7.4.2 Cystic Lesions

Indications for endoscopic surgery in intracranial cystic lesions include colloid cysts, choroid plexus cysts, and arachnoid cysts [2, 3, 11, 23, 37]. The surgical goal is the removal or broad fenestration of the cyst wall. In the majority of arachnoid cysts, the cyst wall is adherent to the surrounding structures and has a tough consistency. Therefore, endoscopic cyst fenestration is the preferred method in order to create a wide communication between the cyst and the CSF-containing spaces. Especially in suprasellar arachnoid cyst, endoscopic fenestration is the preferred treatment.

7.4.3 Intraventricular Tumors

Endoscopes have been used in different ways in patients with intraventricular tumors [5]. The most useful technique is endoscopic biopsy. Other procedures include endoscopic tumor resection and endoscopic implantation of radioactive material. Special ultrasonic aspiration probes have been developed for use through the endoscope, to facilitate endoscopic tumor removal. The advantages of endoscopic procedures for this indication are the ability to look and work around the corner and the brilliant visualization and illumination of the structures in depth, especially in patients with hydrocephalus due to a tumorous lesion of the posterior third ventricle. Endoscopes enable definite treatment of hydrocephalus and histological verification of tumors during the same procedure through a single burr hole approach.

Standard open microneurosurgery also has seen developments towards smaller access, e.g., with Vycor Medical's ViewSite™ Brain Access System (Vycor Medical, Boca Raton, FL, USA) or the 11.5-mm endoscopic port, known as the Neuroendoport® (UPMC, Pittsburg, PA, USA), developed by Amin Kassam and Johnathan Engh in Pittsburgh. Here we can see that open microneurosurgery and endoscopy are coming closer together.

7.4.4 Aneurysm Surgery

Although nowadays endovascular procedures are used in the majority of aneurysm cases, the microneurosurgical clipping has also changed over the past two decades. One of the developments was the introduction of the endoscope to facilitate dissection of the aneurysm and control around the aneurysm after the clipping without the need of additional retraction [17, 29, 34, 43]. The concept of endoscope-assisted microneurosurgery was pioneered by Professor Axel Perneczky in the early 1990s and has made a great change especially in surgery for posterior circulation aneurysms that usually are more difficult to reach due to the deep and confined location [7, 14, 32, 34–36].

7.4.5 Pituitary Surgery

Transphenoidal surgery through a transeptal or sublabial microscopic approach has been the standard for decades with excellent results. The introduction of the endoscopic endonasal approach has brought the view directly into the sphenoid sinus without the need of septal or sublabial dissection [33, 41]. The excellent view provided by the endoscope has allowed to move into more extended and expanded approaches to skull base lesion, like frontobasal meningiomas, craniopharyngiomas, and clival chordomas [4, 15, 22, 24, 25, 31, 39].

7.4.6 Microvascular Decompression

Treatment of cranial nerve compression syndrome like trigeminal neuralgia and hemifacial spasm by microvascular decompression is a highly successful procedure, albeit with some inherent risks. One of the godfathers of this technique, Peter Jannetta, described the moment of "turning the corner" (the retraction of the cerebellum to visualize the vascular conflict) as the most dangerous part of the procedure. The use of a 30° optic allows visualization without the need of retraction, making this procedure safer [19].

7.5 Future Developments

We can envisage the development of a new modular system of different shafts, the so-called working trocars for brain access with different diameters and shapes, according to the need and indication, e.g., a small trocar for one optic and one working instrument for endoscopic third ventriculostomy but a wider and larger trocar for the removal of an intraventricular tumor or colloid cyst, and further expanding towards the already available portal systems described above.

There will be an ongoing need for new instruments for neuroendoscopic surgery. Most instruments that are available nowadays are more or less miniaturized microsurgical instruments. We will need more versatile instruments that will make endoscopic dissection, tissue removal, and hemostasis more easy and safe. We should work towards the development of multimodality instruments, the so-called smart tools that have more than one function.

When we learn and understand more of neurooncology, neurodegenerative diseases, and CSF dynamics and its disturbances, the targets and demand for endoscopic procedures will change accordingly. Telemanipulated neurosurgery, with supervisory-controlled robotic systems, or shared control systems or even fully robotic telesurgery as well as the development in nanotechnology will be needed to address future indications for minimally or even ultramicro-access neurosurgery.

Disclosure Dr. Andre Grotenhuis is a member of the advisory board for Neurosurgery for B. Braun/Aesculap AG, Tuttlingen, Germany.

References

1. Beems T, Grotenhuis JA (2004) Long-term complications and definition of failure of neuroendoscopic procedures. Childs Nerv Syst 20(11–12):868–877
2. Boogaarts HD, Decq P, Grotenhuis JA, Le Guérinel C, Nseir R, Jarraya B, Djindjian M, Beems T (2011) Long-term results of the neuroendoscopic management of colloid cysts of the third ventricle: a series of 90 cases. Neurosurgery 68(1):179–187
3. Boogaarts H, El-Kheshin S, Grotenhuis JA (2011) Endoscopic colloid cyst resection: technical note. Minim Invasive Neurosurg 54(2):95–97
4. Cappabianca P, Cavallo LM, Esposito F, De Divitiis O, Messina A, De Divitiis E (2008) Extended endoscopic endonasal approach to the midline skull base: the evolving role of transsphenoidal surgery. Adv Tech Stand Neurosurg 33:151–199
5. Cappabianca P, Cinalli G, Gangemi M, Brunori A, Cavallo LM, de Divitiis E, Decq P, Delitala A, Di Rocco F, Frazee J, Godano U, Grotenhuis JA, Longatti P, Mascari C, Nishihara T, Oi S, Rekate H, Schroeder HW, Souweidane MM, Spennato P, Tamburrini G, Teo C, Warf B, Zymberg ST (2008) Application of neuroendoscopy to intraventricular lesions. Neurosurgery 62(Suppl 2):575–598
6. Cinalli G, Cappabianca P, de Falco R, Spennato P, Cianciulli E, Cavallo LM, Esposito F, Ruggiero C, Maggi G, de Divitiis E (2005) Current state and future development of intracranial neuroendoscopic surgery. Expert Rev Med Devices 2(3):351–373
7. Fries G, Perneczky A (1998) Endoscope-assisted brain surgery: part 2 – analysis of 380 procedures. Neurosurgery 42(2):226–232
8. Fries G, Perneczky A (1999) Intracranial endoscopy. Adv Tech Stand Neurosurg 25:21–60
9. Gangemi M, Donati P, Maiuri F, Longatti P, Godano U, Mascari C (1999) Endoscopic third ventriculostomy for hydrocephalus. Minim Invasive Neurosurg 42(3):128–132
10. Gerzeny M, Cohen AR (1998) Advances in endoscopic neurosurgery. AORN J 67(5):957–961, 963–965
11. Greenfield JP, Souweidane MM (2005) Endoscopic management of intracranial cysts. Neurosurg Focus 19(6):E7
12. Griffith HB (1986) Endoneurosurgery: endoscopic intracranial surgery. Adv Tech Stand Neurosurg 14:2–24
13. Grotenhuis JA (1995) Manual of endoscopic procedures in neurosurgery. Machaon, Nijmegen
14. Grotenhuis JA (1998) Endoscope-assisted microneurosurgery. A concise guidebook. Machaon, Nijmegen
15. Grotenhuis JA (1998) The use of endoscopes during surgery in the suprasellar region. In: Hellwig D, Bauer B (eds) Minimally invasive techniques for neurosurgery. Current status and future perspectives. Springer, Berlin, pp 107–110
16. Grotenhuis JA (2000) How to avoid complications of endoscopic third ventriculostomy. In: Ferrer E (ed) Proceedings of the 4th international congress on minimally invasive neurosurgery. Monduzzi Editore, Bologna, pp 43–49
17. Grotenhuis JA (2000) Angioscopy-assisted aneurysm clipping. Neurosurgery 47(3):792–793
18. Grotenhuis JA (2001) Endoscopische neurochirurgie. Ned T Neurologie 4(6):452–457
19. Grotenhuis JA (2001) The use of the endoscope in microvascular decompression surgery. Oper Tech Neurosurg 4(3):162–165
20. Grotenhuis JA, Vandertop WP (1998) Indications, techniques and results of pediatric neuroendoscopy. In: Bax E (ed) Endoscopic surgery in children. Springer, Berlin, pp 443–462
21. Hellwig D, Grotenhuis JA, Tirakotai W, Riegel T, Schulte DM, Bauer BL, Bertalanffy H (2005) Endoscopic third ventriculostomy for obstructive hydrocephalus. Neurosurg Rev 28(1):1–38
22. Holzmann D, Reisch R, Krayenbühl N, Hug E, Bernays RL (2010) The transnasal transclival approach for clivus chordoma. Minim Invasive Neurosurg 53(5–6):211–217
23. Hopf NJ, Perneczky A (1998) Endoscopic neurosurgery and endoscope-assisted microneurosurgery for the treatment of intracranial cysts. Neurosurgery 43(6):1330–1337
24. Jarrahy R, Shahinian HK, Young J, Berci G (1999) Endoscopic skull base surgery II: a new animal model for surgery of the posterior fossa. J Invest Surg 12(6): 335–339
25. Jho HD, Ha HG (2004) Endoscopic endonasal skull base surgery: part 1 – the midline anterior fossa skull base. Minim Invasive Neurosurg 47(1):1–8
26. Jones RF, Kwok BC, Stening WA, Vonau M (1994) The current status of endoscopic third ventriculostomy in the management of non-communicating hydrocephalus. Minim Invasive Neurosurg 37(1): 28–36
27. Jones RF, Stening WA, Brydon M (1990) Endoscopic third ventriculostomy. Neurosurgery 26(1):86–92
28. Kassam A, Horowitz M, Welch W, Sclabassi R, Carrau R, Snyderman C, Hirsch B (2005) The role of endoscopic assisted microneurosurgery (image fusion technology) in the performance of neurosurgical procedures. Minim Invasive Neurosurg 48(4):191–196
29. Kato Y, Sano H, Nagahisa S, Iwata S, Yoshida K, Yamamoto K, Kanno T (2000) Endoscope-assisted microsurgery for cerebral aneurysms. Minim Invasive Neurosurg 43(2):91–97

30. Kellnar S, Boehm R, Ring E (1995) Ventriculoscopy-aided implantation of ventricular shunts in patients with hydrocephalus. J Pediatr Surg 30(10): 1450–1451
31. Locatelli D, Castelnuovo P, Santi L, Cerniglia M, Maghnie M, Infuso L (2000) Endoscopic approaches to the cranial base: perspectives and realities. Childs Nerv Syst 16(10–11):686–691
32. Menovsky T, Grotenhuis JA, de Vries J, Bartels RHMA (1999) Endoscope-assisted supraorbital craniotomy for lesions of the interpeduncular fossa. Neurosurgery 44:106–112
33. Netea-Maier RT, van Lindert EJ, den Heijer M, van der Eerden A, Pieters GF, Sweep CG, Grotenhuis JA, Hermus AR (2006) Transsphenoidal pituitary surgery via the endoscopic technique: results in 35 consecutive patients with Cushing's disease. Eur J Endocrinol 154(5):675–684
34. Perneczky A, Boecher-Schwarz HG (1998) Endoscope-assisted microsurgery for cerebral aneurysms. Neurol Med Chir (Tokyo) 38 Suppl:33–34
35. Perneczky A, Fries G (1998) Endoscope-assisted brain surgery: part 1 – evolution, basic concept, and current technique. Neurosurgery 42(2):219–225
36. Reisch R, Fries G, Patonay L, Perneczky A (2003) Biportal neuroendoscopy of the prepontine cisterns. Ideggyogy Sz 56(3–4):76–81
37. Schroeder HW, Gaab MR (1999) Intracranial endoscopy. Neurosurg Focus 6(4):e1
38. Schroeder HW, Wagner W, Tschiltschke W, Gaab MR (2001) Frameless neuronavigation in intracranial endoscopic neurosurgery. J Neurosurg 94(1): 72–79
39. Stamm AM (2006) Transnasal endoscopy-assisted skull base surgery. Ann Otol Rhinol Laryngol Suppl 196:45–53
40. Teo C (1997) Neuroendoscopy: current applications and future directions. Surg Technol Int 6:327–333
41. van Lindert EJ, Grotenhuis JA (2005) New endoscope shaft for endoscopic transsphenoidal pituitary surgery. Neurosurgery 57(1 Suppl):203–206
42. van Lindert EJ, Grotenhuis JA, Beems T (2004) The use of a head-mounted display for visualization in neuroendoscopy. Comput Aided Surg 9(6):251–256
43. van Lindert EJ, Perneczky A, Fries G, Pierangeli E (1998) The supraorbital keyhole approach to supratentorial aneurysms: concept and technique. Surg Neurol 49(5):481–490

Integrating Endoscopy in the Technological Environment of the Modern Neurosurgical Operating Room

8

Dieter Hellwig

8.1 Introduction

With their aim of minimising surgical trauma, so-called minimally invasive neurosurgical procedures have gained in popularity over the last years. In this context, neuroendoscopy has undergone a renaissance following the development of suitable flexible, steerable fibrescopes as well as highly developed rigid endoscopes. The refinement of supplementary instruments, such as forceps, scissors, dissectors, balloon catheters, laser technology and electrosurgery, has opened a wide indication spectrum for neuroendoscopic interventions, both in intracranial and intraspinal spaces [1]. The main indications for neuroendoscopic interventions are procedures in preformed intracranial spaces, such as the ventricular [21], subarachnoid [4, 26] or subdural [18] compartments, and in pathological cavities as brain cysts, intracerebral haematomas [13] and brain abscesses. In the last years also endoscopy through the nasal cavity for pituitary processes [2] and skull base lesions [27] has been standardised. This report gives an overview of my own experiences from 1989 [15] to 2009 [5] to integrate neuroendoscopy into the environment of a modern operating room.

The evolution of endoscopic techniques is based on the specific description of the topographical anatomy of preformed intracranial spaces and the development of useful endoscopes as well as supplementary working instruments. The design and application of electrosurgical devices has been another milestone to establish this technique in daily operative routine. Furthermore, three-dimensional approach planning using digital fluoroscopy, CCT or MRI stereotactic guidance and neuronavigation offer a high grade of safety and precision. All these components have contributed to make neuroendoscopic interventions acceptable as an alternative treatment option in well-defined indications. More than 500 neuroendoscopic interventions have been performed by the author for treatment of intracranial pathologies. The main indications were endoscopic interventions on hydrocephalus [19, 24], biopsy for unclarified space-occupying lesions [8, 9, 30], fenestration and evacuation of intracranial cysts [12, 29], evacuation of intracranial haematoma [13] and brain abscesses [14] and evacuation of septated chronic subdural haematoma [11].

8.2 Topographic Anatomy

Knowledge of the so-called endoscopic anatomy is a prerequisite and essential, because the endoscopic operative technique is different from the microsurgical approach [22]. Microsurgical preparation is performed from outside through different anatomical layers into cavities, whilst the endoscopic approach is performed from a preformed space into solid structures (Fig. 8.1).

D. Hellwig, MD, PhD
Stereotactic and Functional Neurosurgery,
International Neuroscience Institute Hannover,
Hannover, Germany
e-mail: hellwig@ini-hannover.de

S. Sgouros (ed.), *Neuroendoscopy*,
DOI 10.1007/978-3-642-39085-2_8, © Springer-Verlag Berlin Heidelberg 2014

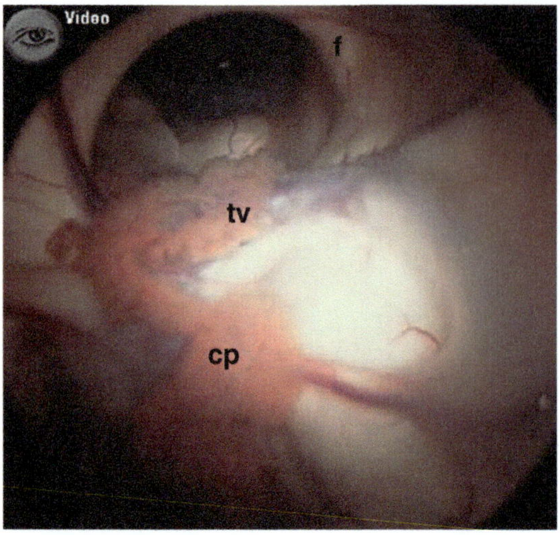

Fig. 8.1 Typical anatomic landmarks around the foramen of Monro – choroid plexus (*cp*), thalamostriate vein (*tv*), fornix (*f*)

All these structures are tissue covered and sometimes not well identifiable, which can make endoscopic interventions risky.

"Learning by doing" can have fatal consequences because the possibility to manage intraoperative complications such as haemorrhage using the endoscope is limited. This means that an optimal targeting is essential without harming delicate structures.

8.3 Endoscopes

Various rigid and flexible, steerable endoscopes (encephaloscopes, ventriculoscopes and spinaloscopes) are available [10]. The specifications vary according to the planned operative application. The optimal neuroendoscope has not yet been developed. It should have the flexibility and the steerability of fibrescopes, combined with the optic resolution of Hopkins optics and optimal light transmission. Furthermore, it needs the integration of two or more working channels for bimanual preparation and the option for adaption to modern neuronavigation systems. The advantage of the rigid lens scope is the brilliant and bright optical quality; however, the working space is limited due to the straight predetermined trajectory. The field of action can be enlarged by the use of different angled optics, which vary from 5° to 120°, depending on the endoscopic system. These angled endoscopes can also be used during endoscopy-assisted microsurgical interventions, such as cerebellopontine angle surgery, pituitary surgery or aneurysm surgery.

Despite a lower optical quality, flexible endoscopes offer the opportunity to "look around corners" and have a high degree of manoeuvrability, especially in the ventricular system. Ultrathin flexible endoscopes can be used as "baby" endoscopes through larger endoscope working channels.

A new and very sophisticated technique, which will become available in the future, will integrate the third dimension into neuroendoscopes. We have tested several prototypes of rigid and flexible 3D endoscopes with Hopkins optics. These endoscopes give a high quality of field of depth and will provide a higher level of accuracy for neuroendoscopic interventions.

As a result of the long experience with different neuroendoscopes, we designed a new ventriculoscope. The ventriculoscope has a working length of 180 mm. The outer diameter is 6.5 mm. The direction of view is 5°. There are three channels, one for instrumentation (2.8 mm), one for suction (1.4 mm) and one for irrigation (1.4 mm) (Fig. 8.2).

8.4 Fixation and Guiding Systems

To avoid uncontrolled movements during neuroendoscopic procedures and to free the endoscopist from fatigue, different fixation devices have been developed and are available. The Marburg neuroendoscopy fixation and guiding system consists of a retaining arm with joints, which allows movements of the instrument in all spatial directions. It provides the necessary stability to the whole endoscopic system during the operative procedure. The working depth is regulated by micrometre screws. The system is compatible to various stereotactic and microsurgical holding devices [20].

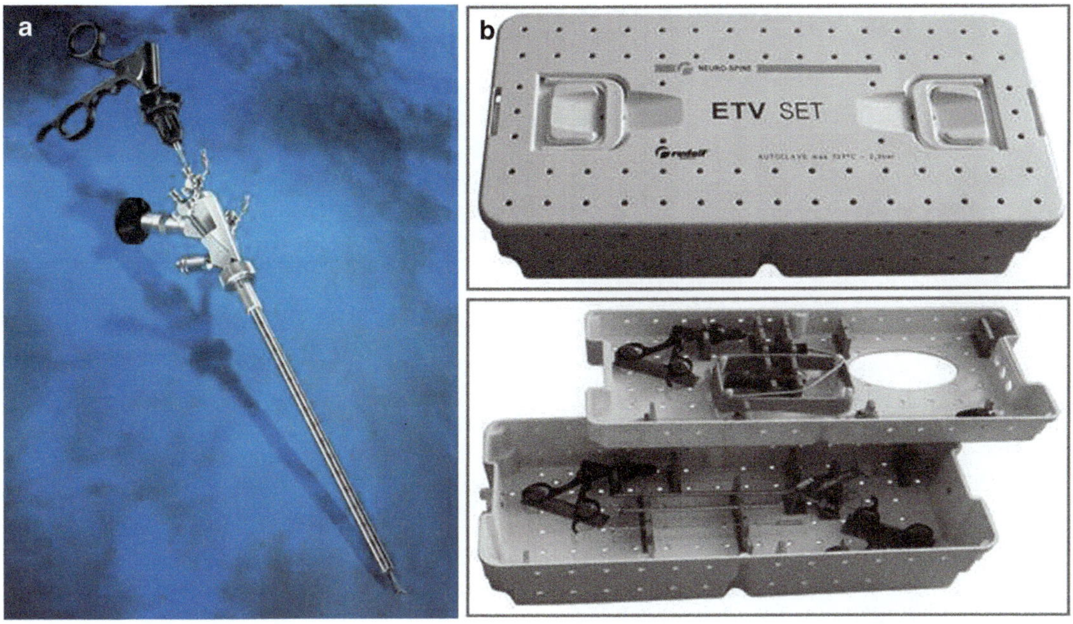

Fig. 8.2 (**a**) Multipurpose ventriculoscope according to Hellwig and (**b**) ETV-SET (Rudolf Medical Co.)

8.5 Video Camera System

Different light sources and camera systems are available with the newly developed charge couple device (CCD) technology. We use the Monolith Line ® Video Camera System with extremely light-sensitive 3xHD 1/3″ CCD sensors. *The camera head* has special features: 2× multifunctional remote buttons preconfigured for simultaneous control up to six special camera functions directly via camera head, standard c-mount connector and a high-quality optical zoom coupler (*f*=21–36 mm). *The camera control unit* has a full HDTV resolution of 1920–1080 pixel, 10× user application presets – 3 of these user settings are in addition individually programmable, excellent visual characteristics and a high-contrast colour reproduction.

8.6 Picture Distribution and Video Transmission System

The 44 HD SDI OR-MATRIX ® is, due to its function range, picture distribution from one or more OR camera systems to various diagnosis, monitoring or operation monitors respectively documentation systems, which may be operated separately or simultaneously, as well as real-time transmission of surgical interventions through an enabled LAN network (e.g. intranet), a useful additional equipment for each operation room used for minimally invasive or open surgery. It combines high-definition video routing in full HDTV resolution of 1920×1080 pixel, system oriented, throughout continuous HD signal chain; latest H.264-based video transmission via LAN; programming and storage of video routes; live transmission from the operating theatre via LAN; and an IT-based solution for interactive consultation.

8.7 Documentation System

The Monolith Line HDTV Documentation System (1080 HD SDI Controltec®) meets the demands for a simple yet comprehensive documentation of the course of operations, both of open and minimally invasive surgeries, and it is also a solution based on the latest imaging and data storage. The features of this system are based on a consequent implementation of a consistent HD video chain.

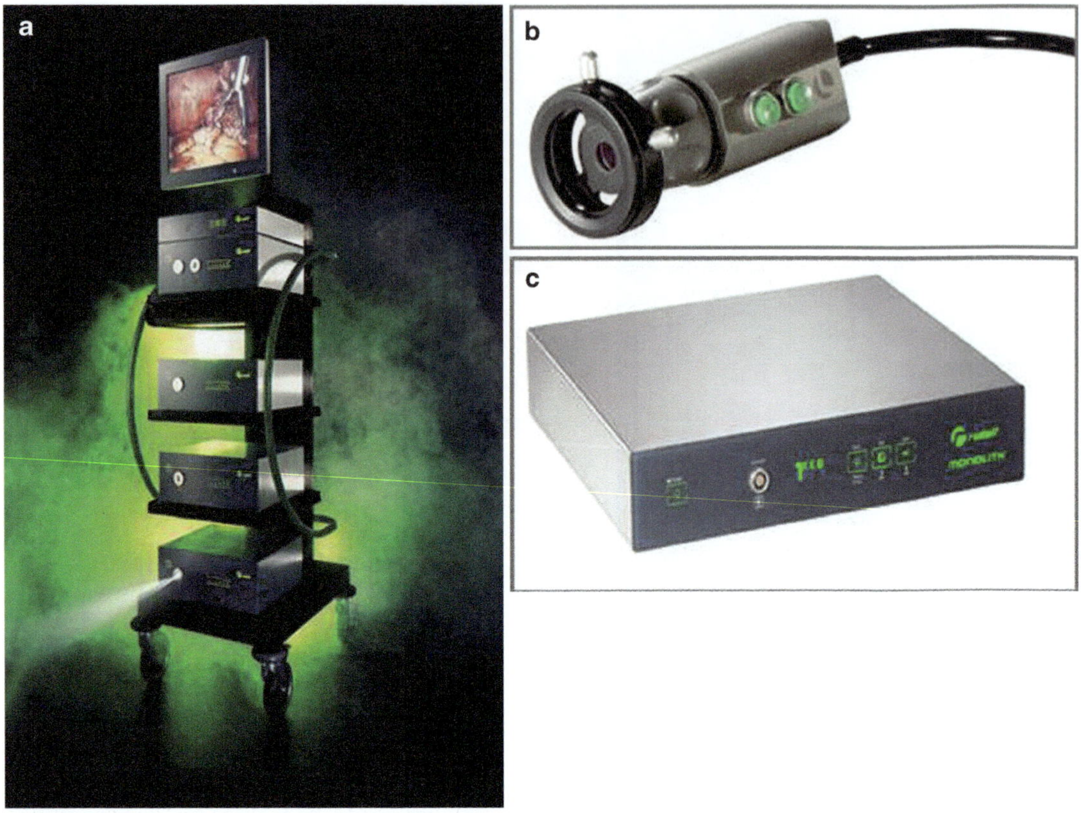

Fig. 8.3 (**a**) Complete Monolith Line System, (**b**) camera head, (**c**) camera control unit

It uses digital video signals only, which provide a complete HDTV resolution. The information storage is in HDTV format. Consistent picture quality with a resolution of 1080 TV lines from the source or pictures up to their recording and saving is guaranteed. There are optional extension tools like network functioning. Figure 8.3 shows all the components of the Monolith Line System.

8.8 Supplementary Instruments

Moving endoscopes and instrumentation within preformed spaces through small working channels demands training. The working instruments enter the viewing field at the tip of the endoscope anteriorly, posteriorly or laterally. It may be difficult to watch the instruments; if the endoscope is too close to the target area, injury of brain tissue is possible. It is advisable to have a safe distance of 5 mm, when the working instrument enters the region of interest.

A variety of supplementary working instruments for neuroendoscopic interventions are now available (Fig. 8.4).

Flexible instruments for fibrescopes have the peculiarity that they do not open gradually. They snap with a short delay between the action of the hand and the effect at the tip of the instrument. This is different from the action of rigid instruments and also needs familiarisation.

8.9 Electrosurgery

8.9.1 Electrosurgical Unit (ESU)

Like in microsurgery the further development of electrosurgery contributed to the successful introduction of endoscopy into neurosurgical techniques. Together with the technical development and increasingly frequent use, there has been demand for more precise instruments and generators [17]. The technical problem has been the

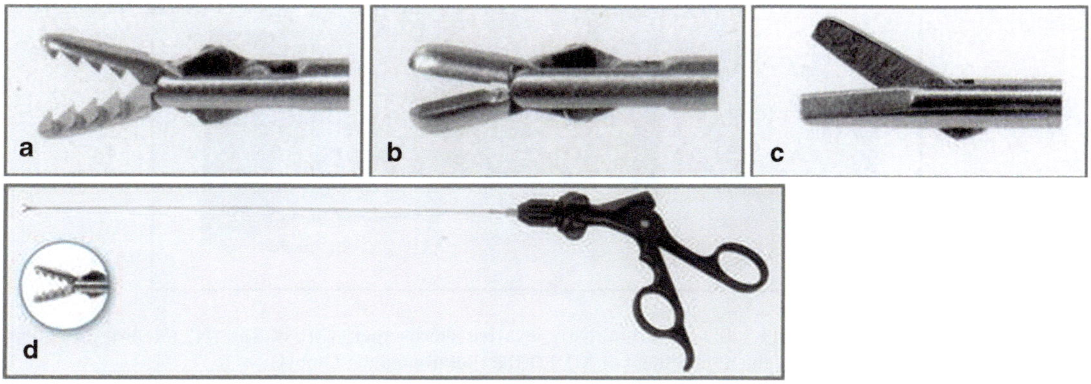

Fig. 8.4 (**a**) Grasping forceps, (**b**) biopsy forceps and (**c**) microscissors with diameters from 1.6 for ETV, tumour biopsy and dissection of membranes and cyst walls. These instruments are detachable and rotatable (**d**) (Rudolf Medical Co.)

regulation of the cutting depth, cutting speed, electrode size and cutting quality of differing tissues. In practice, this often meant that an insufficiently low-power setting would deliver a less desirable cut and a rather mechanical "pulling up" of the tissue. This led to the use of a higher output power in order to ensure a safe cut. When a superficial cut was then made, the electrical voltage was too high, i.e. the applied power was too high for cut. The consequence was either carbonisation during incision or after cut, or the tip of the fine instrument could burn out.

An insufficient power setting for coagulation could result in insufficient haemostasis; a power setting that was too high resulted in the electrode sticking to the tissue, which could also lead to bleeding, when the electrode was removed. Another unintended effect was that carbonisation could occur. These problems were solved by the development of an automatically controlled electrosurgical unit (ESU) and precise instruments made of novel materials. Thus, for the first time, it was possible to achieve reproducible cutting and coagulation qualities even using differing instruments. Modern microprocessor-controlled solid-state bipolar coagulating and cutting systems contribute significantly to the performance of major microsurgical and neuroendoscopical procedures, decreasing operative time and blood loss whilst facilitating outcome.

Recently an automatically controlled generator was designed where the output voltage and spark intensity remain constant, forming the basis for reproducible cut. According to the latest research, voltage regulation in neurosurgery is more relevant than spark regulation. Voltages can be preselected within a useful range, i.e. no voltages below 200 V can be set which would make it physically impossible to cut, and no excessively strong carbonisation and metallic erosion of the active electrodes can occur. Once the surgeon has preselected his individual setting, the preselected effects will automatically be held constant. By means of such regulation, the cutting quality remains reproducible. Due to the voltage regulation, it is possible to achieve good cutting qualities with a relatively low voltage level. This is the prerequisite to being able to use the finest instruments as described below.

Different principal modes of coagulation are distinguished, of which soft coagulation is an extremely gentle coagulation mode. The electric voltage is relatively low (less than 190 V), so that there is no electric arc between active electrode and tissue. This results in the following advantages: no unintended cutting effect, no carbonisation and significantly reduced sticking effect between active electrode and tissue. These advantages are particularly useful in neurosurgery.

In addition to "the soft coagulation", there is the function "soft coagulation with auto stop". In this mode, a sensor measures the optimal coagulation point occurring when intracellular and extracellular liquids are converted to vapour. The generator switches off automatically before carbonisation or sticking of electrodes to the tissue can occur.

In summary, the described electrosurgical unit *VIO 300D-2* (Fig. 8.5) provides optimal conditions for neuroendoscopic procedures.

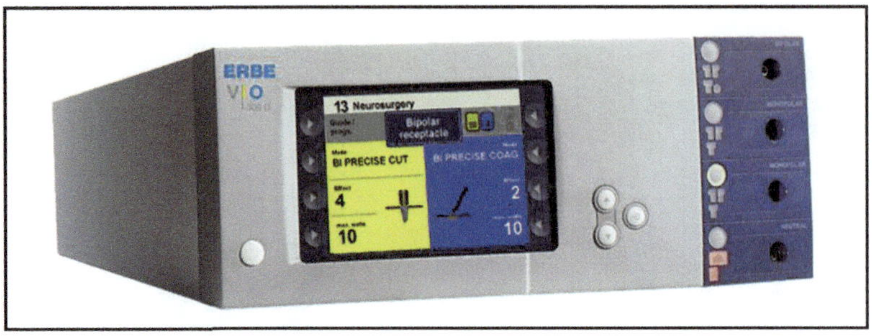

Fig. 8.5 Electrosurgical unit VIO 300D-2 for minimally invasive neurosurgery (MIN). The "N" (Neuro) programme provides finest power tunings for the requirement of MIN (Erbe Elektromedizin GmbH)

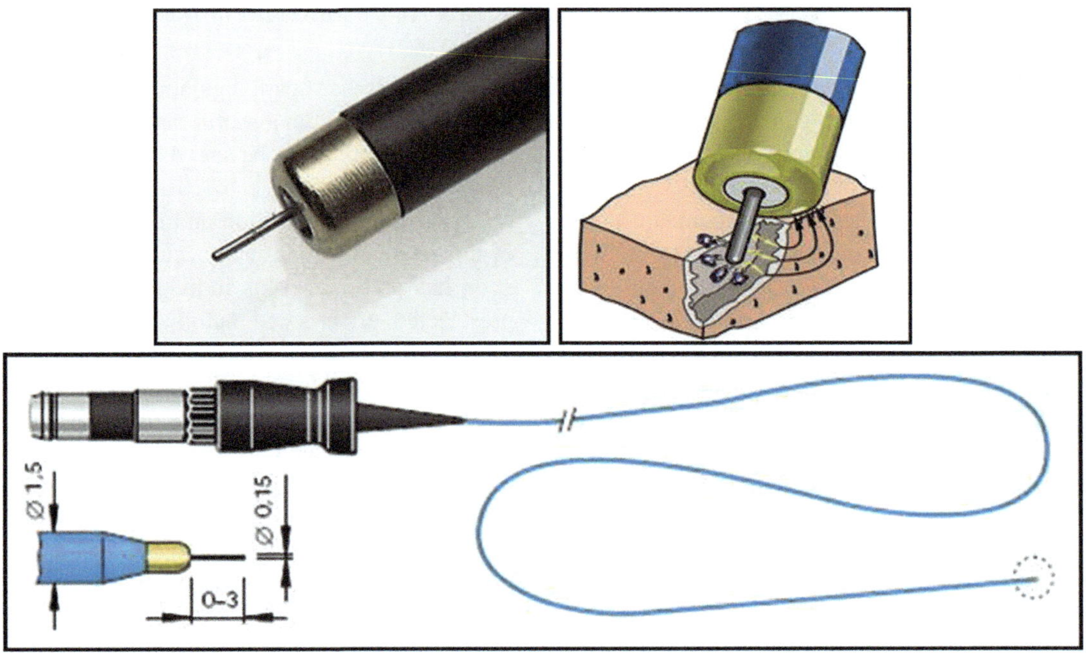

Fig. 8.6 Flexible Marburg® bipolar cutting and coagulation probe (Erbe Elektromedizin GmbH) Specifications: diameter 0.9 mm, working length 600 mm, insulated, needle length adjustable from 0 to 3 mm, maximal operating voltage 500 Vp

8.9.2 Bipolar Microprobes for Endoscopic Neurosurgery

Due to technological advantages offered by automatically controlled ESUs, it is possible to use finest bipolar instruments at a much higher safety level. These microprobes operate according to the *Plug and Act principle*. With the help of the automatic instrument recognition of the *VIO 300D-2*, the probes are immediately ready for use after connection to the system including automatic adjustment to the particular parameters of the unit coagulated and then cut with the same instrument (Fig. 8.6). The unique bipolar microforceps (Fig. 8.7) is another newly developed instrument for ETV and endoscopic microdissection. The branches can be opened by 5–6 mm without deformation of the metal because the device is made of nickel–titanium alloy, which is characterised by extremely high elastic elongation of

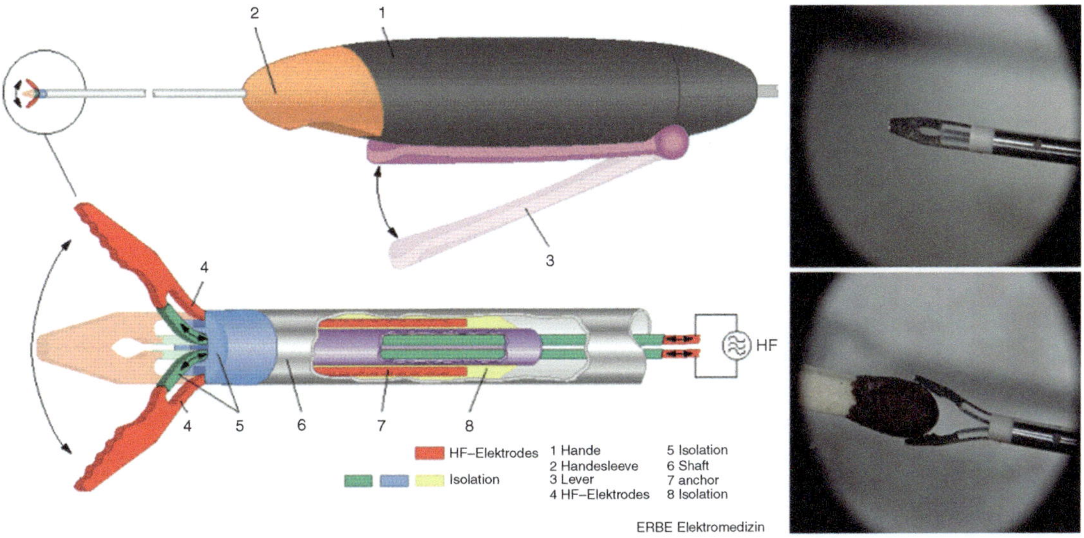

Fig. 8.7 Novel multipurpose bipolar instrument for endoscopic neurosurgery

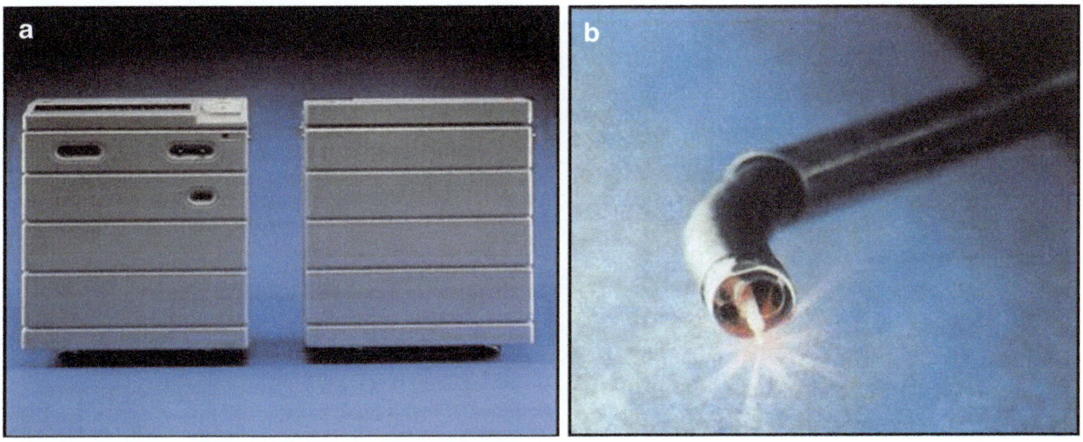

Fig. 8.8 (**a**) Neodymium–YAG laser, (**b**) bare laser fibre forwarded to the working channel of the flexible, steerable endoscope

10 %. All moving parts of the microforceps are located in the internal lumen of the sheath [25].

8.10 Laser Application

Thin laser probes and ultrathin bare laser fibres can be used either for different purposes in endoscopic neurosurgery [3]. The main indications are ETV, septostomy and membranectomy [16]. When we started our neuroendoscopic activities, we preferred bare laser fibres adapted to a Neodymium–YAG laser system (Fig. 8.8). However, the use of laser energy can have the disadvantage of uncontrolled energy delivery, which can give disastrous thermal effects to the brain. After developing the above-mentioned new microdevices for ESU, we abandoned using lasers for neuroendoscopic interventions. This is in contrast to others who have reported their results from using laser technology in endoscopic neurosurgery recently without complications. They claim that with the new LASER technology a controlled application is possible [20].

8.11 Intraluminal Ultrasound and Navigated Ultrasound

Intraluminal ultrasound has its main applications in endovascular, intraurethral and intrabiliary interventions. In 1996 the first use of intraluminal ultrasound for endoscopic neurosurgery in cases of intracerebral space-occupying lesions has been published [20]. The ultrasonic system consisted of the Siemens Sonoline SI 450, combined with the CVIS intravascular ultrasonic system. The ultrasonic probe has a 5F diameter and a length of 90 cm. The frequency is 30 Hz and the maximal radial penetration depth 15 mm. The ultrasonic probe is directed intraoperatively to the centre of the lesion under endoscopic control. In small solid or in cystic lesions, we are able to measure the diameter of the intracerebral lesion and to define its relationship to normal brain tissue. For the future ultrasound-navigated neuroendoscopy through a burr hole could also be an option in diagnosis and treatment of hydrocephalus (Fig. 8.9).

8.12 Three-Dimensional Approach Planning and Intraoperative Orientation

Different technologies can be applied for approach planning and intraoperative orientation.

Frame-based stereotaxy for neuroendoscopy was described by us the first time in 1990 [7] (Fig. 8.10). Today it is replaced by frameless neuronavigational guidance [28].

The exact three-dimensional approach planning, localisation of the burr-hole approach, trajectory and localisation of the target point or region, as well as the maintenance of the trajectory during endoscopy, reduce the risk of inadvertent damage of vital structures [9]. Especially in patients with large ventricles and in cases with bloody or blurry CSF or small foramen of Monro, image guidance using stereotactic techniques is very helpful (Fig. 8.11).

In specific pathologies intraoperative dynamic digital subtraction ventriculography is a useful tool for intraoperative quality control of interventions in the ventricular system. With DDSV we are able to show in real-time mode the restoration of CSF flow in obstructive hydrocephalus after third ventriculostomy or the improvement of CSF circulation in multiloculated hydrocephalus after septostomy.

Intraoperative fluoroscopy is also helpful in cases with ventriculomegaly or multiloculated hydrocephalus, where intraoperative navigation through the distorted ventricular system is difficult (Fig. 8.12).

8.13 BrainSUITE

The so-called BrainSUITE integrates all facets of modern neurosurgery. Neuronavigation, operation microscope and intraoperative MRI can be

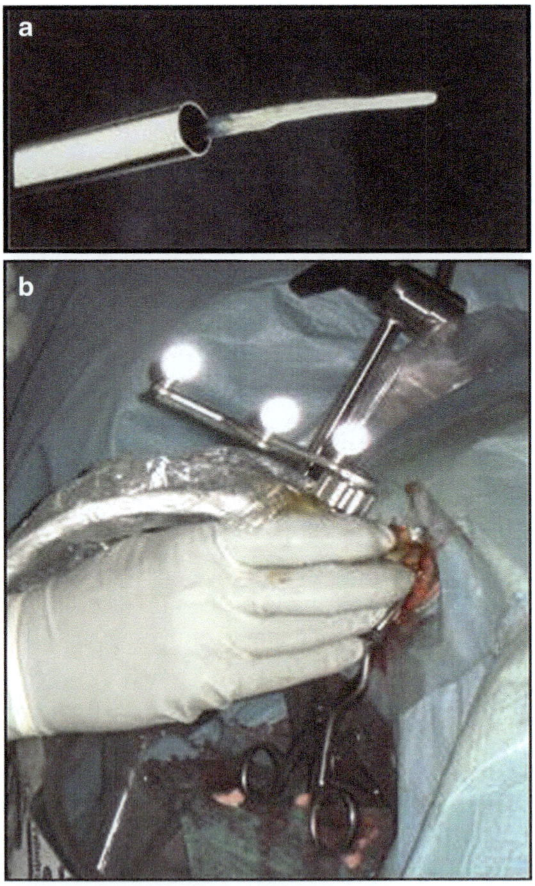

Fig. 8.9 (a) Siemens Sonoline probe (SI 450) for application of intraluminal ultrasound (b) and (c) navigated ultrasound in endoscopic treatment of hydrocephalus

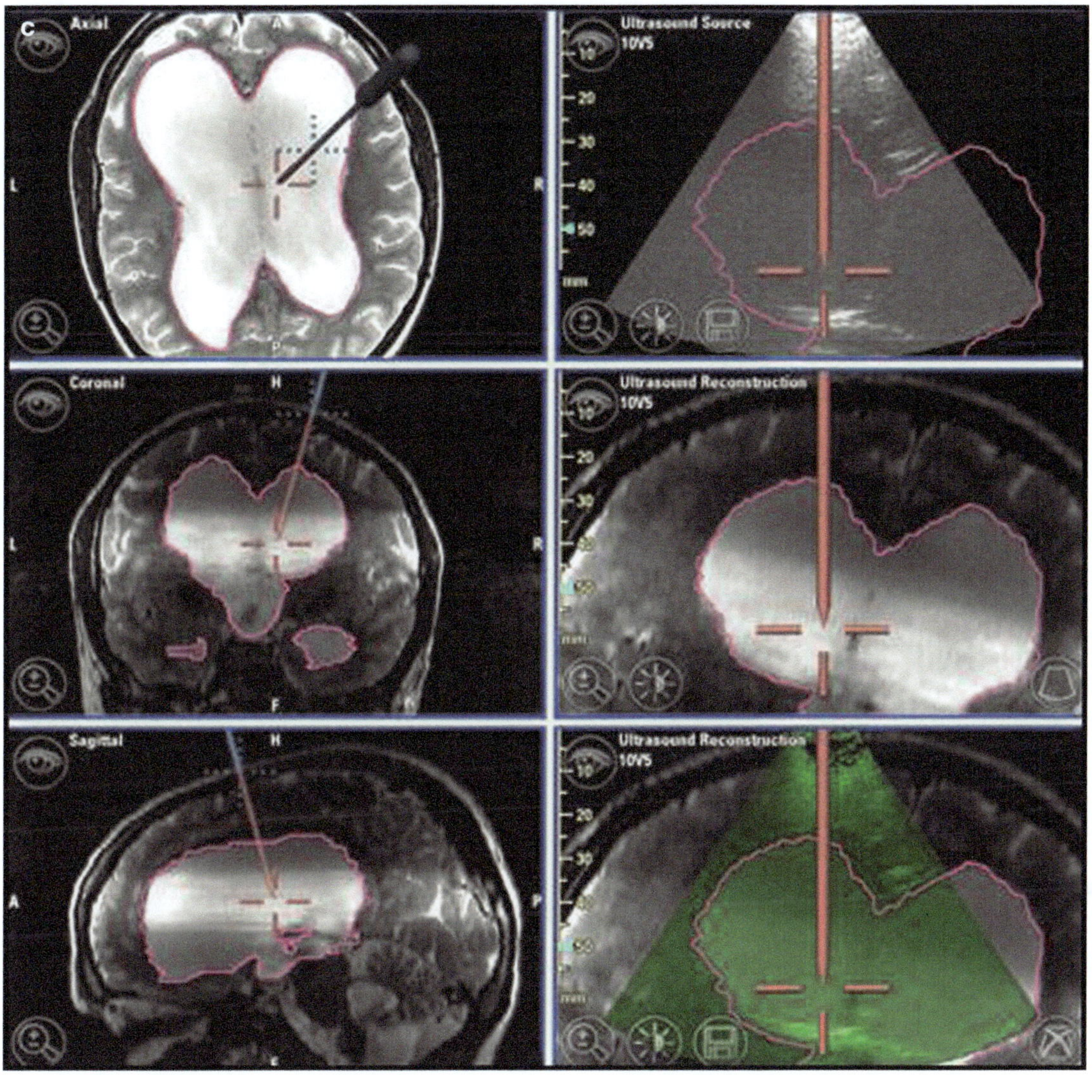

Fig. 8.9 (continued)

combined with neuroendoscopy. This is of special value for brain tumour biopsy and pituitary surgery (Fig. 8.13).

8.14 Virtual Reality Simulation

Advances in computer technology have permitted virtual reality images of the ventricular system. To determine the relevance of these images, we have compared virtual reality simulations of the ventricular system with endoscopic findings. The virtual fly-through can be simulated after definition of waypoints. Flight objects of interest can be viewed from all sides. Important drawbacks are that filigree structures may be missed and blood vessels cannot be distinguished clearly [6, 22, 23]. However, virtual endoscopy can presently be used as a planning tool or for training and has future potential in neurosurgery (Fig. 8.14).

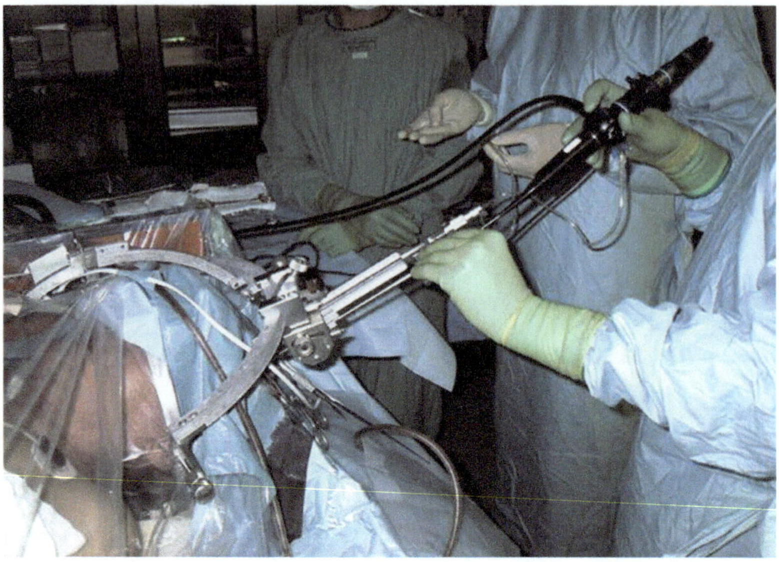

Fig. 8.10 Stereotactic neuroendoscopy: the flexible endoscope is forwarded stereotactically into the ventricular system

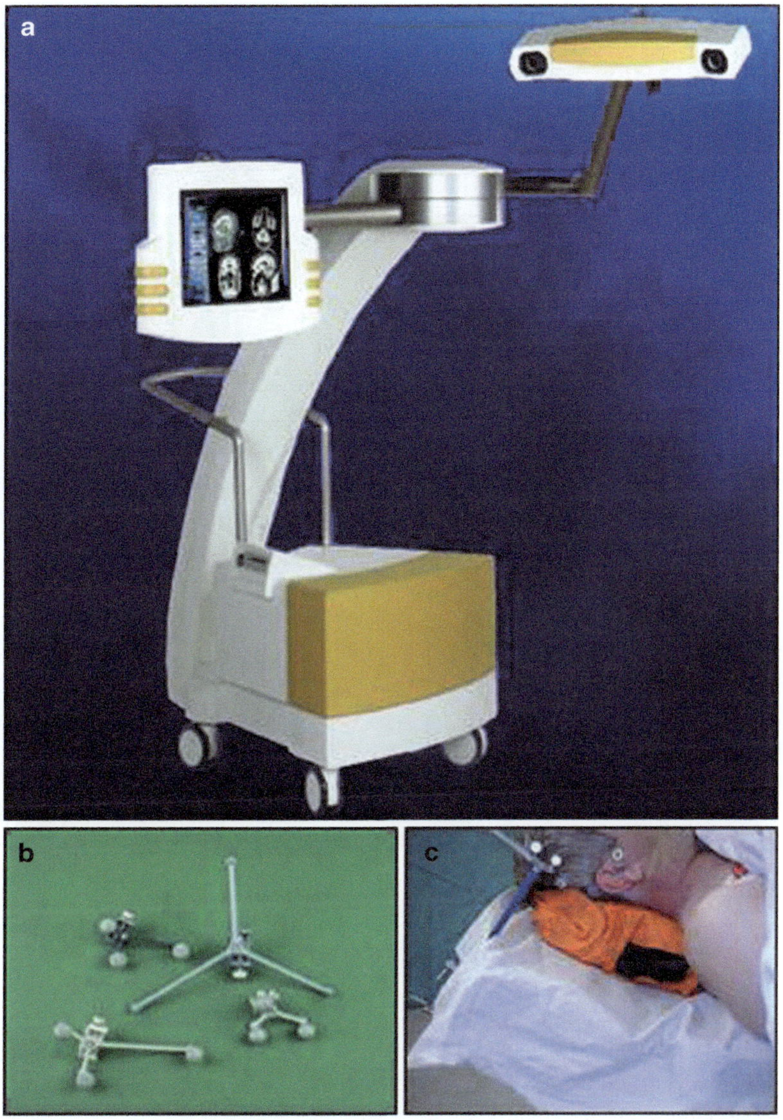

Fig. 8.11 Neuronavigation: (**a**, **b**) Brainlab System, (**c**) vacuum head rest, (**d**) three-dimensional planning of the operative trajectory for a cystoventriculostomy

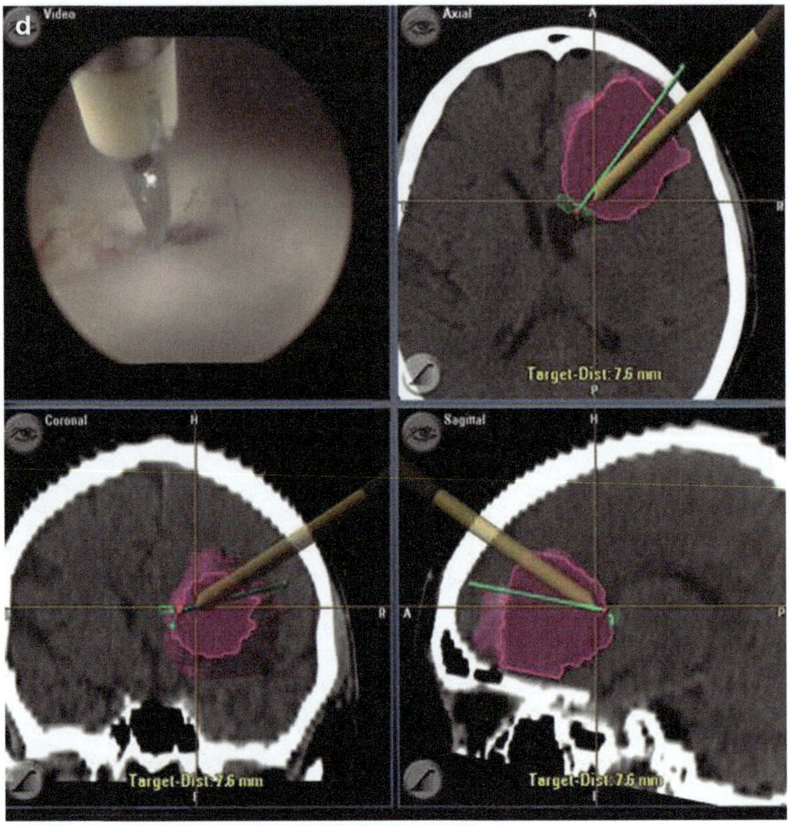

Fig. 8.11 (continued)

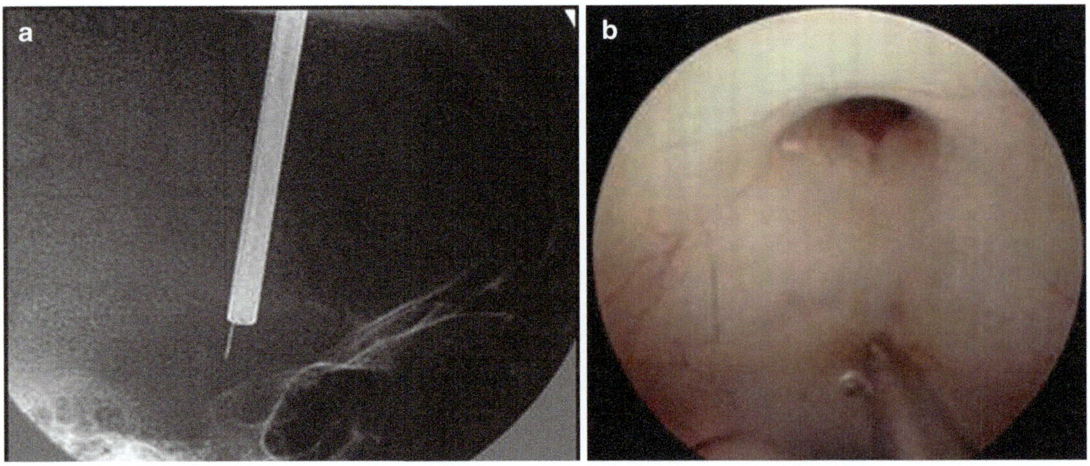

Fig. 8.12 Intraoperative fluoroscopy – ETV: (**a**) posterior clinoid process as a bony landmark, (**b**) bipolar microelectrode touching the floor of the third ventricle, (**c**) ventriculography shows an obstruction of the aqueduct (*red arrow*), (**d**) strong CSF flow into the interpeduncular cistern after ETV (*yellow arrow*)

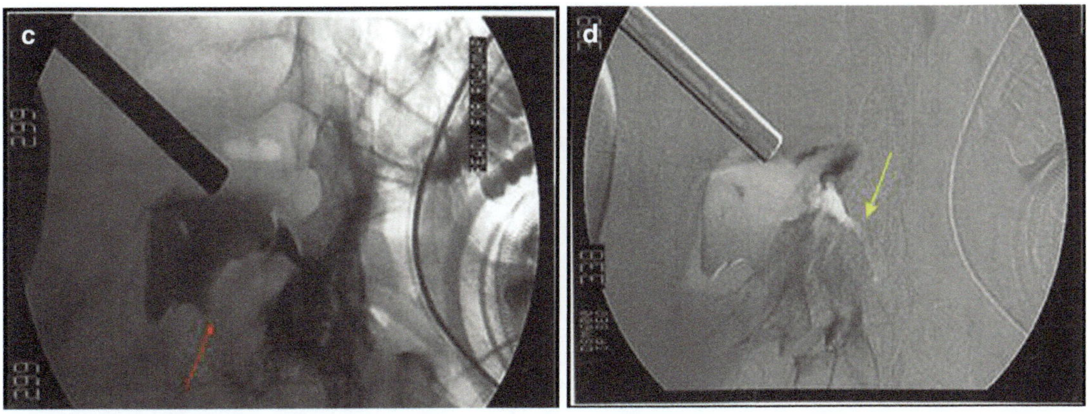

Fig. 8.12 (continued)

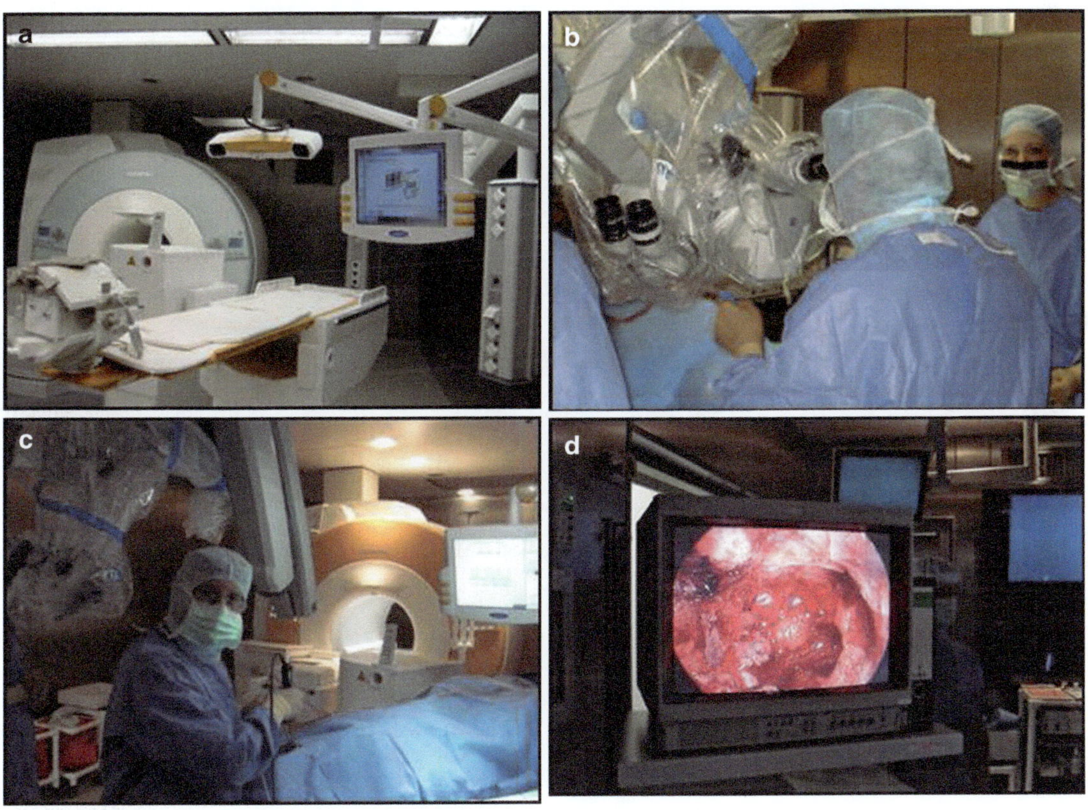

Fig. 8.13 BrainSUITE: (**a**) intraoperative MRI, (**b**) microscope, (**c**) neuroendoscope, (**d**) screen

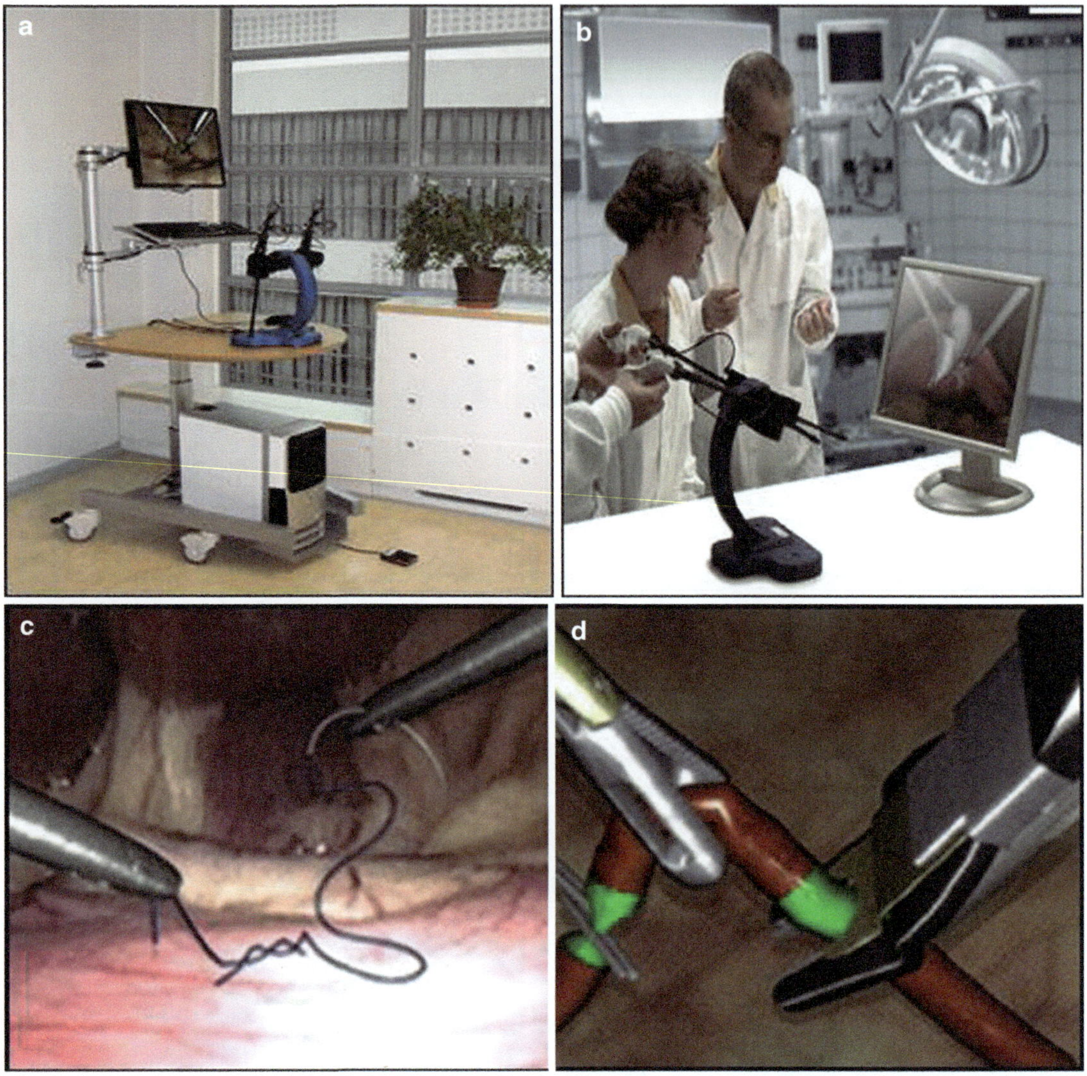

Fig. 8.14 (**a**) LapSim® – device with the Immersion Medical interface, a graphic design of the sewing (**b**) and clip application task (**c**) (Courtesy of Dr. Iyad Haasan)

Conclusion

Today, after a long developmental period, endoscopy is well integrated in the environment of the modern neurosurgical operating room. Neuronavigation and microsurgery as well as intraoperative MRI or ultrasound are compatible techniques in special indications. However, these technologies are cost-intensive and very sensitive and tend to break. Knowledge of the endoscopic topographical anatomy and the availability of basic and useful instruments are therefore indispensable prerequisites.

References

1. Bauer BL, Hellwig D (1994) Minimally invasive neurosurgery – a survey. Acta Neurochir Suppl 61: 1–12
2. Ghandi CD, Christiano LD, Eloy JA, Pestigiacomo CJ, Post KD (2009) The historical evolution of transsphenoidal surgery: facilitation by technological advances. Neurosurg Focus 27(3):E8
3. Goebel KR (1994) Fundamentals in laser science. Acta Neurochir Suppl 61:20–33
4. Grotenhuis JA (1998) Endoscope-assisted microneurosurgery – a concise guidebook. Uitgeverij Machaon, Nijmegen

5. Grunert P, Gaab MR, Hellwig D, Oertel JMK (2009) German neuroendoscopy above the skull base. Neurosurg Focus 27(3):E7
6. Hassan I, Kappus C, Gerdes B, Rothmund M, Hellwig D (2006) Comparison of minimally invasive surgical skills of neurosurgeons versus general. Surgeons: is there a difference in the first exposure to a virtual reality simulator? Minim Invasive Neurosurg 50:1–4
7. Hellwig D, Eggers F, Bauer BL, Likoyiannis A (1990) Endoscopic stereotaxis: preliminary results. Stereotactic Funct Neurosurg 54+55:418
8. Hellwig D, Bauer BL, List-Hellwig E, Mennel HD (1991) Stereotactic-endoscopic procedures on processes of the cranial midline. Acta Neurochir Suppl 53:23–32
9. Hellwig D, Bauer BL (1992) Endoscopic procedures in stereotactic neurosurgery. Acta Neurochir Suppl 52:30–32
10. Hellwig D, Bauer BL (1992) Minimally invasive neurosurgery by means of ultrathin endoscopes. Acta Neurochir Suppl 54:62–68
11. Hellwig D, Kuhn TJ, Bauer BL, List-Hellwig E (1996) Endoscopic treatment of septated chronic subdural hematoma. Surg Neurol 45:271–277
12. Hellwig D, Bauer BL, List-Hellwig E (1995) Stereotactic endoscopic interventions in cystic brain lesions. In: Advances and functional neurosurgery 11. Acta Neurochir Suppl 64:59–63
13. Hellwig D, Riegel T (1998) Chapter 13. Endoscopic evacuation of intracerebral and septated chronic subdural hematoma. In: Jimenez DF (ed) Intracranial endoscopic neurosurgery. AANS-Neurosurgical Techniques, Lebanon, pp 186–197
14. Hellwig D, Riegel T (1998) Chapter 14. Stereotactic-endoscopic treatment of brain abscess. In: Jimenez DF (ed) Intracranial endoscopic neurosurgery. AANS-Neurosurgical Techniques, Lebanon, pp 199–207
15. Hellwig D, Benes L, Bertalanffy H, Bauer BL (1997) Endoscopic stereotaxy – an eight year's experience. Stereotact Funct Neurosurg 68:90–97
16. Hellwig D, Riegel T, Bertalanffy H (1998) Neuroendoscopic techniques in treatment of in intracranial lesions. Minim Invasive Ther Allied Technol 7(2):123–135
17. Hellwig D, Haag R, Bartel V, Riegel T, Eggers F, Becker R, Bertalanffy H (1999) Application of new electrosurgical devices and probes in endoscopic neurosurgery. Neurol Res 21:67–72
18. Hellwig D, Heinze S, Riegel T (2000) Neuroendoscopic treatment of loculated chronic subdural hematoma. Neurosurg Clin N Am 11:525–534
19. Hellwig D, Grotenhuis A, Tirakotai W, Riegel T, Schulte DM, Bauer BL, Bertalanffy H (2005) Endoscopic third ventriculostomy for obstructive hydrocephalus. Neurosurg Rev 28:1–34
20. Hellwig D, Bauer BL, Schulte D, Gatscher S, Riegel T, Bertalanffy H (2008) Neuroendoscopic treatment for colloid cysts of the third ventricle: the experience of a decade. Neurosurgery 62(Suppl): 1101–1108
21. Ludwig HC, Kruschat T, Knobloch T, Teichmann HO, Rostasy K, Rohde V (2007) First experiences with ta 2.0-microm near infrared laser system for neuroendoscopy. Neurosurg Rev 30(3):195–201
22. Riegel T, Hellwig D, Bauer BL, Mennel HD (1994) Endoscopic anatomy of the third ventricle. Acta Neurochir Suppl 61:54–56
23. Riegel T, Retsch R, Shiratori V, Hellwig D, Bertalanffy H (2000) Relationships of virtual reality neuroendoscopic simulations to actual imaging. Minim Invasive Neurosurg 43:176–180
24. Riegel T, Alberti O, Hellwig D, Bertalanffy H (2001) Operative management of third ventriculostomy in cases of thickened, non-translucent third ventricular floor: technical note. Minim Invasive Neurosurg 44: 65–69
25. Riegel T, Freudenstein D, Alberti O, Duffner F, Bartel V, Bertalanffy H (2001) Novel multipurpose bipolar instrument for endoscopic neurosurgery. Neurosurgery 51:270–274
26. Rohlfs J, Riegel T, Khalil M, Iwinska-Zelder J, Mennel HD, Bertalanffy H, Hellwig D (2005) Enlarged perivascular spaces mimicking multicystic brain tumors. Report of two cases and review of literature. J Neurosurg 102:1142–1146
27. Snyderman CH, Carrau RL, Prevedello DM, Gardner P, Kassam AB (2009) Technological innovations in neuroendoscopic surgery. Otolaryngol Clin North Am 42(5):883–890
28. Tirakotai W, Riegel T, Sure U, Bozinow O, Hellwig D, Bertalanffy H (2004) Clinical application of neuronavigation in a series of single burr-hole procedures. Zentralbl Neurochirur 65:57–64
29. Tirakotai W, Schulte DM, Bauer BL, Bertalanffy H, Hellwig D (2004) Neuroendoscopic surgery of intracranial cysts in adults. Childs Nerv Syst 20: 842–851
30. Tirakotai W, Hellwig D, Bertalanffy H, Riegel T (2007) The role of solid or solid-cystic intra- and periventricular tumours. Childs Nerv Syst 23: 653–658

9 Endoscopic Treatment of Hypothalamic Hamartomas

Harold L. Rekate

9.1 Introduction

Hypothalamic hamartomas (HH) are rare nonneoplastic congenital malformations consisting of masses of ectopic neuronal tissue that arise from the inferior hypothalamus or the tuber cinereum [1, 2]. Hypothalamic hamartomas are often associated with an epileptic syndrome which usually begins in early childhood with gelastic seizures and continues with generalized epileptic encephalopathy, infantile spasms, cognitive decline, and behavioral disorders [3, 4]. They are associated also with rage attacks, emotional liability, precocious puberty, and mental retardation [5]. Once the behavioral and cognitive problems appear, they usually become progressive. The epilepsy due to HH is usually refractory to antiepileptic drugs and if left untreated evolves into more sinister epileptic patterns as the child grows [6, 7]. In these cases the video EEG monitoring is of limited benefit and may lead to wrong conclusions. For this reason, the HH should be properly treated, often using more than one therapeutic option.

H.L. Rekate, MD
Institute of Cushing Neuroscience,
Hofstra Northshore LIJ College of Medicine,
611 Northern Blvd, Suite 150,
Great Neck, NY 11021, USA
e-mail: hrekate@nshs.edu

9.2 Classification

The HH are classified anatomically according to the Delalande classification based on size and amount of and laterality of attachment to the hypothalamus [8]. Type I has a horizontal infiltration plane and may be lateralized on one side. Type II has vertical insertion plane and intraventricular location (Fig. 9.1). Type III is a combination of I and II. Type IV includes all giant hamartomas (Fig. 9.2).

Depending on the anatomical position, the surgeon has to choose the correct approach or a combination [9]. In most cases, the HH is primarily attached to the hypothalamus on one side. Less often, an equal bilateral attachment is present. Apart from the cases presenting only with precocious puberty that can be treated medically, all other patients usually demand a more invasive method [10, 11].

9.3 Management Options

The various treatment options include surgical excision or disconnection through transcallosal interforniceal approach, orbitozygomatic approach or endoscopic approach, gamma knife, stereotactic radiofrequency ablation, stereotactic laser ablation, and deep brain stimulation [12, 13]. Usually the surgery of HH is a multistep surgery [14]. No single approach is the best or is appropriate in all cases [15, 16]. It is important to remember that a HH cannot be distinguished from normal hypothalamus under microsurgical

S. Sgouros (ed.), *Neuroendoscopy*,
DOI 10.1007/978-3-642-39085-2_9, © Springer-Verlag Berlin Heidelberg 2014

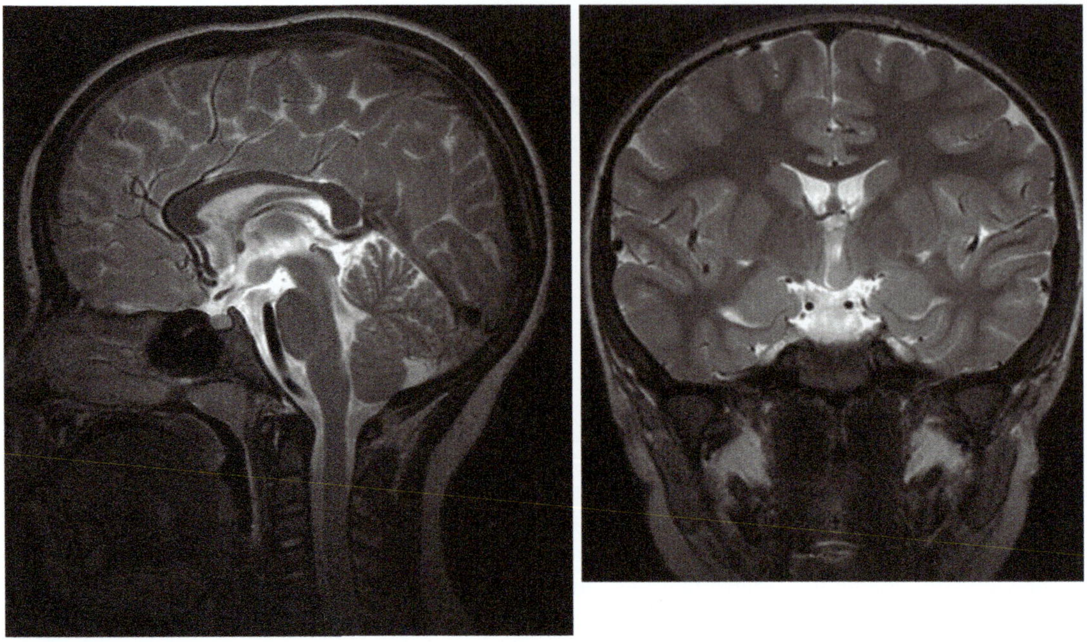

Fig. 9.1 Example of a small type II hamartoma suitable for endoscopic treatment. T-2-weighted sagittal (*left*) and coronal (*right*) MR images showing a hypothalamic hamartoma with vertical insertion plane and intraventricular location (Used with permission from Barrow Neurological Institute)

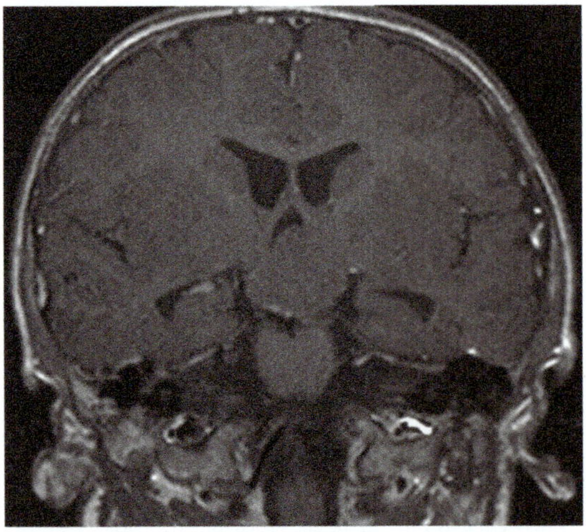

Fig. 9.2 Example of a big type IV hamartoma requiring multiple-step surgery. T-1-weighted coronal MR image showing a giant hamartoma with wide insertion bilaterally and an intraventricular extension

view. Only the abnormal anatomy that it forms allows the surgeon to determine where to stop resection. Hence, assistance from image guidance is of paramount importance, regardless of surgical technique and approach.

The transcallosal, interseptal, interforniceal approach is the preferred approach for large HHs with a significant intraventricular component located superior to the level of the optic tracts [17] (Fig. 9.2). This approach can be used alone to treat large type II lesions. Many type III and IV lesions require a staged approach. If the lesion is entirely medial to the line of sight down the wall of each hypothalamus, then a large type III or IV lesion can be disconnected during one operation. In young patients (<6 years old) and in patients with a small residual cavum septum, the leaves of the septum pellucidum are easily separated. This feature facilitates safe separation of the fornices. As the patient ages, the interforniceal dissection becomes more difficult (used until 12 years of age). It is a long reach to the inferior margin of large type III and IV HHs and often requires working at the tips of the microsurgical instruments with a reduced amount of control. A typical disadvantage of this approach is that the removal of very large lesions carries high risk of severe problems with sodium, but it is useful in moderate lesions in children especially when attached on both sides. Another problem

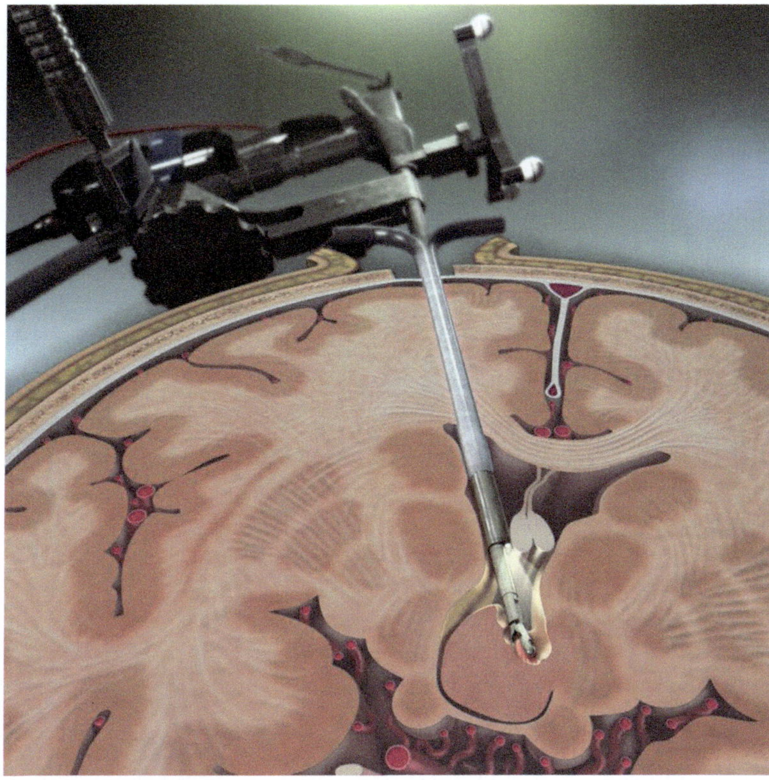

Fig. 9.3 Graphic illustration showing the endoscopic approach of disconnection of hypothalamic hamartoma (Used with permission from Barrow Neurological Institute)

of this method is with adults who have been on anticonvulsants all their lives and they have very thick skulls adherent to sagittal sinus.

The modified orbitozygomatic craniotomy is another valid surgical option because it can maximize working space and light, minimize brain retraction, and achieve as low and lateral of an angle as possible to lesions with bilateral attachment [18, 19]. The key to successful visualization of the inferior hypothalamus, mammillary body, optic tract, and pituitary stalk is achieving a very flat or even upward-looking trajectory. This trajectory is best obtained through a supraorbital craniotomy by extradural drilling of the ridges formed by the orbital part of the anterior skull base. In the case of the orbitozygomatic approach, it is performed by removing the orbital rim and orbital roof. The modified orbitozygomatic approach and a wide sylvian fissure dissection allow the most lateral and upward angle for disconnection of lesions with bilateral attachments. Standard subfrontal dissection and wide splitting of the proximal sylvian fissure are performed.

Endoscopic resection is preferred as the stand-alone surgical treatment for small type II HHs (Fig. 9.1) and as a stage in the treatment of small type III HHs [20, 21]. Stereotactic guidance is required in these cases for three reasons. The entry point is chosen based on using the trajectory views provided by the stereotactic software. The trajectory of resection is determined by tracking the end of the endoscope and again, using the trajectory views to best estimate the course of the HH/normal hypothalamus interface (Fig. 9.3). Endoscopic entry into a small ventricle is often aided by stereotaxy. The entry point is determined by finding the point on the scalp that is intersected by a line drawn from the anterior edge of the side of HH attachment to the hypothalamus and the anterior edge of the contralateral Monro foramen. This is easily done using the trajectory views provided by the stereotactic software. Thus, a right-sided HH will be approached from the patient's left side (Fig. 9.4). Once the entry point is chosen, a generous burr hole is made, and the dura is coagulated and opened.

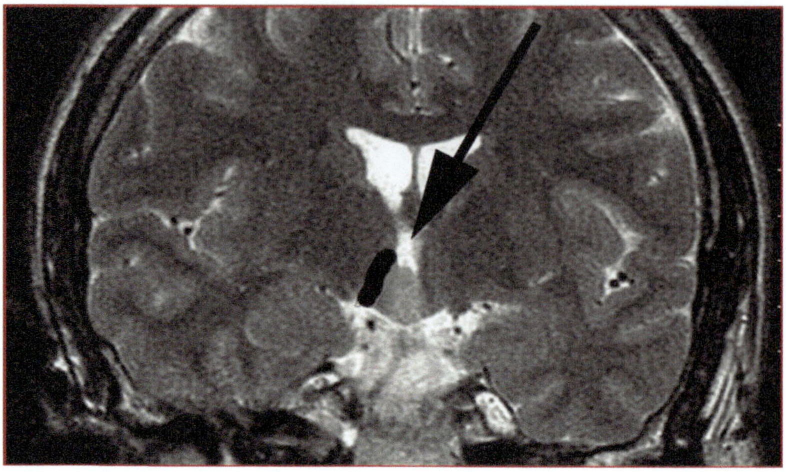

Fig. 9.4 T-2-weighted coronal MR image showing a type II hypothalamic hamartoma. The *black line* and *arrow* show the ideal path of the endoscope and the site of the proposed disconnection. Such a path is designed with the neuronavigation software, to facilitate surgery planning and execution. Comparison can be made with the illustrative image of Fig. 9.3. Reprinted from Wait SD, Abla AA, Killory BD, Nakaji P, Rekate HL: Surgical approaches to hypothalamic hamartomas, *Neurosurg Focus*, 30(2): E2, 2011, with permission from the American Association of Neurological Surgeons

The pia is also coagulated and opened. We then place a peel-away sheath into the brain along the appropriate trajectory and stop just short of the ventricle. Most patients do not have hydrocephalus, and blindly placing a sheath in a small ventricle is challenging. Once the sheath is placed, we use a stereotactically tracked 30° endoscope and endoscopic visualization to advance the tip of the scope into the ventricle. Once the ventricle is entered, gentle irrigation is infused to induce mild ventriculomegaly, and the sheath is advanced over the endoscope until it is just inside the lateral ventricle. Placement of the sheath in the ventricle relieves the ventriculomegaly and leaves a small space within which to work. The choroid plexus and anatomy of the ventricular venous system guide the endoscope through the Monro foramen and into the third ventricle. Care must be exercised to avoid forcefully impinging on the fornix at the anterior margin of the foramen. While the tip of the endoscope is in the third ventricle, the fornix is not visible. The entry point is chosen as described above because the fornix will not tolerate anterior "windshield wiping" of the endoscope. Gentle posterior "windshield wiping" movements are better tolerated but should be minimized. Once the third ventricle has been accessed, gentle irrigation will separate the walls enough to provide a clear view of the anterior and posterior margins of attachment. The endoscope is secured in place using a robotic manipulator arm. We then obtain microelectrode recordings in the HH for research purposes. A distinct cleft or indentation marks the border of the HH attachment to the hypothalamus (Fig. 9.5). Using this cleft as the starting point, we use the stereotactic trajectory view to determine the angle of the disconnection. The resection begins by using a grasper through the working port of the

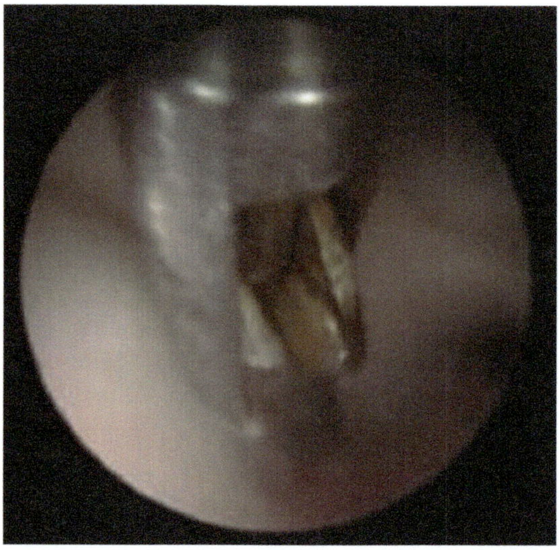

Fig. 9.5 Endoscopic view of a biopsy forceps ready to take a biopsy from a hypothalamic hamartoma. A distinct cleft or indentation (*upper left part of image*) marks the border of the HH attachment to the hypothalamus

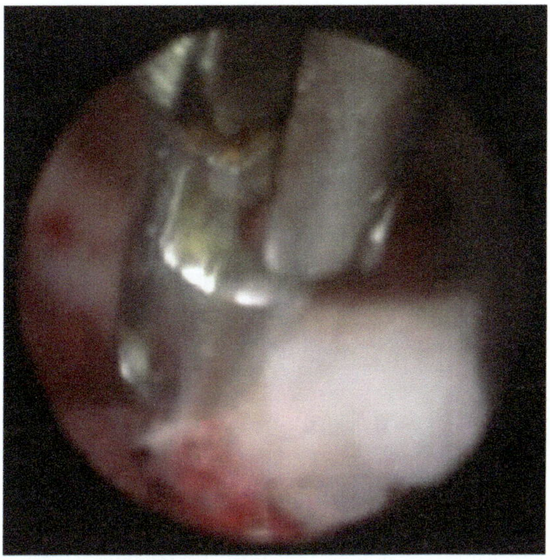

Fig. 9.6 Endoscopic view of hypothalamic hamartoma removal

endoscope (Fig. 9.6). We start at the posterior edge of the HH and work anteriorly. This cycle is repeated until the pial surface on the deep side of the HH is reached. As the disconnection proceeds deeper, the remaining disconnected HH falls away medially from its hypothalamic attachment. We resist the temptation to pull out large chunks of the HH as it is disconnected. Doing so makes the interface swing laterally and increases the difficulty in disconnecting the most inferolateral attachment. Once the HH is disconnected, it is grasped and the endoscope/grasper complex is removed from the ventricle in one piece. If the HH is too large to fit through the foramen, it is morcellized before it is removed. Irrigation with or without coagulation is used to stop any bleeding. A ventriculostomy catheter is typically left in place and removed the next day. One surgical pearl needs to be emphasized: The HH cannot reliably be distinguished from the hypothalamus based on the difference in the color or consistency. Hence, such clues cannot be relied upon to guide resection. It is best to think of the resection as a straight-line disconnection guided by the initial angle determined by stereotaxy and proceed down that line until the deep pia/arachnoid surface is reached or the inferior margin of the lesion as determined by neuronavigation is reached. By not breaching the pial surface, deeper structures such as the optic tract and perforating vessels remain beyond the reach of the instruments. Breaching this surface and damaging the perforating arteries can result in small infarctions of the basal ganglia and internal capsule. Such infarctions are often, but not always, clinically silent. If any part of the HH is positioned superior to the mammillary body, the disconnection must be shallow over the mammillary body to avoid its injury [22]. However, many of these patients are so clinically and socially impaired that clinically significant damage to a mammillary body or fornix would not be evident. For this reason, it is reasonable to be more aggressive in pursuing resection or disconnection and in tolerating damage to relieve epilepsy in severely affected patients.

Gamma knife surgery (GKS) can be also a valid alternative treatment [23–26]. It is more suitable for small lesions where it is more likely to succeed. The usual dose is 17 Gy centered on the interface with the hypothalamus. The optic chiasm and tract should possibly be avoided and it can only tolerate 8 Gy. Another advantage of this method is that it can be repeated and it can be used as an adjunct to an incomplete tumor resection. The results are promising since one out of three is seizure-free at 2 years' follow-up.

9.4 Results of Surgery

Recently we reviewed 165 cases of symptomatic HH [15]. Of the 165 patients with symptomatic HHs, 14 underwent skull base approaches as their initial surgery. Of those 14 patients, 3 required a second approach (endoscopic disconnection of residual HH). GKS was performed in 14 patients as their initial treatment; three of these patients had subsequent endoscopic approaches. Ninety patients underwent endoscopic approaches as their initial surgery. Seven patients had additional procedures (GKS for residual HHs after orbitozygomatic craniotomy in 1 and transcallosal approach in 6). Overall we have had a 70 % rate of complete seizure freedom and 140/165 (89 %) with >90 % reduction in total seizure frequency. Six patients were not relieved despite complete tumor resection. The complications were diabetes insipidus in 30 patients (permanent in 8), 1 patient with basal ganglia injury from scope, and 1 death from injury of the superior sagittal sinus.

Conclusion

Usually the surgery of HH is a multistep surgery. The goal should always remain though the total resection, even if the disconnection leads to improvement of seizure frequency. Because of the catastrophic behavior of precocious puberty even without seizures and the nature of epileptic encephalopathy, early intervention must be warranted. The use and the planning of one or more approaches depend on the characteristics of each lesion and can provide satisfactory results. The endoscopic disconnection of HHs seems to be safer and more effective than other modalities but requires a learning curve from a neurosurgeon familiar with endoscopic techniques.

References

1. Coons SW, Rekate HL, Prenger EC, Wang N, Drees C, Ng YT et al (2007) The histopathology of hypothalamic hamartomas: study of 57 cases. J Neuropathol ExpNeurol 66:131–141
2. Striano S, Santulli L, Ianniciello M, Ferretti M, Romanelli P, Striano P (2012) The gelastic seizures-hypothalamic hamartoma syndrome: facts, hypotheses, and perspectives. Epilepsy Behav 24(1):7–13. Epub 2012 Apr 11
3. Téllez-Zenteno JF, Serrano-Almeida C, Moien-Afshari F (2008) Gelastic seizures associated with hypothalamic hamartomas. An update in the clinical presentation, diagnosis and treatment. Neuropsychiatr Dis Treat 4(6):1021–1031
4. Berkovic SF, Arzimanoglou A, Kuzniecky R, Harvey AS, Palmini A, Andermann F (2003) Hypothalamic hamartoma and seizures: a treatable epileptic encephalopathy. Epilepsia 44(7):969–973
5. Luo S, Li C, Ma Z, Zhang Y, Jia G, Cheng Y (2002) Microsurgical treatment for hypothalamic hamartoma in children with precocious puberty. Surg Neurol 57:356–362
6. Frazier JL, Goodwin CR, Ahn ES, Jallo GI (2009) A review on the management of epilepsy associated with hypothalamic hamartomas. Childs Nerv Syst 25(4):423–432. Epub 2009 Jan 20
7. Palmini A, Chandler C, Andermann F, Costa Da Costa J, Paglioli-Neto E, Polkey C et al (2002) Resection of the lesion in patients with hypothalamic hamartomas and catastrophic epilepsy. Neurology 58: 1338–1347
8. Delalande O, Fohlen M (2003) Disconnecting surgical treatment of hypothalamic hamartoma in children and adults with refractory epilepsy and proposal of a new classification. Neurol Med Chir (Tokyo) 43:61–68
9. Pati S, Abla AA, Rekate HL, Ng YT (2011) Repeat surgery for hypothalamic hamartoma in refractory epilepsy. Neurosurg Focus 30(2):E3
10. Addas B, Sherman EM, Hader WJ (2008) Surgical management of hypothalamic hamartomas in patients with gelastic epilepsy. Neurosurg Focus 25(3):E8
11. Shim KW, Chang JH, Park YG, Kim HD, Choi JU, Kim DS (2008) Treatment modality for intractable epilepsy in hypothalamic hamartomatous lesions. Neurosurgery 62(4):847–856; discussion 856
12. Kuzniecky RI, Guthrie BL (2003) Stereotactic surgical approach to hypothalamic hamartomas. Epileptic Disord 5(4):275–280
13. Régis J, Scavarda D, Tamura M, Nagayi M, Villeneuve N, Bartolomei F, Brue T, Dafonseca D, Chauvel P (2006) Epilepsy related to hypothalamic hamartomas: surgical management with special reference to gamma knife surgery. Childs Nerv Syst 22(8):881–895. Epub 2006 Jun 29
14. Ng YT, Rekate HL (2011) Successful third surgery for a case of status gelasticus: lessons learned after nearly 200 cases of hypothalamic hamartoma surgical resection. Epilepsia 52(1):e1–e3. doi:10.1111/j.1528-1167.2010.02921.x
15. Wait SD, Abla AA, Killory BD, Nakaji P, Rekate HL (2011) Surgical approaches to hypothalamic hamartomas. Neurosurg Focus 30(2):E2
16. Sgouros S, Natarajan K, Walsh AR, Rolfe EB, Hockley AD (1998) Computer simulation of a neurosurgical operation: craniotomy for hypothalamic hamartoma. Childs Nerv Syst 14(7):322–327
17. Rosenfeld JV, Feiz-Erfan I (2007) Hypothalamic hamartoma treatment: surgical resection with the transcallosal approach. Semin Pediatr Neurol 14(2): 88–98
18. Abla AA, Rekate HL, Wilson DA, Wait SD, Uschold TD, Prenger E, Ng YT, Nakaji P, Kerrigan JF (2011) Orbitozygomatic resection for hypothalamic hamartoma and epilepsy: patient selection and outcome. Childs Nerv Syst 27(2):265–277. Epub 2010 Aug 10
19. Feiz-Erfan I, Horn EM, Rekate HL, Spetzler RF, Ng YT, Rosenfeld JV, Kerrigan JF 3rd (2005) Surgical strategies for approaching hypothalamic hamartomas causing gelastic seizures in the pediatric population: transventricular compared with skull base approaches. J Neurosurg 103(4 Suppl):325–332
20. Ng YT, Rekate HL, Prenger EC, Wang NC, Chung SS, Feiz-Erfan I et al (2008) Endoscopic resection of hypothalamic hamartomas for refractory symptomatic epilepsy. Neurology 70:1543–1548

21. Procaccini E, Dorfmüller G, Fohlen M, Bulteau C, Delalande O (2006) Surgical management of hypothalamic hamartomas with epilepsy: the stereoendoscopic approach. Neurosurgery 59(4 Suppl 2):ONS336–ONS344; discussion ONS344–346
22. Stabell KE, Bakke SJ, Egge A (2012) Cognitive neurological sequelae after stereoendoscopic disconnection of a hypothalamic hamartoma. A case study. Epilepsy Behav 24(2):274–278. Epub 2012 Apr 28
23. Abla AA, Shetter AG, Chang SW, Wait SD, Brachman DG, Ng YT et al (2010) Gamma Knife surgery for hypothalamic hamartomas and epilepsy: patient selection and outcomes. Clinical article. J Neurosurg 113:207–214
24. Mathieu D, Deacon C, Pinard CA, Kenny B, Duval J (2010) Gamma Knife surgery for hypothalamic hamartomas causing refractory epilepsy: preliminary results from a prospective observational study. J Neurosurg 113(Suppl):215–221
25. Romanelli P, Muacevic A, Striano S (2008) Radiosurgery for hypothalamic hamartomas. Neurosurg Focus 24(5):E9
26. Régis J, Scavarda D, Tamura M, Villeneuve N, Bartolomei F, Brue T, Morange I, Dafonseca D, Chauvel P (2007) Gamma knife surgery for epilepsy related to hypothalamic hamartomas. Semin Pediatr Neurol 14(2):73–79

Endoscopic Management of Intraventricular Brain Tumors in Children

10

Mark M. Souweidane

10.1 Introduction

Endoscopic surgery for intraventricular brain tumors is a logical application of endoscopic technology. Because of the central and deep location of many childhood brain tumors intraventricular, conventional neurosurgical approaches have a relative increase in potential morbidity. The location of intraventricular tumors being within a CSF compartment affords excellent light and image transmission. The fact that most children with intraventricular tumors have concomitant hydrocephalus makes endoscopic surgery particularly attractive since simultaneous procedures can be employed both for CSF diversion and tumor management. In addition, the inherent benefits of minimally invasive techniques including reduced surgical time, improved cosmetic results, shortened hospital stay, and reduced cost also factor into the appeal of neurosurgical endoscopy for children with intraventricular tumors. Endoscopic procedures for children with brain tumors can be categorized into the main topics of tumor cyst fenestration, tumor biopsy, tumor removal, and metastatic assessment.

10.2 Patient Selection

Patient selection is critical in optimizing the desired surgical goal, avoiding unnecessary procedures, and minimizing surgical morbidity. The intended surgical goal must be carefully established prior to surgery. Many children that can undergo endoscopic surgery may not be logical candidates since they will ultimately require conventional surgical tumor removal or no surgery. In selecting patients, the less experienced surgeon should begin with less demanding cases (septal fenestration and endoscopic third ventriculostomy) and eventually incorporate more complex cases (colloid cyst and solid tumor resection). Although endoscopic surgery can be accomplished in patients with normal-sized ventricles, concomitant hydrocephalus affords easier ventricular cannulation and intraventricular navigation [1].

10.3 Endoscopic Procedures

10.3.1 Endoscopic Fenestration

Tumor cyst fenestration is an appealing therapeutic option when a patient's symptoms can be relieved by cyst decompression and when aggressive tumor resection may be avoided. Craniopharyngiomas, hypothalamic/chiasmatic astrocytomas, and suprasellar germ cell tumors are examples of such tumors (Fig. 10.1) [2, 3].

M.M. Souweidane, MD, FAAP, FACS
Neurological Surgery, Weill Cornell Medical College,
New York, NY, USA
e-mail: mmsouwei@med.cornell.edu

S. Sgouros (ed.), *Neuroendoscopy*,
DOI 10.1007/978-3-642-39085-2_10, © Springer-Verlag Berlin Heidelberg 2014

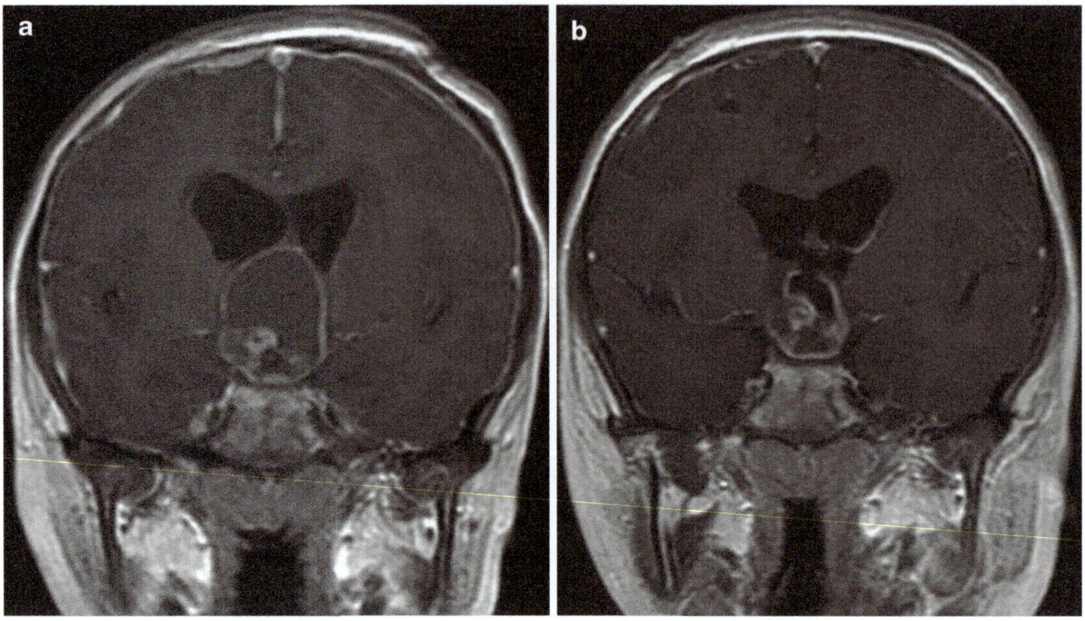

Fig. 10.1 Contrast-enhanced MRI from a patient with a recurrent cystic craniopharyngioma who presented with visual deterioration. The preoperative image (**a**) demonstrates the large dimension and mass effect from the tumor cyst. The postoperative MRI (**b**) after a right transventricular endoscopic fenestration reveals the reduction in size and mass effect of the cyst

Transventricular endoscopic cyst decompression is a minimally invasive method for temporarily or permanently alleviating obstructive hydrocephalus or visual loss.

For most cystic tumors causing obstructive hydrocephalus at the level of the third ventricle, a standard coronal approach is an ideal trajectory. Tumor cysts in the region of the posterior third ventricle, typically being benign mesencephalic tumors, need to be approached from a far-precoronal entry similarly used for biopsy or removal of pineal region tumors (Fig. 10.2).

Regardless of tumor position, one should attempt to create the largest fenestration possible to reduce any future occlusion of the opening (Fig. 10.3). Unlike a technique used for endoscopic third ventriculostomy, energy sources such as bipolar coagulation or laser are used to generously cut through the tumor cyst membrane. Although rare, inflammatory changes in the CSF from cyst contents are reduced with preoperative corticosteroids and continuous irrigation.

10.3.2 Tumor Biopsy

Endoscopic tumor biopsy is a well-established method for sampling intraventricular brain tumors. The results of these minimally invasive techniques can have a profound impact on the management of children with intraventricular brain tumors [4–7]. The diagnostic yield is high and the risk is low [8, 9]. In the author's current series of 80 patients who have undergone endoscopic biopsy, the diagnostic yield was 98 % (78/80 diagnostic samples) with a 1.3 % risk of postoperative permanent neurologic morbidity. Endoscopic tumor biopsy is of particular importance in patients in which the overall oncologic management may not require an aggressive or total tumor removal. Thus, a patient in whom the potential diagnosis includes a germ cell tumor, infiltrative hypothalamic/optic pathway glioma, and Langerhans cell histiocytosis would be an ideal candidate for a minimally invasive endoscopic diagnostic sampling. Given that the majority of these tumor types occur in young patients, age is quite influential in the decision-making process regarding the role of endoscopic tumor biopsy.

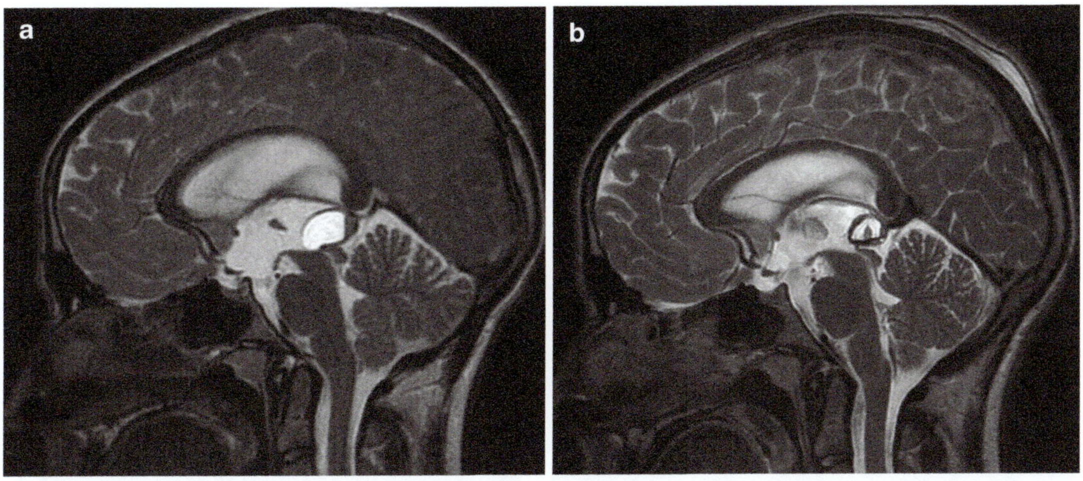

Fig. 10.2 Sagittal T2-weighted MRI before (**a**) and after (**b**) endoscopic fenestration of a cystic tumor at the rostral mesencephalon. This adolescent male required no further therapy for a biopsy-proven low-grade glial tumor

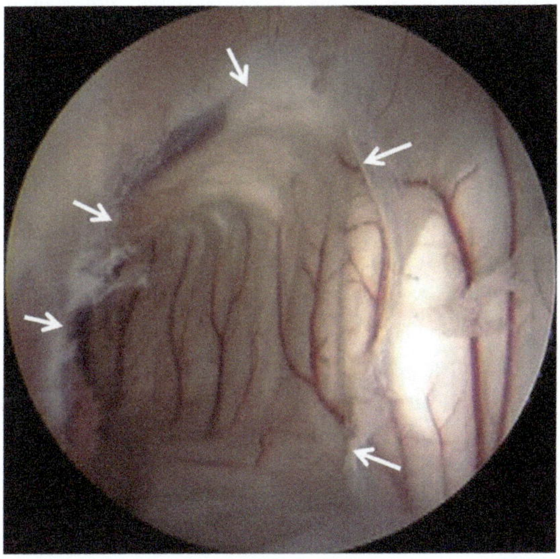

Fig. 10.3 Endoscopic view through a large fenestration created in a cyst of the right lateral ventricle. The wide margins of the fenestration (*arrows*) minimizes the potential for subsequent occlusion

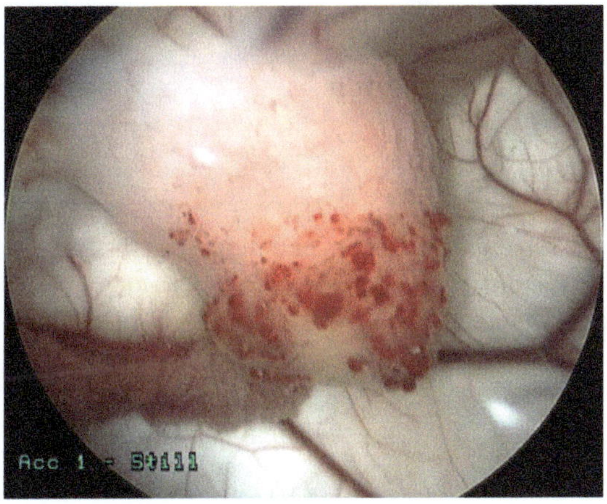

Fig. 10.4 Endoscopic view into the frontal horn of the lateral ventricle demonstrates an ideal tumor for endoscopic biopsy or removal. The tumor is exophytic into the ventricular compartment and distinct from the ependymal surface

A patient with a clinical suspicion of CNS germ cell tumor with positive serum tumor markers (βHCG, αAFP) represents a relative contraindication for endoscopic tumor sampling. The tumor morphology also plays a role in assessing the potential for safe endoscopic biopsy. In short, only tumors that exhibit an exophytic component into the ventricle are logical candidates for endoscopic tumor biopsy (Fig. 10.4). Subependymal tumors that do not present into the ventricular system even though they may distort the ventricular walls can be difficult to locate intraoperatively and alternative methods of tumor sapling should be considered.

Surgical planning with navigational guidance will result in less torque on cortical and subcortical tissues and hence is an important adjunct for endoscopic tumor biopsy [10, 11]. Once the tumor is visualized, cupped biopsy forceps are used to

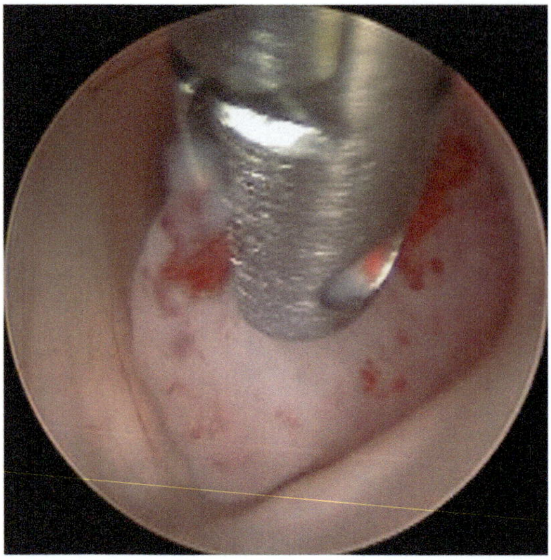

Fig. 10.5 Cupped biopsy forceps are used for tumor sampling in this posterior third ventricular/pineal region tumor. The tumor is clearly distinguished from the walls of the hypothalamus

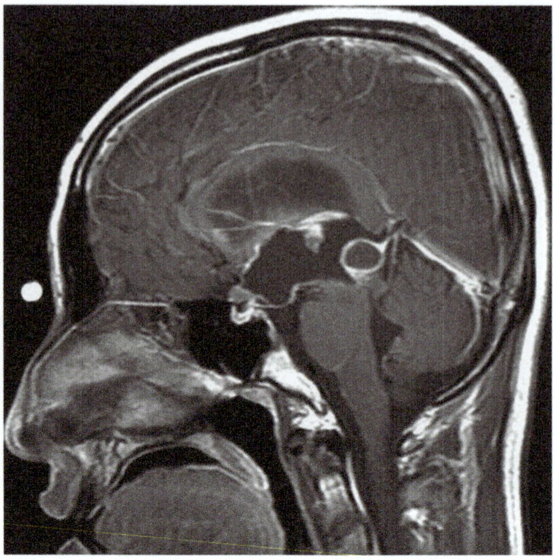

Fig. 10.6 Sagittal T1-weighted MRI after administration of contrast agent reveals a cystic enhancing tumor in the pineal region. This adolescent male who presented with symptoms of hydrocephalus had no detectable serum markers (AFP, HCG) and thus underwent a simultaneous endoscopic third ventriculostomy and tumor biopsy. He was subsequently treated for a pure germinoma with no further surgery

sample the tumor (Fig. 10.5). Sites of sampling are chosen that most likely represent pathologic tissue, are relatively avascular, and require as little torque as possible. The small samples of tissue obtained with cupped forceps are challenging for accurate pathologic interpretation, and every attempt should be made to minimize artifact from electrocautery. Therefore, the use of coagulation on the tumor surface, as logical as that may seem, should be avoided prior to sampling. Varying degrees of venous hemorrhage invariably occur with cupped biopsy forceps. This degree of hemorrhage will typically be controlled with continuous irrigation, balloon tamponade, or electrocautery. The number of samples should be governed by frozen specimen interpretation and no more tissue than is absolutely necessary is taken in an effort to reduce intraventricular hemorrhage.

10.3.3 Simultaneous Tumor Biopsy and Endoscopic Third Ventriculostomy

The prominence of pineal region tumors in children coupled with the high frequency of tumors that may not necessitate aggressive surgical resection converges nicely with endoscopic applications [12–15]. Notably, primary central nervous system germ cell tumors (CNS GCT), both pure germinomas and nongerminomatous germ cell tumors, can be effectively treated without radical resection. Thus, children who present with noncommunicating hydrocephalus with a pineal region tumor should always be considered for primary endoscopic management by way of ETV and tumor biopsy (Fig. 10.6). Serum biochemical analysis for alpha-fetoprotein (AFP) and human chorionic gonadotropin (HCG) should always precede endoscopic biopsy since marker-positive GCT should be initially managed with neo-adjuvant chemotherapy.

While the child with a pineal region tumor and noncommunicating hydrocephalus represents one of the best surgical candidates for endoscopic surgery, the situation can represent a challenging procedure. Navigating the endoscope into the limited space of the posterior third ventricle and sampling tumors that are variably hemorrhagic contribute toward this challenge. Since the optimal trajectory for ETV (coronal entry) and pineal region tumor biopsy (frontal-precoronal entry) is distinct, a single or dual entry site will need to be chosen if a rod lens endoscope is used (Fig. 10.7). It is advised to choose a technique that best suites the individual patient based upon the ventricular size, the relative position of the tumor, the dimension of the massa intermedia, and the surgical goal. Typically, a combined approach through a single burr hole mandates that the entry site be located midway between the optimal entry sites for either separate procedure. This single approach is best used when the tumor presents anterior to the massa intermedia, when the massa is small, when the degree of ventriculomegaly is severe, or when the tumor size obviates any consideration for total tumor removal. Alternatively, when tumors that are recessed behind the massa intermedia, when the degree of ventriculomegaly is moderate, when tumors may be amenable to total removal (<2 cm), or when the massa intermedia is large, two sites of entry are advocated; one being optimal for the tumor biopsy and the other being optimal for the ETV (Fig. 10.8). Although fiberoptic or steerable endoscopes are ideally suited for this combined procedure, the smaller working channels, the greater potential for disorientation, and the decreased image resolution associated with these endoscopes all have limited their widespread appeal.

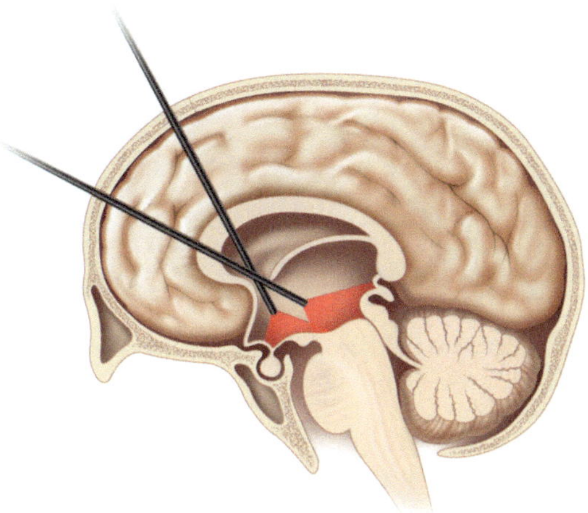

Fig. 10.7 This illustration depicts the ideal and separate trajectories for endoscopic third ventriculostomy (precoronal entry) and a pineal region tumor approach (frontal-precoronal). The use of a single or dual entry is determined by the characteristics of the tumor and the third ventricular anatomy (Illustration provided by Thom Graves of Thom Graves Media, New York, New York.)

When performing simultaneous ETV and tumor biopsy, it is preferred to perform the ETV prior to tumor biopsy. This order is advocated since the most pressing clinical condition of noncommunicating hydrocephalus should be defini-

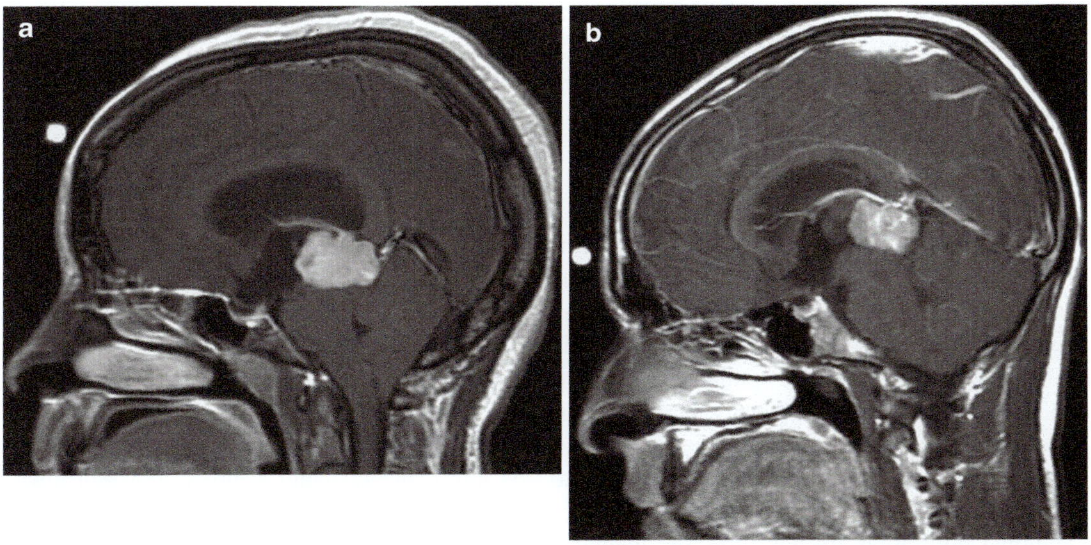

Fig. 10.8 Sagittal MRI of two different patients that underwent simultaneous ETV and tumor biopsy for hydrocephalus and a pineal region tumor. Tumors that extend anterior to the massa intermedia in patients with significant ventriculomegaly (**a**) are good candidates for a single trajectory while smaller tumors or less hydrocephalus (**b**) may require two different approaches

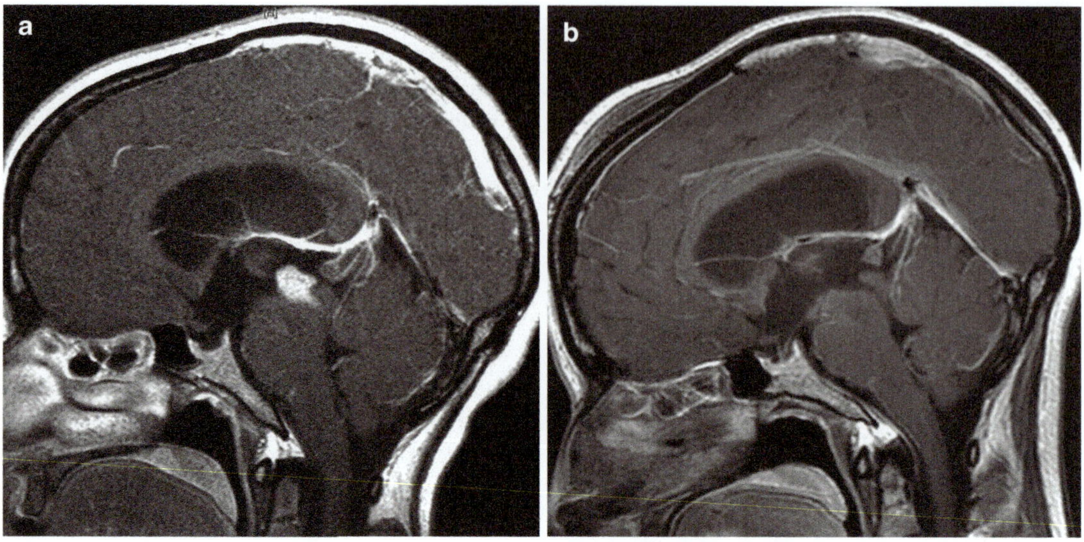

Fig. 10.9 Sagittal MRI with contrast administration prior (**a**) and after (**b**) endoscopic total removal of a posterior third ventricular ependymoma

tively addressed prior to any visual potential obscuration by hemorrhage that invariably occurs with tumor biopsy. Thus far, the hypothetical concern of tumor dissemination from the intraventricular compartment to the subarachnoid space following this simultaneous procedure has not been supported by retrospective clinical series [16]. However, metastatic spread of tumor at the endoscopic path has been documented and thus the actual risk of tumor spread remains undefined [17, 18].

10.3.4 Solid Tumor Resection

Solid tumor removal, although a logical application of endoscopic techniques, is somewhat limited due to the inadequacy of compatible instrumentation and the small caliber of current endoscopic portals. The success of endoscopic tumor removal is dependent upon the tumor characteristics including size, density, and vascularity. Tumors larger than 2 cm, those that have appreciable calcification on computed tomography (CT), and those that have significant subependymal infiltration are not currently amenable to endoscopic removal. Variables that can limit complete endoscopic tumor removal are nearly impossible to predict based on current imaging techniques. When a patient is being considered for purely endoscopic tumor removal, noncontrast CT can be used to estimate the degree of mineralization based on the presence or absence of solid calcifications.

Thus far, most descriptions for tumor removal have focused on the colloid cyst, a rare tumor of childhood. The colloid cyst, unlike solid tumors, lends itself to endoscopic removal given the primarily cystic nature of that mass [19–23]. However, children with small, non-mineralized, and avascular tumors are excellent candidates for primary endoscopic removal (Fig. 10.9) [24–30]. Larger tumors that are pedunculated at the ependymal surface are also good candidates for endoscopic removal (Fig. 10.10). In this situation, the pedunculated aspect of the tumor is first controlled with coagulation and sharp dissection followed by removal of the tumor in a piecemeal fashion or by delivering the tumor in total through the scope pathway.

Integrated stereotactic navigational guidance is important to obtain a direct approach toward the tumor surface (Fig. 10.11). An angled rigid lens system is preferred to the variability in viewing angles within a restricted field. The optimal surgical plan is obtained through careful

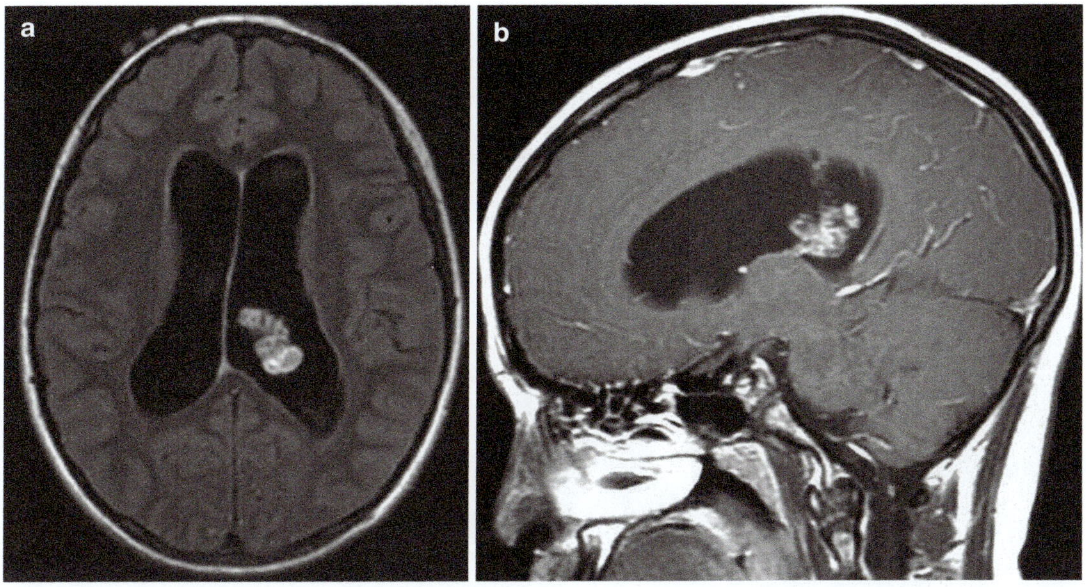

Fig. 10.10 Axial (**a**) and sagittal (**b**) MRI of a 14-year-old male with an intraventricular choroid plexus papilloma. The small pedunculated attachment at the base of the tumor is an appealing feature for endoscopic removal

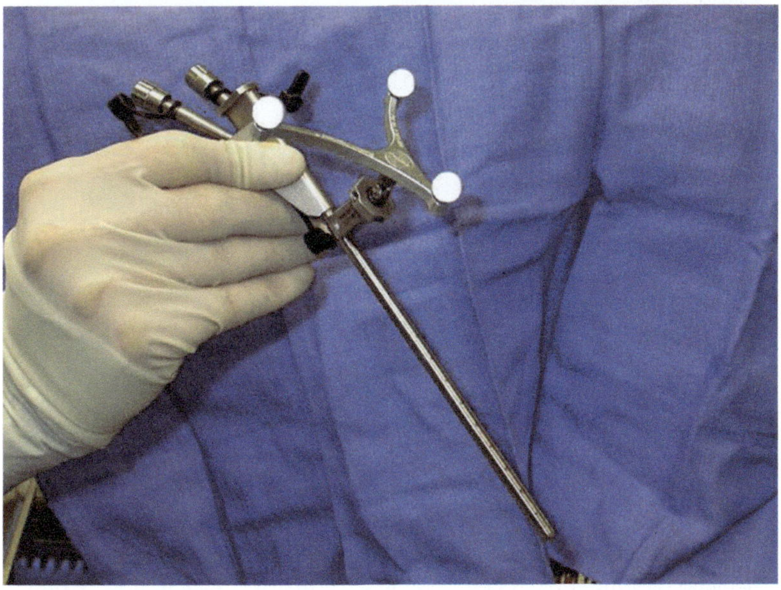

Fig. 10.11 Most endoscopes are easily integrated for use with navigational guidance. This image demonstrates how the reflecting spheres for optically-guided stereotaxy are positioned away from the working channels of the sheath

inspection of high-resolution MRI scans in three dimensions. The T2-weighted sequences are very helpful in delineating tumor margins and potential sites of tumor attachment. For third ventricular and pineal region tumors, the laterality of the entry is governed by any asymmetry of the ventricular size or relative eccentricity of the tumor within the third ventricle. If the tumor favors one side of the third ventricle, it is best to plan on a contralateral entry site to optimize visualization of the tumor and tumor-brain interface (Fig. 10.12).

At the time of tumor exposure, cupped biopsy forceps should be utilized initially prior to the application of any energy source to ensure the best opportunity for pathologic interpretation.

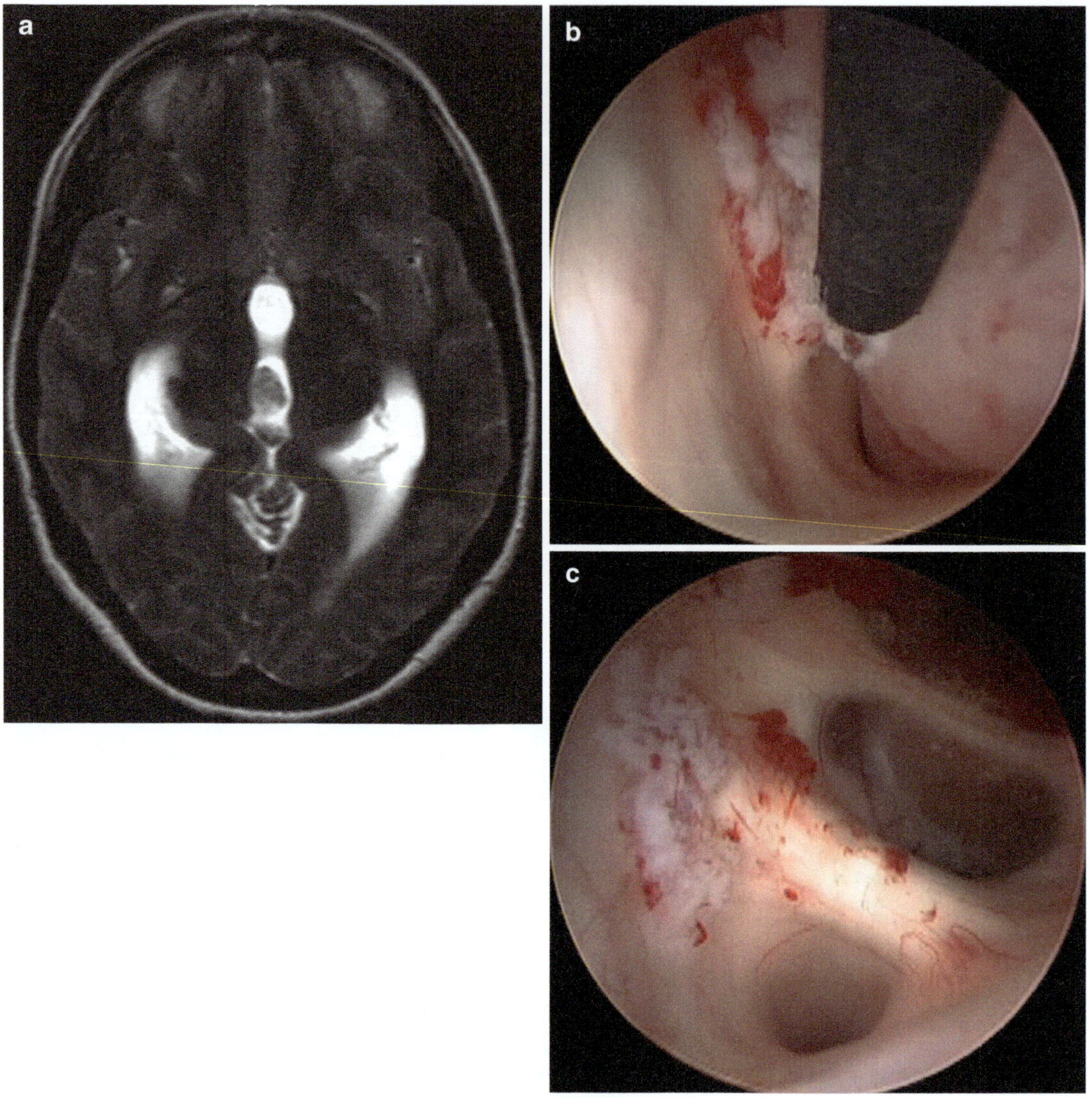

Fig. 10.12 This axial T2-weighted MRI (**a**) illustrates a pedunculated third ventricular tumor attached to the right hypothalamus. A left frontal entry site was used to offer direct visualization of the tumor-brain interface (**b**). The endoscopic view into the back of the third ventricle confirms a total removal of an ependymoma (**c**)

Once the specimen has been obtained for histologic diagnosis, the tumor is then removed sequentially, utilizing electrocautery or laser, cupped biopsy forceps, and suction aspiration. The application of electrocautery or laser within the tumor parenchyma alters the consistency of the tumor, so as to allow aggressive suction aspiration. Again, suction should only be applied once the aspirator is placed within the parenchyma of the tissue, so as to avoid CSF evacuation. Continuous irrigation is utilized to maintain a clear visual field. Hemostasis is maintained as discussed above. Once the entire solid tumor has been removed, electrocautery is utilized at the site of ependymal attachment to decrease any potential for microscopic residual tumor. The use of a ventricular drain is decided on an individual basis depending upon the degree of hemorrhage and preoperative condition of the patient.

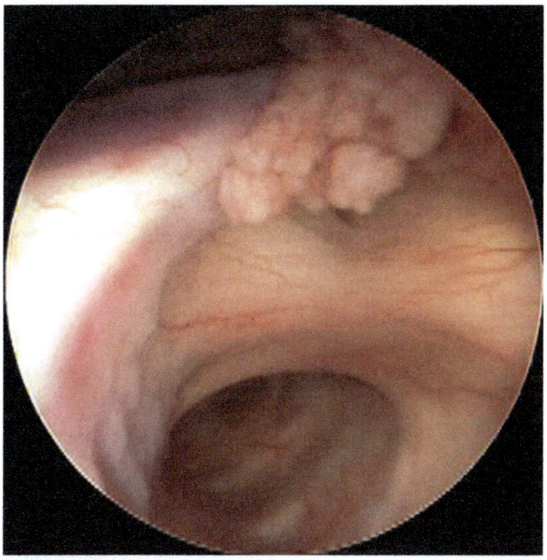

Fig. 10.13 An endoscopic view into the right foramen of Monro illustrates probable tumor dissemination of the lateral aspect of the foramen as irregularities of the ependymal surface

10.3.5 Disease Staging

An important and unique physiologic feature of primary pediatric brain tumors is the potential for cerebrospinal fluid dissemination. Only through accurate staging can children be assigned to appropriate therapeutic strategies. The neurosurgeon's role in diagnostic staging is considerable. Preliminary data exists to support the notion of using endoscopic inspection of the intraventricular system in children with certain brain tumors. Tumor dissemination observed during endoscopic surgery has recently been highlighted in patients with germ cell tumors in which the preoperative magnetic resonance imaging failed to exhibit metastatic disease (Fig. 10.13) [31, 32]. This method is awaiting validation through cooperative group studies and may be integrated into future diagnostic protocols in certain conditions.

Conclusion

Endoscopic surgical management for intraventricular brain tumors in children has burgeoned over the past decade to a field with clearly defined surgical indications, dedicated instrumentation, and general acceptance by the neurosurgical community. Patient selection requires a thorough understanding of neuro-oncologic principles and the limitations of neuroendoscopic methods. Endoscopic tumor biopsy has been shown to be highly successful while affording significant advantages over conventional neurosurgical techniques. Simultaneous CSF diversion through ETV at the time of tumor biopsy further contributes to the appeal of endoscopic methods in children with brain tumors. Endoscopic excision of solid intraventricular tumors, although feasible, remains challenging due to technical limitations. Intraoperative stereotactic guidance contributes greatly toward a safer and more efficacious procedure and should be considered as an integral adjunct in patients undergoing endoscopic neurosurgery for third ventricular brain tumors or in patients without hydrocephalus. The potential of endoscopic surgery for intraventricular brain tumors is expected to expand with technological advancements in compatible instrumentation.

References

1. Souweidane MM (2008) Endoscopic surgery for intraventricular brain tumors in patients without hydrocephalus. Neurosurgery 62:1042–1048
2. Pettorini BL, Tamburrini G, Massimi L, Caldarelli M, Di Rocco C (2009) Endoscopic transventricular positioning of intracystic catheter for treatment of craniopharyngioma. Technical note. J Neurosurg Pediatr 4:245–248
3. Burgess C, Jayamohan J (2008) Colloid cyst in a 12-week-old infant treated with endoscopic third ventriculostomy and cyst fenestration. Br J Neurosurg 22:588–590
4. Depreitere B, Dasi N, Rutka J, Dirks P, Drake J (2007) Endoscopic biopsy for intraventricular tumors in children. J Neurosurg 106:340–346
5. Shono T, Natori Y, Morioka T, Torisu R, Mizoguchi M, Nagata S, Suzuki SO, Iwaki T, Inamura T, Fukui M, Oka K, Sasaki T (2007) Results of a long-term follow-up after neuroendoscopic biopsy procedure and third ventriculostomy in patients with intracranial germinomas. J Neurosurg 107:193–198
6. Souweidane MM (2005) Endoscopic management of pediatric brain tumors. Neurosurg Focus 18:E1
7. Ahn ES, Goumnerova L (2010) Endoscopic biopsy of brain tumors in children: diagnostic success and utility in guiding treatment strategies. J Neurosurg Pediatr 5:255–262

8. Luther N, Cohen A, Souweidane MM (2005) Hemorrhagic sequelae from intracranial neuroendoscopic procedures for intraventricular tumors. Neurosurg Focus 19:E9
9. Schroeder HW, Oertel J, Gaab MR (2004) Incidence of complications in neuroendoscopic surgery. Childs Nerv Syst 20:878–883
10. Hellwig D, Bauer BL (1991) Endoscopic procedures in stereotactic neurosurgery. Acta Neurochir Suppl (Wien) 52:30–32
11. Wagner W, Gaab MR, Schroeder HW, Sehl U, Tschiltschke W (1999) Experiences with cranial neuronavigation in pediatric neurosurgery. Pediatr Neurosurg 31:231–236
12. Al-Tamimi YZ, Bhargava D, Surash S, Ramirez RE, Novegno F, Crimmins DW, Tyagi AK, Chumas PD (2008) Endoscopic biopsy during third ventriculostomy in paediatric pineal region tumours. Childs Nerv Syst 24:1323–1326
13. Ellenbogen RG, Moores LE (1997) Endoscopic management of a pineal and suprasellar germinoma with associated hydrocephalus: technical case report. Minim Invasive Neurosurg 40:13–15; discussion 16
14. O'Brien DF, Hayhurst C, Pizer B, Mallucci CL (2006) Outcomes in patients undergoing single-trajectory endoscopic third ventriculostomy and endoscopic biopsy for midline tumors presenting with obstructive hydrocephalus. J Neurosurg 105:219–226
15. Pople IK, Athanasiou TC, Sandeman DR, Coakham HB (2001) The role of endoscopic biopsy and third ventriculostomy in the management of pineal region tumours. Br J Neurosurg 15:305–311
16. Luther N, Stetler WR Jr, Dunkel IJ, Christos PJ, Wellons JC 3rd, Souweidane MM (2010) Subarachnoid dissemination of intraventricular tumors following simultaneous endoscopic biopsy and third ventriculostomy. J Neurosurg Pediatr 5:61–67
17. Choi UK, Cha SH, Song GS, Choi CH, Lee SW, Lim YT, Kim WT (2007) Recurrent intracranial germinoma along the endoscopic ventriculostomy tract. Case report. J Neurosurg 107:62–65
18. Haw C, Steinbok P (2001) Ventriculoscope tract recurrence after endoscopic biopsy of pineal germinoma. Pediatr Neurosurg 34:215–217
19. Schroeder HW, Gaab MR (2002) Endoscopic resection of colloid cysts. Neurosurgery 51:1441–1444; discussion 1444–1445
20. Decq P, Le Guerinel C, Brugieres P, Djindjian M, Silva D, Keravel Y, Melon E, Nguyen JP (1998) Endoscopic management of colloid cysts. Neurosurgery 42:1288–1294; discussion 1294–1296
21. Abdou MS, Cohen AR (1998) Endoscopic treatment of colloid cysts of the third ventricle. Technical note and review of the literature. J Neurosurg 89:1062–1068
22. Lewis AI (1999) Endoscopic management of colloid cysts. Neurosurgery 44:232
23. Rodziewicz GS, Smith MV, Hodge CJ Jr (2000) Endoscopic colloid cyst surgery. Neurosurgery 46:655–660; discussion 660–662
24. Badie B, Brooks N, Souweidane MM (2004) Endoscopic and minimally invasive microsurgical approaches for treating brain tumor patients. J Neurooncol 69:209–219
25. Souweidane MM, Luther N (2006) Endoscopic resection of solid intraventricular brain tumors. J Neurosurg 105:271–278
26. Luther N, Souweidane MM (2005) Neuroendoscopic resection of posterior third ventricular ependymoma. Case report. Neurosurg Focus 18:E3
27. Harter DH, Omeis I, Forman S, Braun A (2006) Endoscopic resection of an intraventricular dysembryoplastic neuroepithelial tumor of the septum pellucidum. Pediatr Neurosurg 42:105–107
28. Gaab MR, Schroeder HW (1998) Neuroendoscopic approach to intraventricular lesions. J Neurosurg 88: 496–505
29. Gaab MR, Schroeder HW (1999) Neuroendoscopic approach to intraventricular lesions. Neurosurg Focus 6:e5
30. Oertel JM, Baldauf J, Schroeder HW, Gaab MR (2009) Endoscopic options in children: experience with 134 procedures. J Neurosurg Pediatr 3: 81–89
31. Reddy AT, Wellons JC 3rd, Allen JC, Fiveash JB, Abdullatif H, Braune KW, Grabb PA (2004) Refining the staging evaluation of pineal region germinoma using neuroendoscopy and the presence of preoperative diabetes insipidus. Neuro Oncol 6: 127–133
32. Wellons JC 3rd, Reddy AT, Tubbs RS, Abdullatif H, Oakes WJ, Blount JP, Grabb PA (2004) Neuroendoscopic findings in patients with intracranial germinomas correlating with diabetes insipidus. J Neurosurg 100:430–436

Neuroendoscopic Treatment of Colloid Cysts

11

Phillipe Decq

11.1 Introduction

Colloid cysts are histologically benign tumors that represent between 0.5 and 2 % of all intracranial neoplasms. They are mostly located at the anterior part of the third ventricle and are able to cause occlusion of the foramen of Monro with resultant obstructive uni- or biventricular hydrocephalus. Because of their obstructive nature, colloid cysts can cause rapid neurological deterioration and even sudden death [1].

The usual symptoms of first presentation are headache, a progressive or fluctuating dementia with or without symptoms of raised intracranial pressure, nausea and vomiting, visual deficit, gait disturbances, seizures, short-term memory deficit (symptoms similar to the triad occurring in normal pressure hydrocephalus), and psychiatric symptoms (see Table 11.1). Sudden death is rare and lumbar puncture might be a precipitating factor [2].

11.2 Management of Asymptomatic Colloid Cysts

The management of the asymptomatic colloid cysts is still very debatable. Many neurosurgeons advise "prophylactic" surgical removal to avoid catastrophic neurological deterioration. However, long-term follow-up study of 68 subjects with asymptomatic colloid cysts suggests that only a few (8 %) subjects go on to develop symptoms at 10 years [3]. To our opinion asymptomatic cyst should be monitored frequently (at least annually), and patients should be encouraged to report symptomatology without delay. Small (less than 1 cm in diameter) asymptomatic cyst without related hydrocephalus can be managed safely conservatively. If related hydrocephalus is present or the cyst is seen to enlarge on subsequent neuroimaging, risk of deterioration and surgical risk should be balanced, taking into account the clinical condition of the patient and personal preferences.

11.3 Management of Symptomatic Colloid Cysts

The management of symptomatic colloid cysts is always surgical, and the choice of the approach depends on the surgeon's preferences. Several surgical approaches can be used. The microsurgical transcortical-transventricular and transcallosal approaches were considered gold standard in the days before endoscopy. For the last two decades, the endoscopic approach developed and gained acceptance as an alternative to microsurgical techniques [4–9]. It remains debatable if it can be considered as the preferential and primary surgical modality. Surgical expertise and preference is a dominant factor. During the last decade, a number of series on endoscopic removal appeared [1, 10–18]. Due to the rarity of the disease, most series

P. Decq, MD
Department of Neurosurgery,
Assistance Publique-Hôpitaux de Paris, Groupe
Hospitalier Henri Mondor, Creteil, France
e-mail: philippe.decq@bjn.aphp.fr

S. Sgouros (ed.), *Neuroendoscopy*,
DOI 10.1007/978-3-642-39085-2_11, © Springer-Verlag Berlin Heidelberg 2014

Table 11.1 Clinical symptoms of a series of 90 patients with colloid cyst of the third ventricle

Symptoms	Pre (*n* patients)	Post (*n* patients)	% (patient free of symptoms)
Headaches	83	22	73
Visual troubles	34	4	88
Sphincter troubles	8	4	50
Gait and balance troubles	22	5	72
Consciousness troubles	21	3	86
Memory troubles	53	23	56

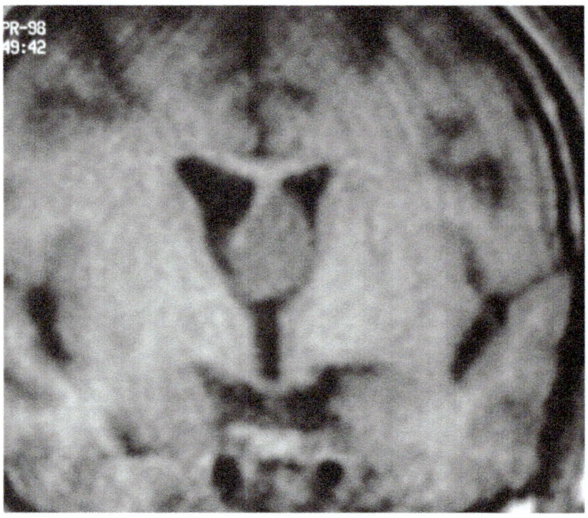

Fig. 11.1 Coronal T1w MR image of a 40-year-old man with persistent headaches. A round mass is seen in the left aspect of the foramen of Monro, causing occlusion of the foramen and unilateral dilatation of the right frontal horn. This is a typical appearance of a colloid cyst

are relatively small and with limited follow-up. However, many surgeons consider the endoscopic removal of colloid cysts as a valid first-line treatment for these lesions [7, 18–21].

11.4 Neuroendoscopic Technique for Removal of Colloid Cysts

Colloid cysts are the ideal tumors for neuroendoscopic removal except of some limitations (Fig. 11.1): (1) the content of the cyst may be very thick and as a result make the removal difficult [22]; (2) the cyst may be firmly attached to the ventricular walls and the ventricular veins, requiring careful dissection; and (3) a part of the cyst may be hidden under ventricular structures and have a difficult identification.

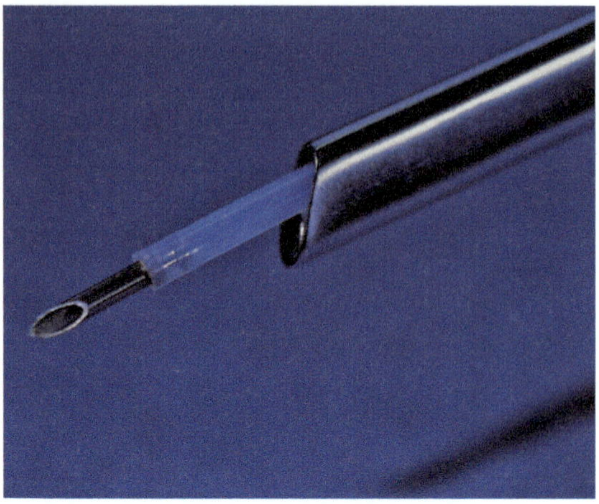

Fig. 11.2 Closeup photograph of the tip of the Storz Decq endoscope, showing the facility to introduce through it a special puncture needle with incorporated aspiration tube. This facilitates the aspiration of the viscous fluid of the colloid cysts

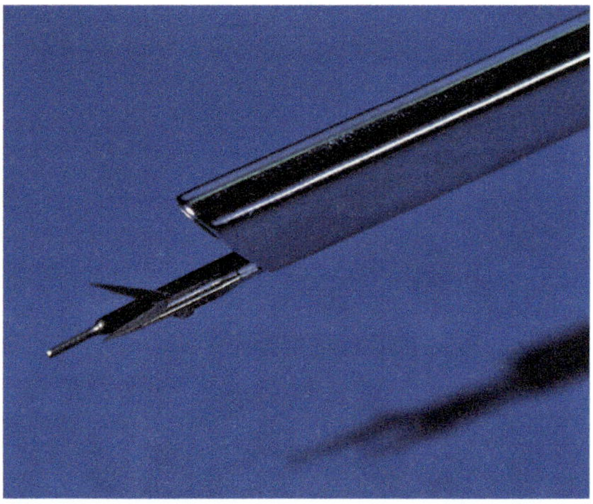

Fig. 11.3 Closeup photograph of the tip of the Storz Decq endoscope, showing the facility to introduce through its two separate working channels a pair of scissors and the monopolar diathermy, simultaneously. This arrangement facilitates greatly the dissection of the cyst capsule from the ventricular walls

With respect to the operative technique, after general endotracheal anesthesia is administered, the patient is positioned supine. We propose the use of an endoscope that takes large instruments (Fig. 11.2) and offers the possibility of simultaneous use of two instruments (Fig. 11.3) and

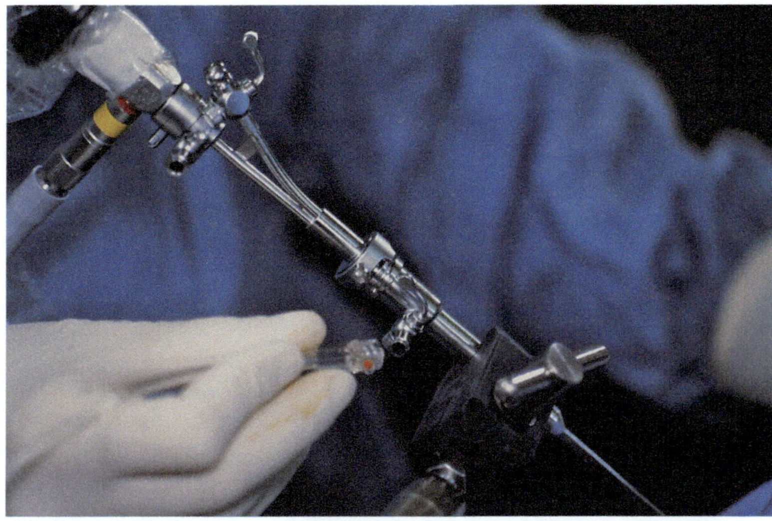

Fig. 11.4 Setting of the Storz Decq endoscope with irrigation system

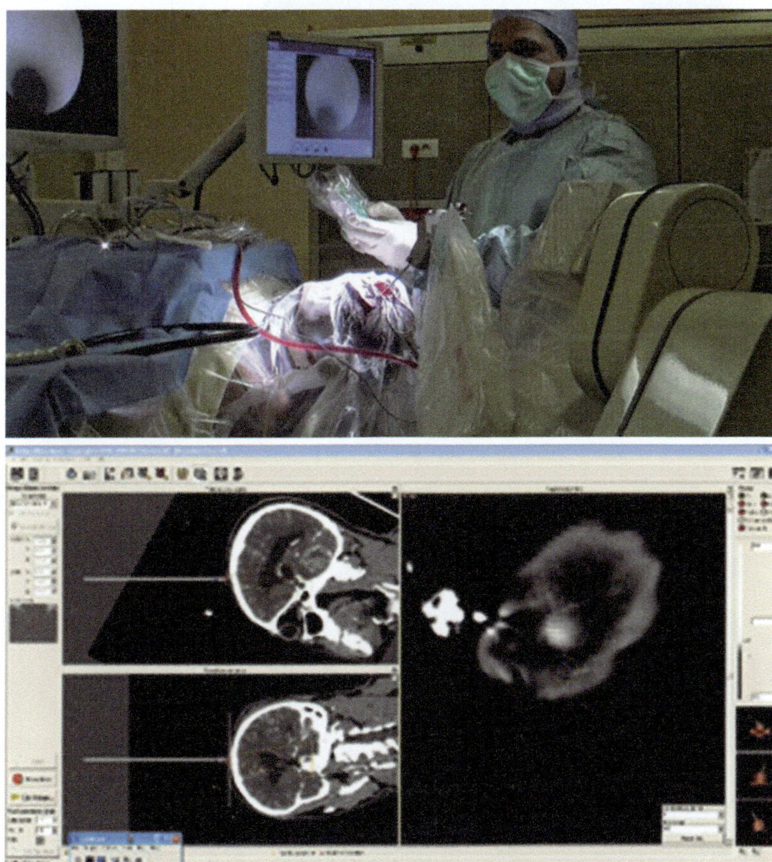

Fig. 11.5 Use of neuronavigation to introduce the endoscope in a small lateral ventricle

irrigation (Fig. 11.4) [23]. The neuroendoscope is introduced into the ventricle under freehand guidance. The cyst is approached through a burr hole placed about 4–5 cm lateral to the midline and 1 cm at least (may be more) in front of the coronal suture depending on the ventricular configuration and cyst location. Neuronavigation or stereotactic guidance is only used when the ventricles are small (see Fig. 11.5) [24]. A right-sided approach is chosen unless the cyst is far more prominent through the left foramen of Monro or the right ventricle is too small. The cyst is exposed, coagulated, and punctured and the content aspirated. When possible, the cyst capsule is coagulated at its attachment site, which is then sectioned or carefully pulled out with a forceps to attempt total removal (depends on surgeon's preference). The use of a supraorbital endoscopic approach to the colloid cysts has been proposed as well, advocating advantages in the visualization of the cyst adhesion to the roof of the third ventricle (Fig. 11.6) [25]. As a surgical advice we would recommend to stay always in the lateral ventricle, avoiding entry into the third ventricle; make safe maneuvering; and always be gentle on grasping and pulling [26].

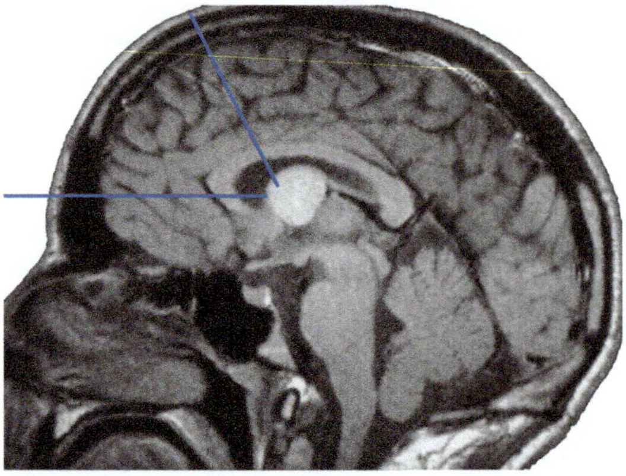

Fig. 11.6 Diagrammatic illustration of the endoscopic approaches for removal of colloid cysts, classic and supraorbital, on a sagittal MR image. Directions of surgical approaches (*blue lines*)

11.5 Results

Recently we published a series of 90 cases between 1994 and 2007 with mean follow-up of 51 months (4, 3 years) [1]. The symptoms can be summarized in Table 11.1, before and after surgery. In this series the Evans' index improved from 0.42 to 0.36, and only 3 % of the patients needed a permanent shunt. The postoperative result was evaluated with MRI and is divided in three groups radiologically: group A with no remnant visible (Fig. 11.7), group B with remnant membrane or cyst (with CSF), and group C with remnant colloid cyst. The results are shown on Table 11.2 and the complications on Table 11.3. The results are considered good, with high cyst removal rate, low reoperation, and complication rate, comparable if not better to the open craniotomy methods. Certainly, memory disturbance is less following endoscopic removal.

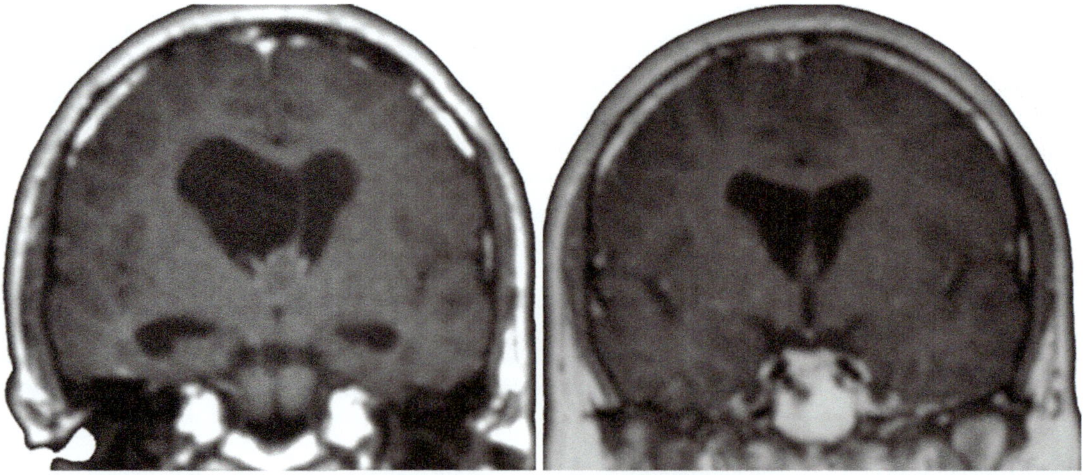

Fig. 11.7 Preoperative (*left*) and postoperative (*right*) coronal T1w MR image of a patient with colloid cyst, which was removed endoscopically

11.6 Discussion

In the last years many papers have been published supporting the efficacy and the safety of the endoscopic approach over to the classical transcallosal approach [5, 14, 21, 27–29] (Fig. 11.8). The endoscopic approach is associated with a shorter operative time, shorter hospital stay, lower infection rate, and lower seizure rate than the transcallosal approach. The only limitation of the endoscopic method is that in some cases there cannot be a total removal of the cyst. For this reason a neurosurgeon must be familiar with both approaches. Given the rarity of the pathology, there is a need to concentrate surgical expertise, whatever the chosen approach is. On the other hand the difficult cases for endoscopy are also difficult cases for microsurgery. Another very important factor for successful endoscopic removal is the right selection of the instruments. As a conclusion we can say that the endoscopic technique can be considered as a first-line option for removal of colloid cysts, with the acceptance that a small number of these patients may need a transcallosal craniotomy to remove residual cysts.

Table 11.2 Postoperative results following endoscopic removal of the colloid cyst (90 patients)

			Reoperations
A	41 (51 %)	46 (57 %)	2
B	5 (6 %)		
C	34 (43 %)		4
			6 (6 %)

Group A: no visible cyst remnant
Group B: remnant of cyst membrane
Group C: remnant of a frank portion of the colloid cyst

Table 11.3 Complications following removal of colloid cyst of the third ventricle (90 patients)

Meningitis	1 (1 %)
Memory deficit	7 (8 %)
Organic psychosyndrome	2 (2 %)
Hemiparesis	1 (1 %)
Visual deficit	2 (2 %)
Pulmonary embolism	1 (1 %)
Wound infection	1 (1 %)
CSF leak	1 (1 %)
Single postop seizure	1 (1 %)

Acknowledgment We would like to thank Dr C. Chamilos, of "Mitera" Children's Hospital, Athens, Greece, for the significant assistance in the writing of this manuscript.

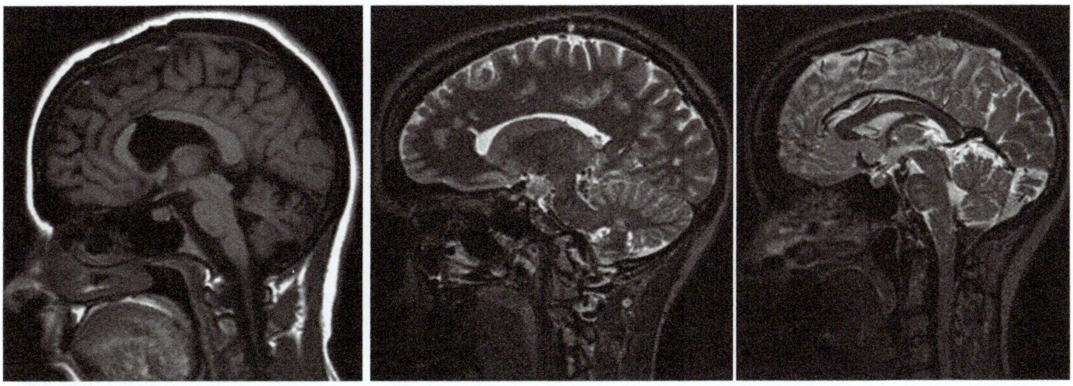

Fig. 11.8 Postoperative sagittal MR images of patients who had colloid cysts of the third ventricle removed with transcallosal approach (*left*) and endoscopic approach (*middle* and *right*)

References

1. Boogaarts HD, Decq P, Grotenhuis JA, Le Guérinel C, Nseir R, Jarraya B, Djindjian M, Beems T (2011) Long-term results of the neuroendoscopic management of colloid cysts of the third ventricle: a series of 90 cases. Neurosurgery 68(1):179–187
2. Pollock BE, Schreiner SA, Huston J III (2000) A theory on the natural history of colloid cysts of the third ventricle. Neurosurgery 46:1077–1081
3. Pollock BE, Huston J III (1999) Natural history of asymptomatic colloid cysts of the third ventricle. J Neurosurg 91:364–369
4. Stachura K, Libionka W, Moskała M, Krupa M, Polak J (2009) Colloid cysts of the third ventricle. Endoscopic and open microsurgical management. Neurol Neurochir Pol 43(3):25–27
5. Horn EM, Feiz-Erfan I, Bristol RE, Lekovic GP, Goslar PW, Smith KA, Nakaji P, Spetzler RF (2008) Treatment options for third ventricular colloid cysts: comparison of open microsurgical versus endoscopic resection. Neurosurgery 62(6 Suppl 3):1076–1083
6. Grondin RT, Hader W, MacRae ME, Hamilton MG (2007) Endoscopic versus microsurgical resection of third ventricle colloid cysts. Can J Neurol Sci 34(2):197–207
7. Charalampaki P, Filippi R, Welschehold S, Perneczky A (2006) Endoscope-assisted removal of colloid cysts of the third ventricle. Neurosurg Rev 29(1):72–79. Epub 2005 Nov 8
8. Kehler U, Brunori A, Gliemroth J, Nowak G, Delitala A, Chiappetta F, Arnold H (2001) Twenty colloid cysts–comparison of endoscopic and microsurgical management. Minim Invasive Neurosurg 44(3):121–127
9. King WA, Ullman JS, Frazee JG, Post KD, Bergsneider M (1999) Endoscopic resection of colloid cysts: surgical considerations using the rigid endoscope. Neurosurgery 44(5):1103–1109; discussion 1109–1111
10. Kwiek S, Kocur D, Doleżych H, Suszyński K, Szajkowski S, Sordyl R, Slusarczyk W, Kukier W, Bażowski P (2012) Endoscopic technique in the treatment of patients with colloid cysts of the third ventricle. Report based on a decade of experience. Neurol Neurochir Pol 46(3):216–223
11. Mishra S, Chandra PS, Suri A, Rajender K, Sharma BS, Mahapatra AK (2010) Endoscopic management of third ventricular colloid cysts: eight years' institutional experience and description of a new technique. Neurol India 58:412–417
12. El-Ghandour NM (2009) Endoscopic treatment of third ventricular colloid cysts: a review including ten personal cases. Neurosurg Rev 32(4):395–402. Epub 2009 Jul 11
13. Hellwig D, Bauer BL, Schulte M, Gatscher S, Riegel T, Bertalanffy H (2008) Neuroendoscopic treatment for colloid cysts of the third ventricle: the experience of a decade. Neurosurgery 62(6 Suppl 3): 1101–1109
14. Levine NB, Miller MN, Crone KR (2007) Endoscopic resection of colloid cysts: indications, technique, and results during a 13-year period. Minim Invasive Neurosurg 50(6):313–317
15. Acerbi F, Rampini P, Egidi M, Locatelli M, Borsa S, Gaini SM (2007) Endoscopic treatment of colloid cysts of the third ventricle: long-term results in a series of 6 consecutive cases. J Neurosurg Sci 51(2):53–60
16. Zohdi A, El Kheshin S (2006) Endoscopic approach to colloid cysts. Minim Invasive Neurosurg 49(5):263–268
17. Longatti P, Godano U, Gangemi M, Delitala A, Morace E, Genitori L, Alafaci C, Benvenuti L, Brunori A, Cereda C, Cipri S, Fiorindi A, Giordano F, Mascari C, Oppido PA, Perin A, Tripodi M (2006) Italian neuroendoscopy group. Cooperative study by the Italian neuroendoscopy group on the treatment of 61 colloid cysts. Childs Nerv Syst 22(10):1263–1267. Epub 2006 Apr 29
18. Schroeder HW, Gaab MR (2002) Endoscopic resection of colloid cysts. Neurosurgery 51(6):1441–1444; discussion 1444–1445
19. Margetis K, Souweidane MM (2013) Endoscopic treatment of intraventricular cystic tumors. World Neurosurg 79:S19
20. Qiao L, Souweidane MM (2011) Purely endoscopic removal of intraventricular brain tumors: a consensus opinion and update. Minim Invasive Neurosurg 54(4):149–154. Epub 2011 Sep 15
21. Greenlee JD, Teo C, Ghahreman A, Kwok B (2008) Purely endoscopic resection of colloid cysts. Neurosurgery 62(3 Suppl 1):51–55; discussion 55–56
22. Schirmer CM, Heilman CB (2011) Complete endoscopic removal of colloid cyst using a nitinol basket retriever. Neurosurg Focus 30(4):E8
23. Bergsneider M (2007) Complete microsurgical resection of colloid cysts with a dual-port endoscopic technique. Neurosurgery 60(2 Suppl 1):ONS33–ONS42; discussion ONS42–43
24. Harris AE, Hadjipanayis CG, Lunsford LD, Lunsford AK, Kassam AB (2005) Microsurgical removal of intraventricular lesions using endoscopic visualization and stereotactic guidance. Neurosurgery 56(1 Suppl):125–132; discussion 125–132
25. Delitala A, Brunori A, Russo N (2011) Supraorbital endoscopic approach to colloid cysts. Neurosurgery 69(2 Suppl Operative):ONS176–ONS182; discussion ONS182–183
26. Boogaarts H, El-Kheshin S, Grotenhuis J (2011) Endoscopic colloid cyst resection: technical note. Minim Invasive Neurosurg 54(2):95–97. Epub 2011 Jun 7
27. Hadjipanayis CG, Schuette AJ, Boulis N, Hao C, Barrow DL, Teo C (2010) Full scope of options. Neurosurgery 67(1):197–203; discussion 203–204
28. Teo C (1999) Complete endoscopic removal of colloid cysts: issues of safety and efficacy. Neurosurg Focus 6(4):e9
29. Decq P, Le Guerinel C, Brugières P, Djindjian M, Silva D, Kéravel Y, Melon E, Nguyen JP (1998) Endoscopic management of colloid cysts. Neurosurgery 42(6): 1288–1294; discussion 1294–1296

12 MRI of Patients with Hydrocephalus

Jérôme Hodel, Alain Rahmouni, and Philippe Decq

12.1 Introduction

Enlargement of the brain ventricles is a common imaging finding: In the daily clinical practice, the challenge is to recognize a pathological ventricular dilatation [1]. Several classifications of hydrocephalus have been proposed [2]. Noncommunicating hydrocephalus (NCH) is related to an obstacle on the CSF pathways, whereas communicating hydrocephalus (CH) concerns a pathological ventricular dilatation without identified obstacle [3]. Some authors [2, 4] consider that the term "obstructive" applies to all types of hydrocephalus as the defective CSF resorption related to a diffuse subarachnoid blockage or a venous obstruction represents an obstacle to CSF flow even if it is not morphologically identifiable. "Normal pressure hydrocephalus" (NPH) is characterized by the clinical triad described by Adams and Hakim [5], namely, a dementia syndrome, gait disorders, and sphincter disorders.

J. Hodel, MD (✉)
Neuroradiologie, CHRU Lille,
2 Avenue Oscar Lambret, Lille 59000, France
e-mail: jerome.hodel@hmn.aphp.fr

A. Rahmouni, MD, PhD
Department of Medical Imaging,
Centre Hospitalo-Universitaire Henri Mondor,
Creteil 94010, France

P. Decq, MD
Department of Neurosurgery,
Assistance Publique-Hôpitaux de Paris,
Groupe Hospitalier Henri Mondor, Creteil, France
e-mail: philippe.decq@bjn.aphp.fr

12.2 CSF Flow-Related Artifacts

The CSF signal is hypointense on T1-weighted sequences, hyperintense on T2-weighted sequences, and cancelled out on FLAIR sequences by using long inversion times. The CSF signal can be altered by flow artifacts such as time-of-flight (TOF) signal loss, entry-slice phenomenon, or intravoxel dephasing [6]. Using T2-weighted spin echo sequences, TOF signal loss is due to protons that do not experience either the initial or the refocusing radiofrequency pulse. Entry-slice phenomenon appears as a flow-related hypersignal due to unsaturated protons flowing into the slice (Fig. 12.1). "Intravoxel dephasing" is observed when flow velocities and directions result in a rapid dephasing and a signal loss (Fig. 12.2): Such a turbulent flow is commonly observed within the cerebral aqueduct.

12.3 Steady-State Free Precession (SSFP) Sequences

Using SSFP sequences, the residual transverse magnetization is conserved, participating in both the signal and the contrast. There are several variants in the family of steady-state echo gradient, according to the type of echo recorded and how the gradients are adjusted [7].

True fast imaging with steady-state precession (true FISP) with dual excitation sequences (constructive interference in steady state (CISS)) is a combination of two true FISP acquisitions, with

S. Sgouros (ed.), *Neuroendoscopy*,
DOI 10.1007/978-3-642-39085-2_12,

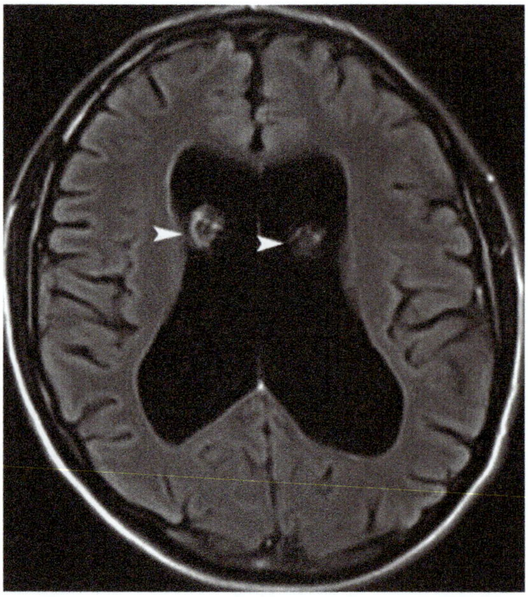

Fig. 12.1 CSF flow artifact. A 42-year-old patient with noncommunicating hydrocephalus. Axial FLAIR image through the lateral ventricles demonstrates the focal increased signal (*arrowheads*) within the lateral ventricles above the foramen of Monro, due to flow-related entry-slice phenomenon

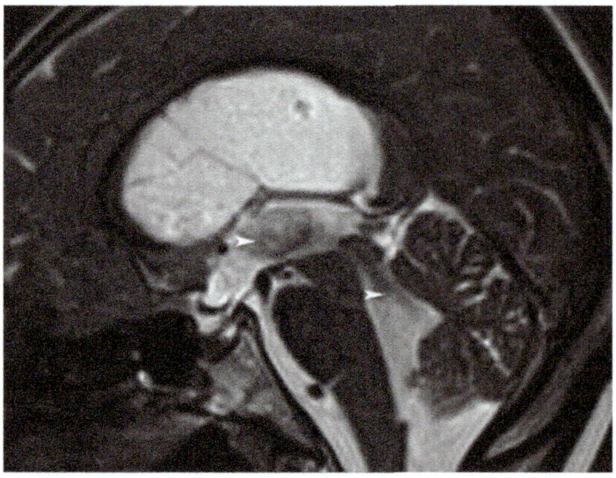

Fig. 12.2 A 65-year-old patient with normal pressure hydrocephalus. Median sagittal T2 TSE with an extensive aqueductal flow-related void sign (*arrowheads*)

and without excitation pulse phase alternation, to eliminate band artifacts. These sequences combine strong T2 weighting, excellent spatial resolution, and little sensitivity to CSF flow [8]. The 3D CISS allows for a multiplanar morphological analysis; its clinical value has been demonstrated

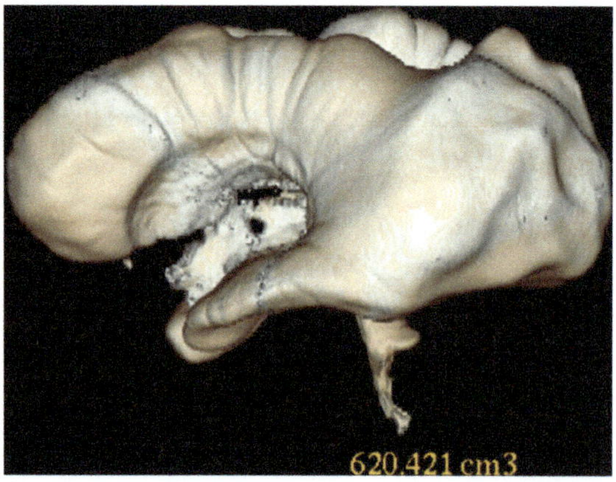

Fig. 12.3 A 37-year-old patient with noncommunicating hydrocephalus due to aqueductal stenosis. Surface reconstruction view obtained from the CISS sequence allowing the ventricular volume to be measured. The whole ventricular volume was 620 cm^3

for the investigation of cerebellopontine and cochleovestibular disorders [8]. With post-processing it is possible to generate volume-rendering views of intracranial CSF, allowing volumetric assessment (Fig. 12.3). The 3D CISS sequence can point to the cause of hydrocephalus and contribute to the preoperative work-up [9].

T2-enhanced SSFP sequences are flow-sensitive 3D sequences [10]. These sequences combine a strong T2 weighting with an excellent spatial resolution. By collecting a stimulated echo (PSIF echo) with an effective TE above the TR [10], the PSIF sequence is highly sensitive to the CSF flow [11]. CSF flow below 2 cm/s yields a void sign [12–14] (Fig. 12.4). This sequence has been reported to be useful for intracranial cysts detection [15] (Fig. 12.5) and endoscopic third ventriculostomy patency assessment [16].

Balanced SSFP sequences (true FISP) use a coherent steady-state technique with a fully balanced gradient waveform to recycle transverse magnetization. Contrast is determined by the ratio of T2 to T1 rather than the inflow effect [17]. Relative to spoiled gradient echo methods, true FISP sequence has an excellent temporal resolution. This sequence allows for the detection of both the brain ventricular wall motion and the CSF flow turbulences [18, 19].

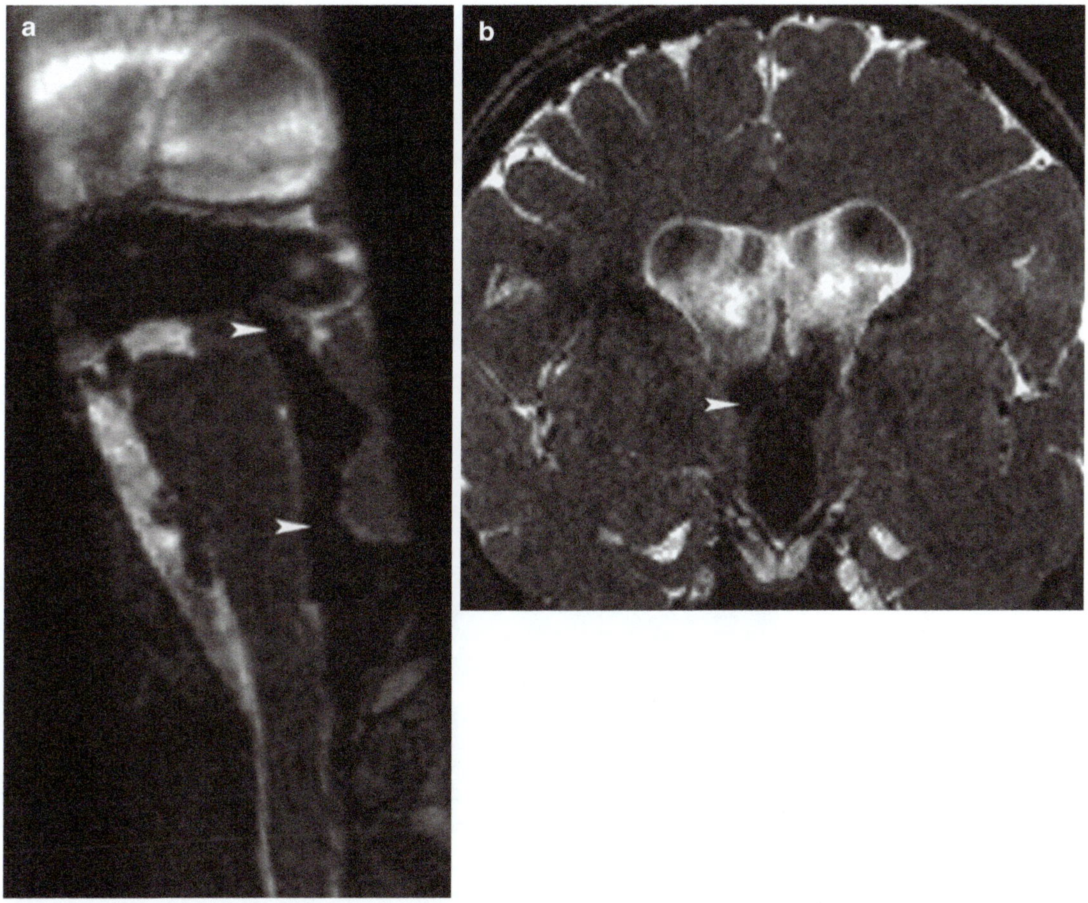

Fig. 12.4 (**a**) A 67-year-old patient with communicating hydrocephalus. Midsagittal PSIF sequence. Note the CSF flow in the third ventricle, the cerebral aqueduct, the fourth ventricle, and the foramen of Magendie, as shown by the flow-related void sign (*arrowheads*). (**b**) A 32-year-old patient with communicating hydrocephalus. Coronal PSIF sequence. Note the CSF flow in the third ventricle and the foramens of Monro (*arrowhead*) reflected by the flow-related void sign

12.4 Phase-Contrast Imaging Sequences

In a constant magnetic field gradient, dephasing occurs between stationary and circulating spins [20]. By using repeated bipolar gradients, a voxel-wise calculation of velocities can be determined during the cardiac cycle [21]. The measured velocities correspond to a projection of the real velocities along the direction of the velocity-encoding gradient that can be perpendicular to the slice (through-plane acquisition) or to one of the two axes defining the plane of the image slice (in-plane acquisition). Through-plane imaging provides a quantitative approach to CSF flow velocity [22], especially at the cerebral aqueduct, but only explores a limited region. In-plane imaging is time effective and covers a large region, but quantitative analysis is prevented by the partial volume effect. The CSF flow is pulsatile: Craniocaudal flow secondary to the cerebral arterial systolic wave is followed by caudocranial flow during diastole. Phase shifts should be within a range of 180° requiring a velocity encoding [23] that determines the highest and lowest detectable velocity encoded. This sequence may also have a predictive value for the surgical treatment of both communicating [22] and noncommunicating [24] hydrocephalus.

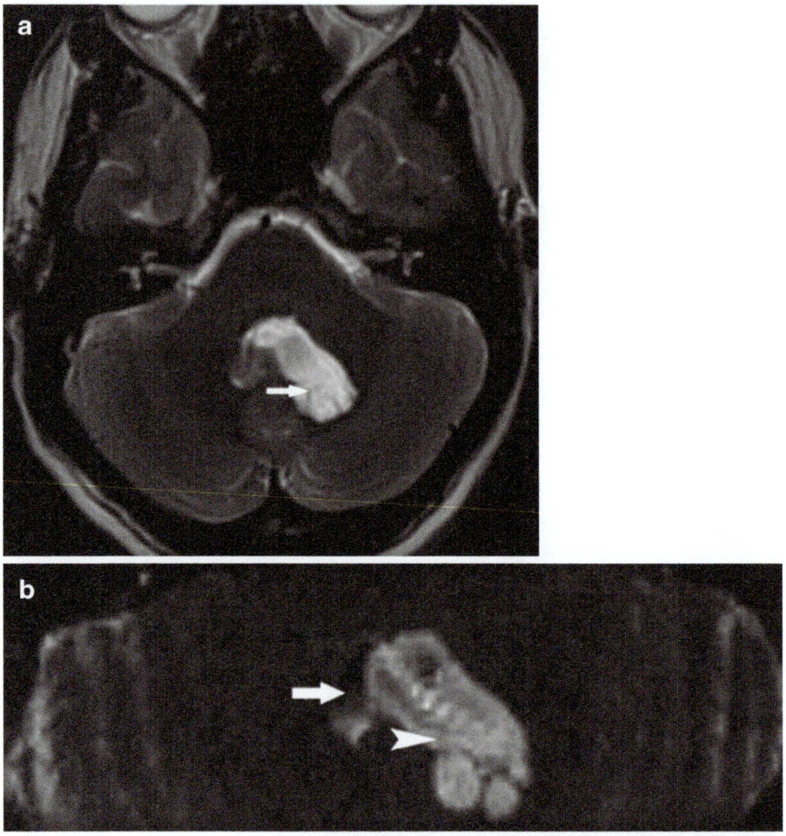

Fig. 12.5 (**a**) A 23-year-old patient with intraventricular cyst. Axial T2 TSE slice showing an asymmetric enlargement of the fourth ventricle (*arrow*). (**b**) A 23-year-old patient with intraventricular cyst. Axial PSIF slice: the noncirculating intraventricular cyst (hyperintense, *arrowhead*) is distinguished from the residual CSF flow in the fourth ventricle (hypointense, *arrow*)

12.5 Imaging Findings

A transependymal resorption consists in the reversal of normal transependymal CSF flow that causes a rim of FLAIR/T2 signal hyperintensity. A thick periventricular resorption tends to reflect rapidly progressive hydrocephalus. MR diffusion imaging may demonstrate a periventricular increase in the ADC value without abnormalities on conventional sequences [25–27]. Brain ventricle recess bulging is a common finding in patients with NCH (Fig. 12.6) [28]. The assessment of pericerebral CSF may also be of use in patients with hydrocephalus: Constricted subarachnoid CSF spaces at the brain midline convexity may be observed in patients with CH [3, 29–32].

The detection of an obstacle that hinders CSF pathways is a clue for the diagnosis of NCH. The 3D CISS sequence [8] allows for the detection of small lesions such as aqueductal membrane (Fig. 12.7). Phase-contrast and T2-enhanced SSFP sequences can be performed to assess the patency of the CSF pathways. Using T2-enhanced

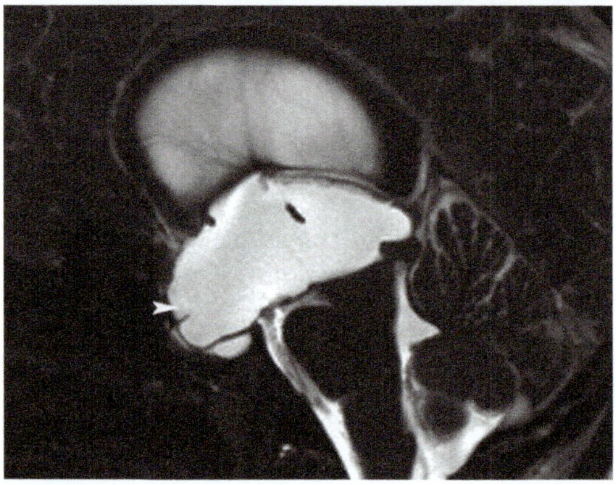

Fig. 12.6 A 36-year-old patient with noncommunicating hydrocephalus due to aqueduct stenosis. Midsagittal slice, true fast imaging. Note the marked dilatation of the anterior (*arrowhead*) and posterior ventricular recesses. Note to the extension of the anterior recesses to the sella turcica, which appears to be widened

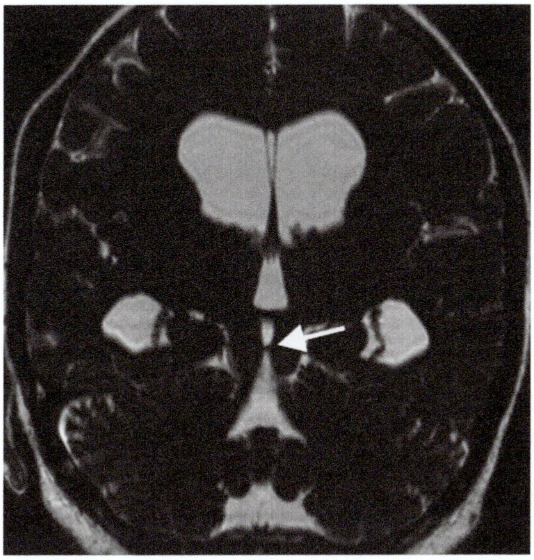

Fig. 12.7 A 31-year-old patient with noncommunicating triventricular hydrocephalus due to an aqueductal stenosis. Oblique plane, CISS sequence that revealed an aqueductal membrane (*arrow*)

SSFP sequences, a lack of CSF flow-related void sign through the cerebral aqueduct can be observed in patients with aqueductal stenosis.

Using gated balanced SSFP sequences, the lack of brain ventricular wall movement assessment appears to be associated with NCH [18]. The patency of a third ventriculostomy can be also assessed using such sequence.

An increased aqueductal flow void is frequently detected on the MR images of patients with CH [33–35]. This artifact is physiological but in NPH would be more extended beyond the aqueduct and foramens of Monro, up to V4. The extent of the flow void on T2-weighted sequences has been correlated with a favorable response to CSF diversion [36]. This artifact is related to the intravoxel dephasing that increases with the intensity of the magnetic field, the echo time, and when spin echo sequences are used [6]. Phase-contrast through-plane sequences can provide information about the CSF flow velocity [22]. Stroke volume, expressed in mL, is defined as the mean CSF volume moving craniocaudad during systole and caudocraniad during diastole. The clinical contribution of stroke volume measurement is controversial, but an increase in stroke volume appears to correlate with a favorable response to ventricular shunting in NPH [22, 37, 38]. Other studies have raised doubts as to its prognostic value [39].

Conclusion

The diagnosis of hydrocephalus relies on MRI. The first step of the diagnostic work-up consists in ruling out NCH using SSFP sequences. Phase-contrast imaging may provide additional information on CSF flow rate and can contribute to the management of patients with CH.

12.6 Imaging Protocol

Data were obtained using 1.5-T MR (Siemens, Avanto, Erlangen, Germany). The MR protocol was as follows:

Gated true FISP MR sequence: midsagittal plane defined on a transverse slice from the center of the lamina terminalis to the cerebral aqueduct; TR/TE, 78 ms/3 ms; number of excitations, 7; flip angle, 82°; field of view, 160 mm; matrix size, 256×256; slice thickness, 2.5 mm; acquisition time from 2 to 4 min; and 20 phases during the R to R interval

Ungated 3D reversed fast imaging with steady-state precession (PSIF): coronal plane; TR/TE, 17 ms/6 ms; number of excitations, 1; flip angle, 30°; field of view, 230 mm; matrix size, 192×256; slice thickness, 1 mm; and acquisition time, 2 min 40 s

Gated cine 2D phase-contrast (cine PC) sequence had the following parameters: through plane; TR/TE, 78 ms/9 ms; number of excitations, 3; flip angle, 30°; field of view, 256 mm; matrix size, 240×256; slice thickness, 5 mm; encoding velocity, 10 cm/s; and acquisition time from 2 to 3 min

3D constructive interference in steady-state (CISS) sequence covering whole ventricular system: TR/TE, 6 ms/3 ms; number of excitations, 1; flip angle, 70°; field of view, 256 mm; matrix size, 303×512; slice thickness, 1 mm; and acquisition time, 5 min 40 s

The diagnostic work-up including MR sequences and findings is summarized Table 12.1.

Table 12.1 MR protocol: 12-min MR protocol proposed to rule out hydrocephalus

MR sequence	Plane	Findings	Acquisition time
FLAIR Diffusion	Axial	Transependymal resorption?	2 min 30 s
True FISP with dual excitation sequences			
CISS	3D covering whole brain	Third ventricle recesses? Obstacle? Pericerebral CSF distribution? CSF volume?	3 min 40 s
Balanced SSFP sequences			
True FISP	Sagittal	Ventricular wall movement?	3 min
3D flow-sensitive sequences			
PSIF	3D covering brain ventricles	CSF pathways patency?	2 min 20 s
Phase-contrast imaging			
Cine PC	Through plane	CSF velocities? Stroke volume?	2 min 10 s

CISS constructive interference in steady state, *true FISP* true fast imaging with steady-state precession, *PSIF* reversed fast imaging with steady-state precession

References

1. Bradley WG Jr (2001) Diagnostic tools in hydrocephalus. Neurosurg Clin N Am 12:661–684, viii
2. Mori K, Shimada J, Kurisaka M et al (1995) Classification of hydrocephalus and outcome of treatment. Brain Dev 17:338–348
3. Barkovich AJ, Edwards MS (1992) Applications of neuroimaging in hydrocephalus. Pediatr Neurosurg 18:65–83
4. Greitz D (2004) Radiological assessment of hydrocephalus: new theories and implications for therapy. Neurosurg Rev 27:145–165; discussion 166–167
5. Adams RD, Fisher CM, Hakim S et al (1965) Symptomatic occult hydrocephalus with "normal" cerebrospinal-fluid pressure. A treatable syndrome. N Engl J Med 273:117–126
6. Lisanti C, Carlin C, Banks KP et al (2007) Normal MRI appearance and motion-related phenomena of CSF. AJR Am J Roentgenol 188:716–725
7. Chavhan GB, Babyn PS, Jankharia BG et al (2008) Steady-state MR imaging sequences: physics, classification, and clinical applications. Radiographics 28: 1147–1160
8. Casselman JW, Kuhweide R, Deimling M et al (1993) Constructive interference in steady state-3DFT MR imaging of the inner ear and cerebellopontine angle. AJNR Am J Neuroradiol 14:47–57
9. Doll A, Christmann D, Kehrli P et al (2000) Contribution of 3D CISS MRI for pre- and post-therapeutic monitoring of obstructive hydrocephalus. J Neuroradiol 27:218–225
10. Bruder H, Fischer H, Graumann R et al (1988) A new steady-state imaging sequence for simultaneous acquisition of two MR images with clearly different contrasts. Magn Reson Med 7:35–42
11. Jolesz FA, Patz S, Hawkes RC et al (1987) Fast imaging of CSF flow/motion patterns using steady-state free precession (SSFP). Invest Radiol 22:761–771
12. Patz S, Hawkes RC (1986) The application of steady-state free precession to the study of very slow fluid flow. Magn Reson Med 3:140–145
13. Schellinger D, LeBihan D, Rajan SS et al (1992) MR of slow CSF flow in the spine. AJNR Am J Neuroradiol 13:1393–1403
14. Brooks ML, Jolesz FA, Patz S (1988) MRI of pulsatile CSF motion within arachnoid cysts. Magn Reson Imaging 6:575–584
15. Hoffmann KT, Hosten N, Meyer BU et al (2000) CSF flow studies of intracranial cysts and cyst-like lesions achieved using reversed fast imaging with steady-state precession MR sequences. AJNR Am J Neuroradiol 21:493–502

16. Hoffmann KT, Lehmann TN, Baumann C et al (2003) CSF flow imaging in the management of third ventriculostomy with a reversed fast imaging with steady-state precession sequence. Eur Radiol 13:1432–1437
17. Francois CJ, Fieno DS, Shors SM et al (2004) Left ventricular mass: manual and automatic segmentation of true FISP and FLASH cine MR images in dogs and pigs. Radiology 230:389–395
18. Hodel J, Decq P, Rahmouni A et al (2009) Brain ventricular wall movement assessed by a gated cine MR trueFISP sequence in patients treated with endoscopic third ventriculostomy. Eur Radiol 19(12):2789–2797
19. Reubelt D, Small LC, Hoffmann MH et al (2009) MR imaging and quantification of the movement of the lamina terminalis depending on the CSF dynamics. AJNR Am J Neuroradiol 30:199–202
20. Moran PR, Moran RA, Karstaedt N (1985) Verification and evaluation of internal flow and motion. True magnetic resonance imaging by the phase gradient modulation method. Radiology 154:433–441
21. O'Donnell M (1985) NMR blood flow imaging using multiecho, phase contrast sequences. Med Phys 12: 59–64
22. Bradley WG Jr, Scalzo D, Queralt J et al (1996) Normal-pressure hydrocephalus: evaluation with cerebrospinal fluid flow measurements at MR imaging. Radiology 198:523–529
23. Lotz J, Meier C, Leppert A et al (2002) Cardiovascular flow measurement with phase-contrast MR imaging: basic facts and implementation. Radiographics 22:651–671
24. Stivaros SM, Sinclair D, Bromiley PA et al (2009) Endoscopic third ventriculostomy: predicting outcome with phase-contrast MR imaging. Radiology 252:825–832
25. Dorenbeck U, Schlaier J, Feuerbach S et al (2005) Diffusion-weighted imaging in the diagnostic evaluation of the hydrocephalus in patients with acute or chronic increase in cerebral pressure. Rofo 177: 99–104
26. Savoiardo M, Grisoli M (2001) Imaging dementias. Eur Radiol 11:484–492
27. Tullberg M, Jensen C, Ekholm S et al (2001) Normal pressure hydrocephalus: vascular white matter changes on MR images must not exclude patients from shunt surgery. AJNR Am J Neuroradiol 22: 1665–1673
28. Segev Y, Metser U, Beni-Adani L et al (2001) Morphometric study of the midsagittal MR imaging plane in cases of hydrocephalus and atrophy and in normal brains. AJNR Am J Neuroradiol 22: 1674–1679
29. Gunasekera L, Richardson AE (1977) Computerized axial tomography in idiopathic hydrocephalus. Brain 100:749–754
30. Sasaki M, Honda S, Yuasa T et al (2008) Narrow CSF space at high convexity and high midline areas in idiopathic normal pressure hydrocephalus detected by axial and coronal MRI. Neuroradiology 50: 117–122
31. Bradley WG Jr, Quencer RM (1999) Hydrocephalus and cerebrospinal fluid flow. Mosby, St. Louis
32. Kitagaki H, Mori E, Ishii K et al (1998) CSF spaces in idiopathic normal pressure hydrocephalus: morphology and volumetry. AJNR Am J Neuroradiol 19: 1277–1284
33. Jack CR Jr, Mokri B, Laws ER Jr et al (1987) MR findings in normal-pressure hydrocephalus: significance and comparison with other forms of dementia. J Comput Assist Tomogr 11:923–931
34. Bradley WG Jr, Kortman KE, Burgoyne B (1986) Flowing cerebrospinal fluid in normal and hydrocephalic states: appearance on MR images. Radiology 159:611–616
35. Quencer RM, Post MJ, Hinks RS (1990) Cine MR in the evaluation of normal and abnormal CSF flow: intracranial and intraspinal studies. Neuroradiology 32:371–391
36. Bradley WG Jr, Whittemore AR, Kortman KE et al (1991) Marked cerebrospinal fluid void: indicator of successful shunt in patients with suspected normal-pressure hydrocephalus. Radiology 178:459–466
37. Luetmer PH, Huston J, Friedman JA et al (2002) Measurement of cerebrospinal fluid flow at the cerebral aqueduct by use of phase-contrast magnetic resonance imaging: technique validation and utility in diagnosing idiopathic normal pressure hydrocephalus. Neurosurgery 50:534–543; discussion 543–544
38. Poca MA, Sahuquillo J, Busto M et al (2002) Agreement between CSF flow dynamics in MRI and ICP monitoring in the diagnosis of normal pressure hydrocephalus. Sensitivity and specificity of CSF dynamics to predict outcome. Acta Neurochir Suppl 81:7–10
39. Relkin N, Marmarou A, Klinge P et al (2005) Diagnosing idiopathic normal-pressure hydrocephalus. Neurosurgery 57:S4–S16; discussion ii–v

Neuroendoscopic Management of Intraparenchymal Lesions

13

Luiz Carlos de Alencastro, Luiz Felipe de Alencastro, Ademir A. Lodetti, and Mário de Barros Faria

13.1 Introduction

The microscope has been the main tool for microsurgical work along the years. For the approach of intraparenchymal lesions, a corridor large enough to bring light and vision from outside has to be created.

In microscope, microsurgical techniques that help to reduce intraoperative retraction of normal intracranial neural and vascular structures contribute to improved postoperative results. The goal must be the reduction or avoidance of retraction of neurovascular structures, which is achieved with bone drilling and extensive dura opening, which, on the other hand, increases operating time and operation-related trauma [1]. The use of endoscopes may help materialize this goal while avoiding extensive bone drilling and dural opening [1].

The approach of deep-seated intracranial lesions, including intraventricular and intraparenchymal pathologies, traditionally has been performed through direct microscopic visualization. Typically, microscope necessitates a cone-shaped access pathway, which will offer vision to the lesion allowing microsurgical dissection [2].

L.C. de Alencastro, PhD (✉) • L.F. de Alencastro, MD
A.A. Lodetti, MD
Department of Neurosurgery, Hospital Moinhos de Vento, Porto Alegre, Brazil
e-mail: lcalencastro@me.com

M. de Barros Faria, MD
Division of Neurovascular, Department of Neurology and Neurosurgery, Hospital de Clínicas de Porto Alegre, Porto Alegre, Brazil

Microscope microsurgical techniques may require brain retraction to maintain the corridor created to reach the lesion. This is essential for optimal visualization throughout the intracranial procedure and enables bimanual dissection by freeing both hands. On the other hand, the occurrence of brain contusions or infarctions after the use of brain retractors is not uncommon. The incidence of brain retraction injury varies from 5 to 10 %, with potential of clinical symptoms [3–5].

As Oi has pointed out [6], neuroendoscopic surgery has become one of the major or leading procedures in "minimally invasive approaches" to intracranial lesions. The indication for neuroendoscopy has been expanded to almost all neurosurgical procedures, as "endoscope-assisted" procedures. This concept was applied mainly to micro-neurosurgical procedures (endoscope-assisted microsurgery). He defined the realistic indication for "pure neuroendoscopic surgery" in many procedures like third ventriculostomy; septostomy; foramen reconstruction; fenestration of septations; removal or biopsy of tumor/cystic lesion, mainly in the intraventricular regions; and removal of hematoma involving the cerebral parenchyma. The author also observed that intraparenchymal or deep-seated intracisternal lesions would also be a realistic indication for "pure neuroendoscopic surgery" when the instruments had further developed in the future [6].

More recently, the use of intraoperative neuronavigation has enabled the surgeon to precisely plan the craniotomy in order to reach lesions

S. Sgouros (ed.), *Neuroendoscopy*,
DOI 10.1007/978-3-642-39085-2_13, © Springer-Verlag Berlin Heidelberg 2014

while traversing the least possible amount of normal and eloquent nervous tissue. Nevertheless, in order to access deep-seated lesions, transcortical approaches require a corticotomy or corticectomy and some degree of dissection of the overlying white matter.

The ability of endoscopes to drive illumination and vision into the area of interest has led to the possibility of working into body cavities through reduced access. In this way, managing lesions inside solid tissues obligates the creation of a working space – just a trajectory where light, vision, and surgical tools come into the working site. The direction and the small diameter of this corridor are critical to minimize brain damage [2].

The concept of a keyhole craniotomy combined with a selected trajectory can enable the approach of intraparenchymal lesions. However, the decision to use endoscopy must be individualized based on the patient, site, and characteristics of the lesion.

Complications associated with minimally invasive tumor neurosurgery have been similar to those associated with conventional neurosurgical approaches [7].

13.2 Evolution of the Technique

There is a large amount of information in the literature regarding many variations of possible techniques for the approach of intraparenchymal lesions. There is a consistent evolution of neuroendoscopic techniques, first aiming at lesions in and around the ventricular system, then progressing naturally to the treatment of intraparenchymal lesions.

Even working with the microscope, the same concept of creating a channel to reach deep-seated lesions was described by Kelly in 2004. He thought that using progressive dilatation of brain parenchyma with a sequence of enlarging diameter tubes to create a working channel would be less harmful to the brain, although a 20-mm-minimum-wide channel would be necessary to let the microscope light come into the target area [8].

This microsurgical technique was modified by Ogura and described as "transcylinder approach." A 0.1-mm transparent polyester film was used to create a cylindrical surgical route. The film was rolled into a thin stick and used to penetrate the brain with a computer-aided navigation system. This technique was employed in 11 cases. By avoiding unnecessary retraction, it significantly reduced the risk of injury to surrounding brain tissue while facilitating precise microsurgical technique, as stated by the author [4].

The early references on endoscopy in the approach of intracerebral lesions are described in the beginning of the 1990s by Hellwig and colleagues. They used a new endoscope prototype that was adapted to a stereotactic frame, performing biopsies of deep-seated lesions and drainage of intracerebral hematomas [9].

The same author in 1992 reinforced the term "minimally invasive neurosurgery," expanding the scope of these approaches to the treatment of subdural hematomas and also to spinal endoscopy. The advantages of this technique were compared to conventional neurosurgical approaches, highlighting the presence of less operative risk and reduced tissue trauma [10].

In 1998, Wan and colleagues developed a special endoscope with a larger working channel so that he could operate on neoplasms and hematomas deep in the brain. They performed surgery in 30 patients, 13 had intracranial tumor, 15 hypertensive intracerebral hematoma, 1 thalamic abscess, and 1 neurocysticercosis, with accurate intraoperative localization, minimal invasion, and good recovery. He concluded that the indications for this intervention were small lesions deep in the brain parenchyma with well-defined boundaries and light vascularity [11]. The same principle was also described by Tirakotai [12].

Fiorindi also reported his experience of endoscopic biopsy of ventricular or paraventricular brain tumors and defined some criteria to use this technique: lesions not suitable for conventional surgical removal or lesions too risky for stereotactic approach. Proper pathological diagnosis was achieved in 19/23 cases [13]. In the other hand, Nakano proposed endoscopic biopsy for solid deep-seated lesions to be considered as the first option in selected cases [14].

Until this moment, mainly biopsies were conducted through pure endoscopic approach. Operating through the endoscope's working channel made clear that the size of the lesion was very important for the success of the technique. Only very small or very soft lesions (e.g., abscesses) would be suitable for endoscopic resection. It was clear that it would be necessary to create a wider channel to approach bigger lesions, so that more instruments could be used in parallel to the endoscope.

In 2000, Nishihara and his colleagues described the use of a transparent sheath for guiding an endoscope, a simple and unique tool for endoscopic surgery, and described the preliminary results of its application in the evacuation of hypertensive intracerebral hematomas. This tube was 10 cm long, made of clear acrylic plastic, which greatly improved visualization of the surgical field through a 2.7-mm nonangled endoscope inserted within it. In nine consecutive cases in which the hematoma was larger than 40 ml in volume, nearly complete evacuation (86–100 %) of the lesion was achieved without complication. The transition between white matter and clot was clearly visible. [15] Chen and colleagues had experienced very similar results [16] with similar technique.

In 2005, Oi and colleagues corroborated this concept of using the endoscope inside an outer sheath, but they applied that only for ventricular lesions. In their system, a rigid scope was used in combination to an elliptic sheath, in order that the endoscope occupied one third of the space inside the sheath, and the other two thirds were used to introduce traditional endoscopic instruments (microscissors, biopsy forceps, grasping forceps, monopolar coagulation, etc.) to resect the lesions in the ventricle [17].

In 2002, the authors of this chapter performed their first endoscopic approach to a deep-seated brain tumor. A metallic tube was conducted to the lesion through neuronavigation. A 0° scope was introduced in parallel with a tumor forceps and/or a suction tube. Rod coagulation was also used whenever was needed. Multifocal biopsies were performed, establishing the diagnosis of lymphoma. Since that time, a total of 90 procedures have been performed, including primary and secondary brain tumors, cavernous angiomas, intraparenchymal hematomas, cerebellar infarctions, sellar tumors, and brain abscess.

Akai and colleagues improved their technique already used for intraventricular and paraventricular lesions. They combined a neuroendoscope to a navigation system and performed a series of three biopsies to intraparenchymal tumors through a transparent sheath. If bleeding was observed, aspiration and monopolar coagulation could be introduced through this sheath, but they discouraged this technique to known rich vascularized lesions [18].

Kassam and his group consolidated their experience with this same technique in 2009. As Nishihara, they used a transparent conduit, performing the surgery in 21 patients (12 metastases, 5 glioblastomas, 3 cavernous malformations, and 1 hemangioblastoma). Image guidance was used to direct the cannulation and resection of all lesions. Total radiographically confirmed resection was achieved in 8 cases, near total in 6 cases, and subtotal in 7 cases [19].

Perneczky and Fries proposed a variation of the technique that could be helpful in many situations. They fixed the scope with retractor arms fixed to the Mayfield headholder. Thus, the surgeon was able to perform microsurgical manipulations with both hands [1].

Navigation systems have a special role in the development of pure endoscopic procedures in brain parenchyma. It undoubtedly contributes to the reduction of brain damage. As mentioned before, the earlier reports of association of the endoscope and stereotactic navigation date from 1991 with Hellwig and colleagues [9]. Endoscopic approach of intraparenchymal lesions often lacks good orientation due to absence of landmarks, so that frameless navigation is specially important in those cases.

Navigation can be used in two different ways. First, as in microsurgery, the navigation probe is used to locate the target and plan the trajectory, so then the endoscope is inserted in the parenchyma. Conversely, in the second option the endoscope itself is connected to navigation system and works as a navigation probe. As the endoscope is inserted in the parenchyma, direct correction of the trajectory can be performed.

In 1998, Rohde reported the combination of the endoscope with a frameless navigation system when performing third ventriculostomies. It was pointed out that this technique allowed to establish an entry point and plan a safe trajectory to the target, avoiding inadvertent damage to vital structures [20]. Hopf and colleagues expanded this concept for patients harboring cystic lesions or intraventricular tumors, with special significance when anatomy distortion was observed [21]. Schroeder had also agreed with those same concepts [22].

Alberti described his experience in the association of neuroendoscopy and neuronavigation. He performed 44 surgeries in different lesions and considered that this association was useful when approaching narrow ventricles and localizing small lesions inside the brain parenchyma [23].

During the last years, ultrasound has been used also as an aid in endoscopic procedures in brain parenchyma. As frameless navigation, ultrasound can orientate the endoscope and sheath towards the lesion in the parenchyma. And this concept is not new. In 1996, Froelich and colleagues used this technique to approach intraparenchymal tumors in two cases. It was described that a clear parenchyma-tumor interface could be well defined, as well as vascular structures along the trajectory could be avoided with transoperative ultrasound imaging [24]. Ultrasound can help overcome the problem of intraoperative brain shift.

In recent years, high-definition fiber tracking has also offered an improvement of intraparenchymal endoscopic procedures. With this information, the trajectory to the target can be performed in order to avoid crossing important projection tracts.

Miranda and colleagues used tractography to plan the endoscopic approach to an intraparenchymal dermoid cyst located in the mesial frontal lobe. Analysis of the proposed initial surgical route was overlaid onto the fiber tracts and was predicted to produce substantial disruption to prefrontal projection fibers (anterior limb of the internal capsule) and the cingulum. Adjustment of the cannulation entry point 1 cm medially was predicted to cross the corpus callosum instead of the anterior limb of the internal capsule or the cingulum. The postop images showed preservation of the fibers in the anterior limb of the internal capsule as planned preoperatively [25].

Ultrasonic aspiration has contributed also to the development of endoscopic resection of intraparenchymal lesions. Although this possibility was described in the late 1990s [26], recent improvement of this technique has been observed with the development of specific ultrasonic probes, narrower and longer than the previous ones, so that they can best be combined to endoscopic procedures. The experience of this technique has been mainly described for intraventricular procedures, but it will obviously get progressively more application in intraparenchymal approaches.

13.3 Technique Description

The patient is carefully investigated through CT and/or MRI scan in order to establish the location of the lesion and understand the relations to the surrounding structures. Then, the approach is planned, determining an ideal entry point and a straight trajectory to the target. Fiber tracking can be very helpful in order to avoid important projection fibers along the trajectory.

The patient is positioned according to the selected trajectory, and the head is placed in a headrest or fixed in Mayfield headrest, depending on the need of neuronavigation or not. Aiming to position the head as to obtain a vertical trajectory to the lesion is helpful in order to prevent collapse of the walls of the tunnel if the cannula is removed. It also helps if gravity produces brain shifting due to CSF drainage or brain shrinking.

A 1.2 cm trepanation is performed, which can be extended to an elliptical shape in order to facilitate some lateral movement of the sheath and endoscope. Dura mater can be incised in a cross or circular shape, so that it can be sutured at the end of the procedure. Brain cortex must be inspected to avoid as much as possible damaging cortical vessels.

The sheath with its internal obturator is then introduced progressively into brain parenchyma, with or without the orientation of a neuronavigation system, depending on each case. Once the target is reached, the sheath can be held in freehand technique or can be secured with Leila retractor arms. As discussed above, different types of sheaths have been used, varying in shape, diameter, length, and material. They have as a common characteristic the possibility to apply a homogenous pressure to the parenchyma around the sheath, minimizing spot pressure and damage.

Once in position, the obturator is removed and the endoscope is introduced to confirm the correct position. In most cases clear differentiation of normal and pathological tissue interface can be observed.

Resection is then performed introducing instruments through the sheath, in parallel to endoscope. Multiple instruments can be used alone or in combination (suction tubes, tumor forceps, microscissors, monopolar or bipolar coagulation) in order to perform resection of the lesion. The number of instruments used at the same time and the maneuvers to be executed will depend on the instrument specifications, the internal diameter of the sheath, and its length. Hemostatic products and cottonoids can also be introduced to control bleeding and clean the surgical field.

Partial or total removal of the lesion may be achieved, depending on its nature and the proposed objectives. Once the intended resection is completed, the sheath is removed progressively with constant endoscopic visualization so that eventual bleeding at the pathway walls can be observed and controlled.

13.4 The Movement-Driven Vision (MDV) Concept

In the recent years the authors have developed a variation of the standard technique, described as the "Movement-Driven Vision (MDV) concept." The technique is described as follows:

Coupling the dissecting, cutting, and suction tools to scopes gives the ability to deal with intracerebral lesions through very narrow corridors, mastering consolidated bimanual microsurgical techniques.

As the vision and light are at the tip of the surgical instrument, the necessary effective working space does not exceed a few cubic centimeters which are accessed through a few-millimeter-width tunnel. The purpose is to drive the surgical tool to the point where action is needed through the narrowest pathway possible. In this way, the vision follows the movement where it is demanded as the endoscope is attached to the dissection tool. The brain structures in the access pathway are preserved maximally.

The tunnel-shaped approach has to be only a few millimeters in width, avoiding brain retraction, and may be performed through small cranial incision and bony opening.

Brain tumors, cavernous angiomas, intraparenchymatous hematomas, abscesses, sellar lesions, and ischemic cerebellar damage are among the lesions that can be managed by this technique. Deep-seated small lesions resection is benefited by frame or frameless stereotactic guidance in addition to the cannular technique.

Bimanual microsurgical dissection is facilitated by strong illumination and vision obtained at the tip of the surgical instrument. The endoscope is attached to suction tubes or dissecting tools. Distinct angled scopes and tool tips give access to structures according to demands of surgery.

The concept design brings a sheath that covers the optical rod putting together vision, illumination, and surgical tool. They are designed to work with 0° and 30° scopes. Different tips give the opportunity to the surgeon to elect the most appropriate instrument for each surgical time.

The sheath provides aspiration at the scope lens tip, keeping it clean and preventing frequent removal of the scope from the operating field. It also houses a sulcus along its superior surface, which allows driving the tools coming from outside the operating field until it gets into the scope vision (Fig. 13.1).

The suction tube may act as a second dissecting tool when the optimized suction intensity control is left opened.

13.5 Surgical Technique

After defining the ideal trajectory, a burr hole is enlarged to 12 mm. For superficial lesion additional removal of 1–2 mm of the inner cortical bone of the skull may ease lateral movements. An arciform dural incision facilitates closure.

Two techniques may be used to create a tunnel to reach the lesion:

1. A cannula with a blunt tip obturator is introduced to the limit between the normal brain and lesion. After removing the obturator, visual identification of abnormal tissue is possible, and sampling for intraoperative histologic confirmation may be obtained. The cannulas vary from 70 to 110 mm in length and have 9-mm external diameter. Dissection can be performed through the cannula, when several instruments may be used simultaneously under endoscopic view. A wider range of movements are obtained by removing the cannula and working through the parenchymal tunnel left, which will remain open with a diameter of 7–8 mm. The maintenance of the opening of the tunnel may be benefited by anesthesia techniques and a vertical trajectory.
2. A direct access by blunt dissection can also lead to the lesion. As mentioned above, working without a cannula gives additional liberty of movements. In this situation typical bimanual neurosurgical microdissection is accomplished under bright illumination and high-definition imaging provided by the scope.

In typical cases, bleeding is very limited, as strong illumination, image amplification, and wide-angle lens allow the vessels to be coagulated before they bleed. When working through a

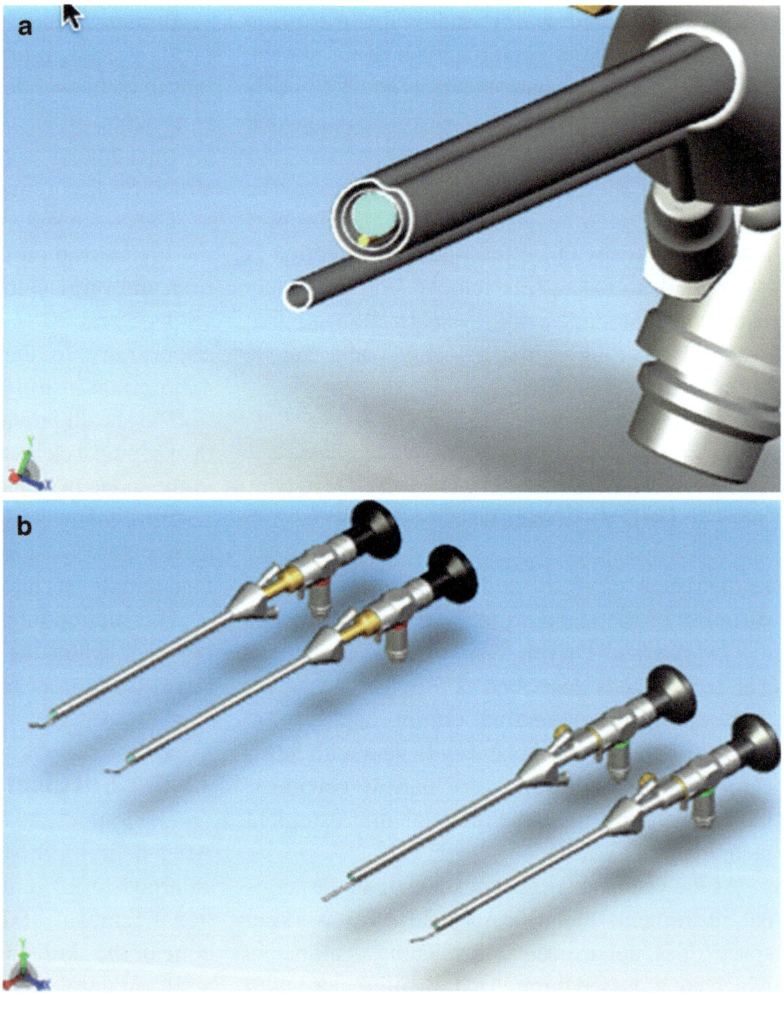

Fig. 13.1 (**a–c**) Depict the sheaths covering the scope harboring suction and dissecting tools constructed for 0° and 30° scopes. The sulcus present in the shaft guides additional instruments to the operating site. Continuous aspiration close to the lens provides clean vision. (**d**) Shows the handle cleft meant to control the suction intensity

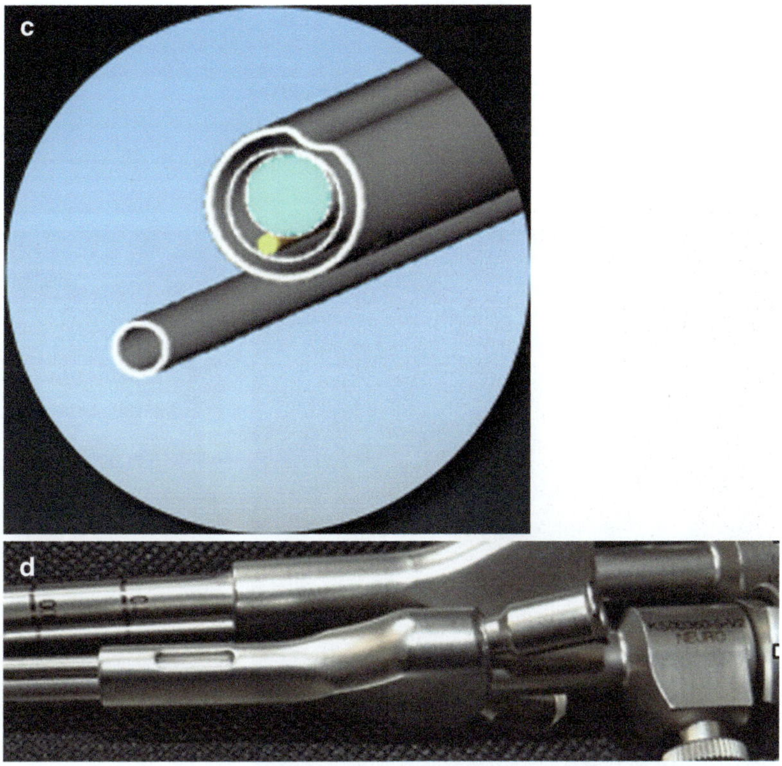

Fig. 13.1 (continued)

bare tunnel, conventional bipolar coagulation ensures safe hemostasis.

This technique reduces incision and damage to the skin, bone, and dura mater, cutting down surgical time and costs, due to opening and closing of surgical wounds.

Once the scope brings light and vision to the tip of the instruments, brain retraction necessary to visualize from outside to the operating field is obviated.

The experience, taken from 81 selected cases, including primary and secondary brain tumors, cavernous angiomas, intraparenchymal hematomas, cerebellar infarctions, sellar tumors, and brain abscess, proves the technique as an accurate and safe procedure. Except for a transient third nerve paresis in a patient with mesial temporal metastasis, no additional neurological deficit was produced in this series of patients.

The patients treated with this method had a shorter ICU and hospital stay when compared to similar cases treated by microsurgical technique by the same group of surgeons.

13.6 Illustrated Cases

13.6.1 Intraparenchymatous Hematoma

13.6.1.1 Case 1 (Fig.s. 13.2, 13.3, 13.4, and 13.5)

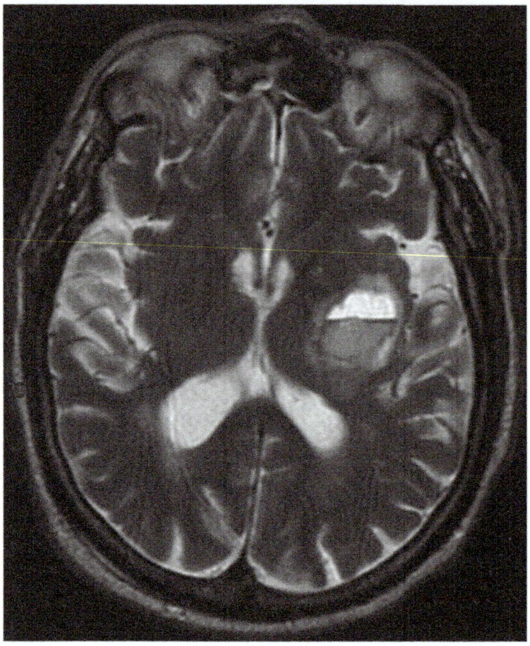

Fig. 13.2 Left putaminal hematoma compressing the posterior limb of the internal capsule

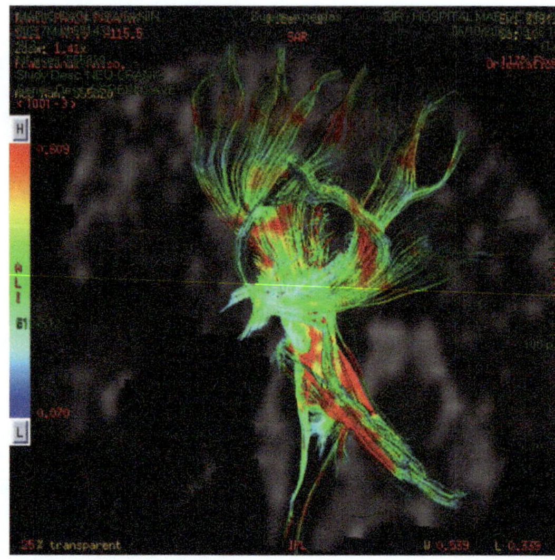

Fig. 13.3 The corticospinal fibers surround the clot. A posterior frontal approach was selected in order to avoid interrupting motor tracts

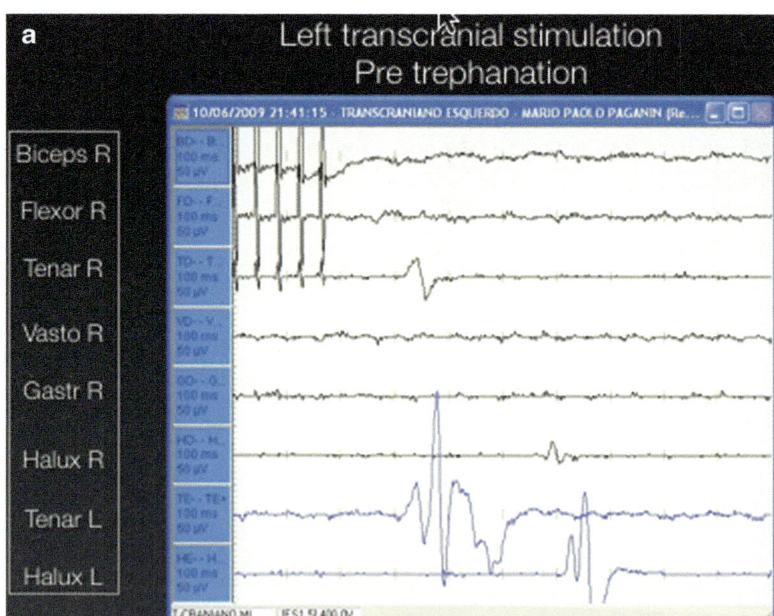

Fig. 13.4 Intraoperative motor monitoring. In (a) there is no motor response to transcranial stimulation. (b) Immediate recordings after clot aspiration demonstrated recovery of the motor responses

Fig. 13.4 (continued)

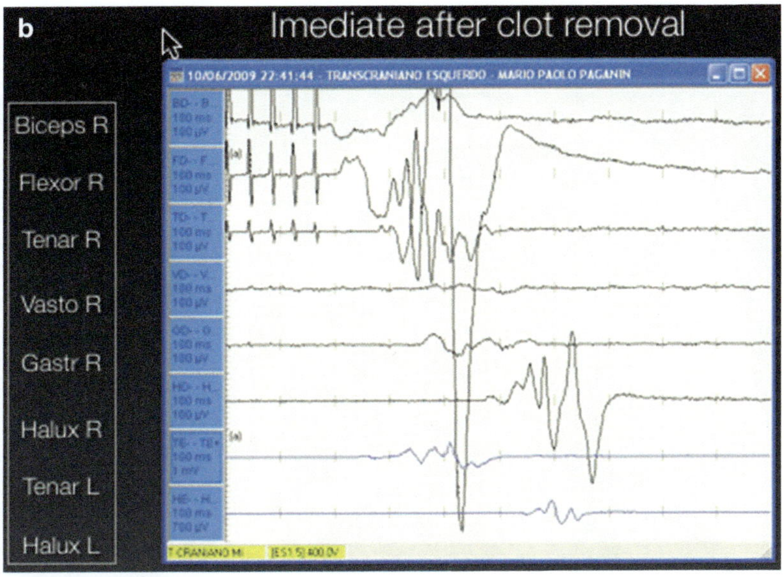

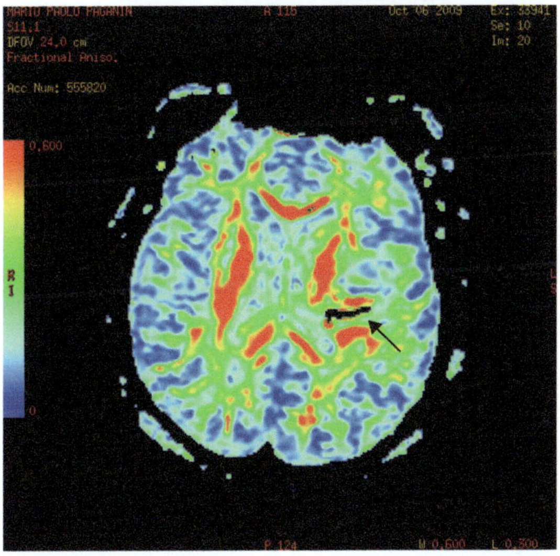

Fig. 13.5 Immediate postop DTI depicts decompression of motor tract. The *black arrow* shows air into the hematoma cavity

13.6.1.2 Case 2 (Fig.s. 13.6, 13.7, and 13.8)

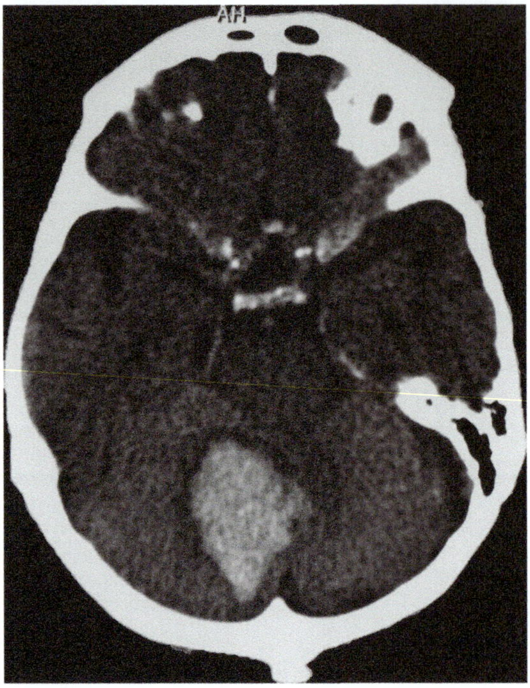

Fig. 13.6 Cerebellar hematoma

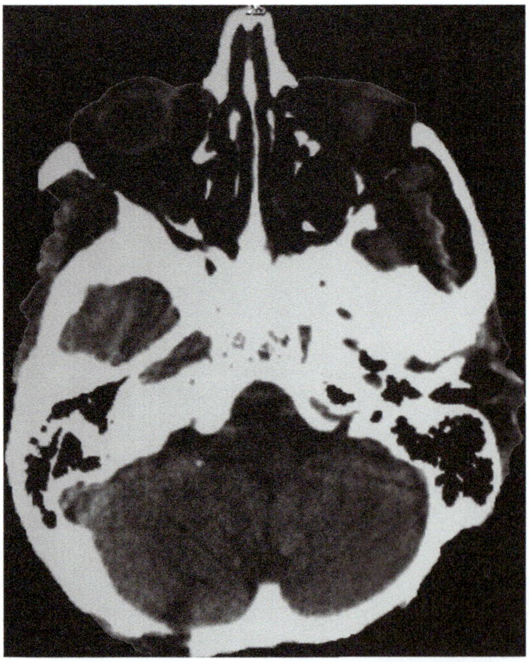

Fig. 13.7 Suboccipital trepanation for hematoma evacuation

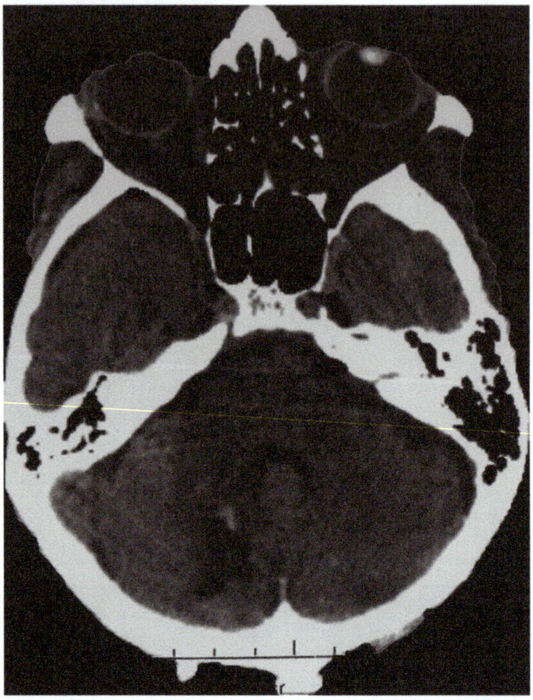

Fig. 13.8 Complete evacuation of hematoma. Decompression of cisterns

13.6.2 **Brain Glioma** (Fig.s. 13.9, 13.10, 13.11, and 13.12)

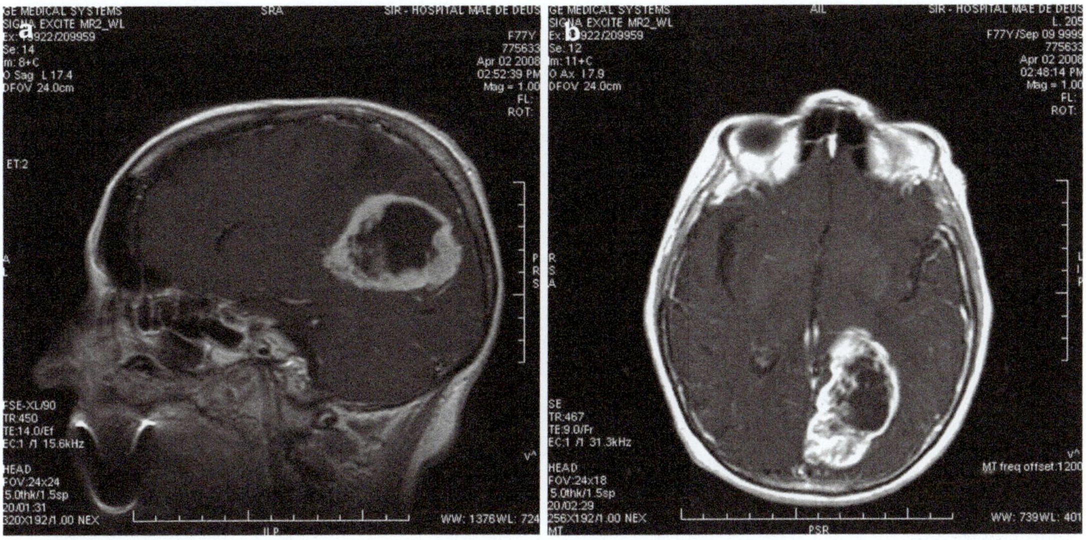

Fig. 13.9 (**a**, **b**) Preoperative images of left occipital GBM

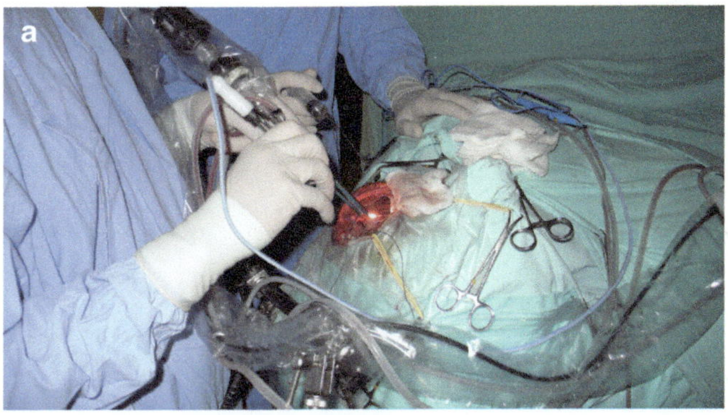

Fig. 13.10 (**a**, **b**, **c**) Intraoperative dissection work: bimanual dissecting. No need for brain retraction

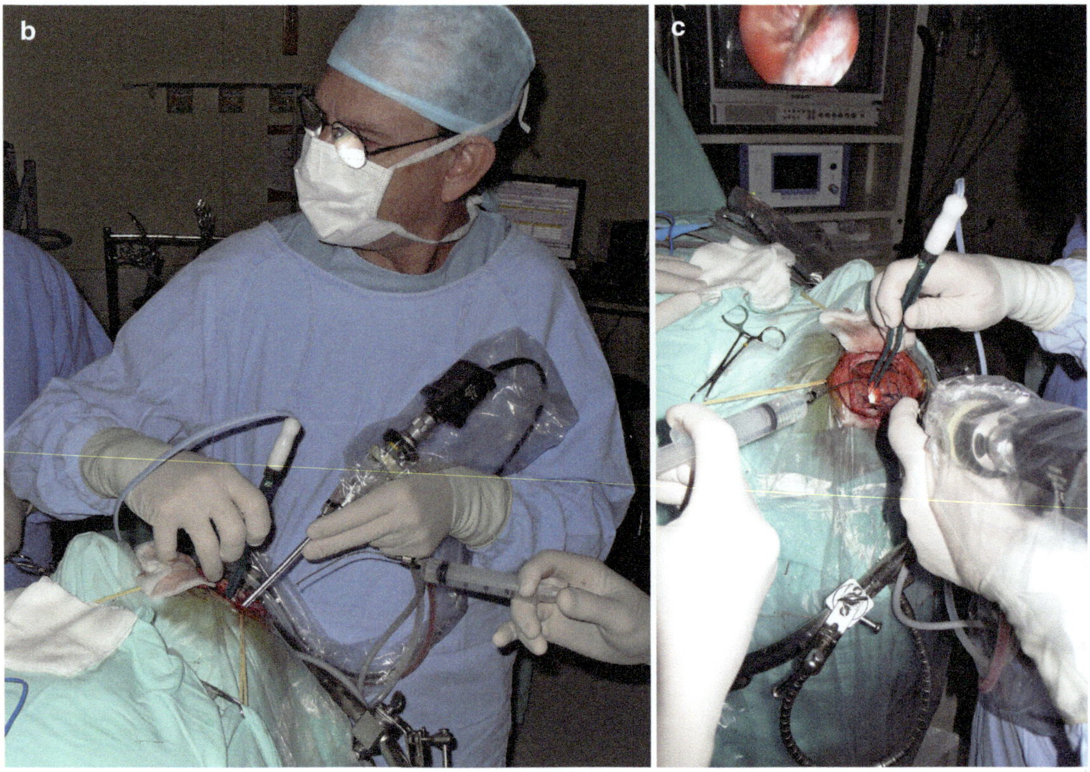

Fig. 13.10 (continued)

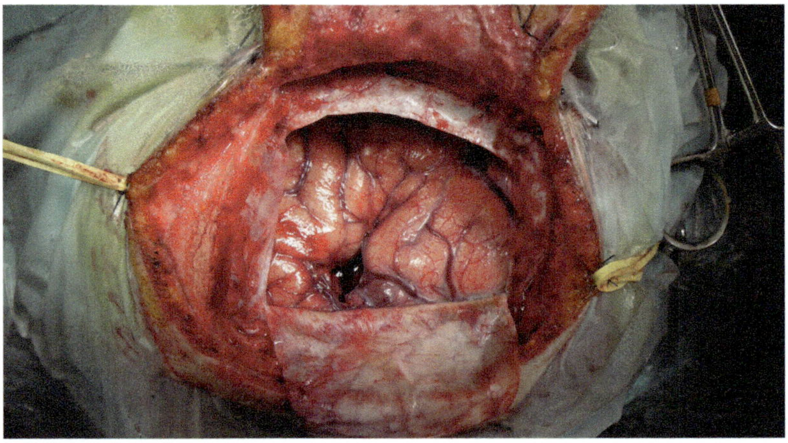

Fig. 13.11 Operating field at the end of surgery showing cerebral decompression and the 1 cm corticotomy needed for tumor removal. No brain retraction was necessary

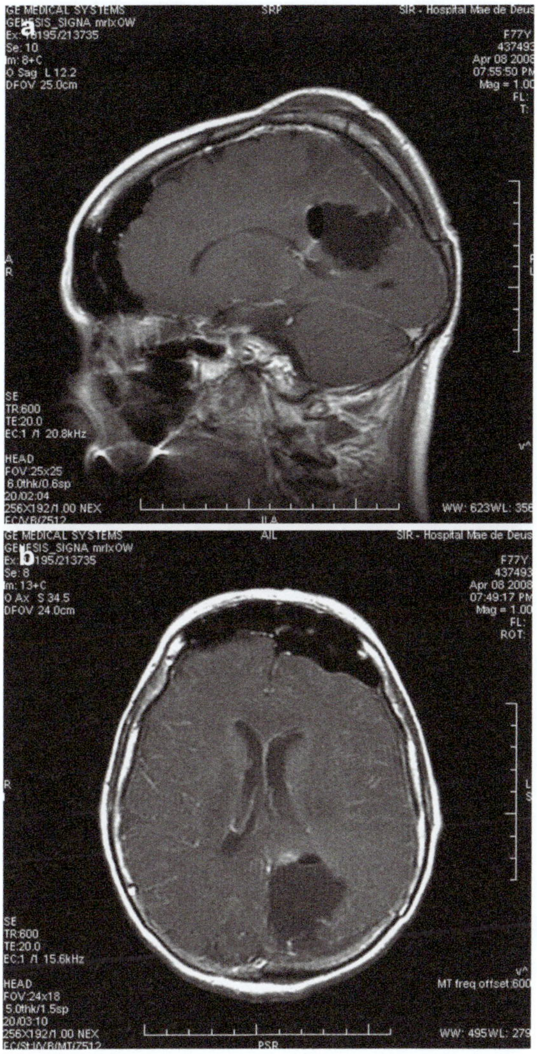

Fig. 13.12 (**a**, **b**) Immediate postop images. A larger craniotomy was performed for safety. Gross total removal was achieved

13.6.3 Cavernous Angioma

13.6.3.1 Case 1 (Fig.s. 13.13, 13.14, and 13.15)

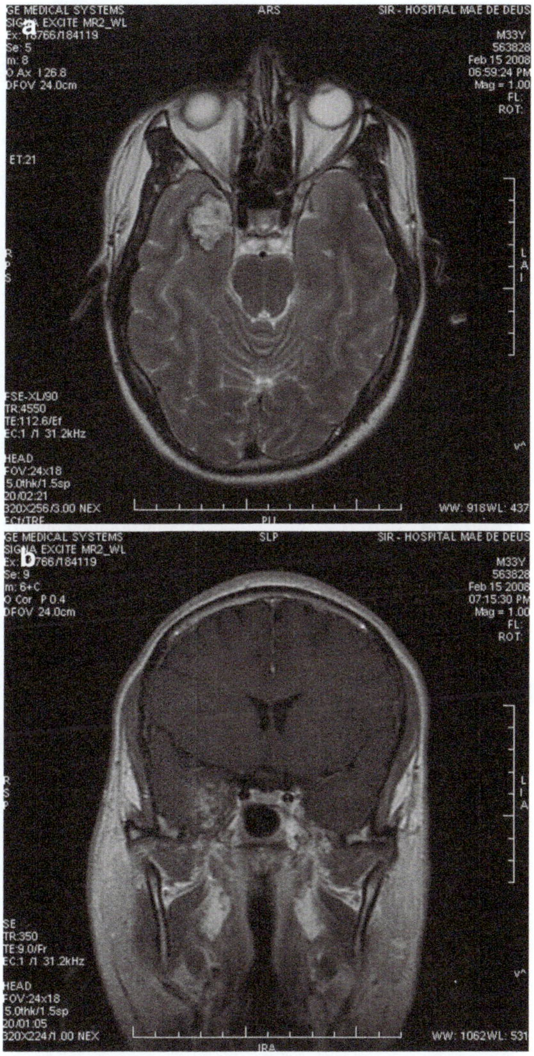

Fig. 13.13 (**a**, **b**) Temporomesial cavernous angioma. Preop images

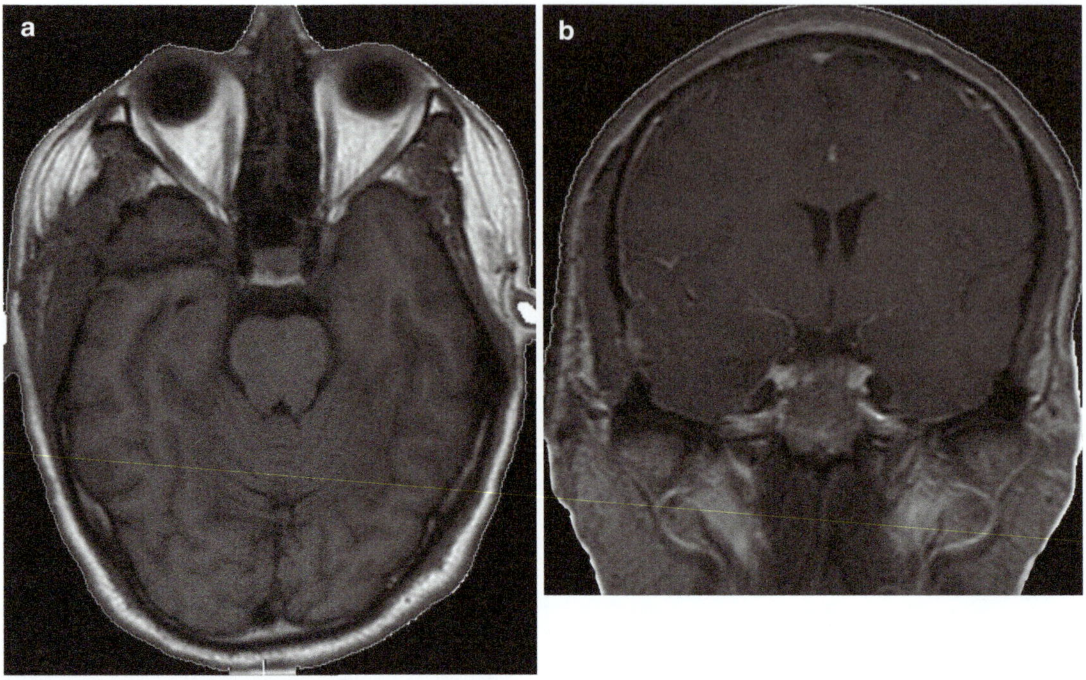

Fig. 13.14 (**a**, **b**) A 12-mm temporal bone opening and the trajectory of the scope to the locus of the cavernoma can be seen

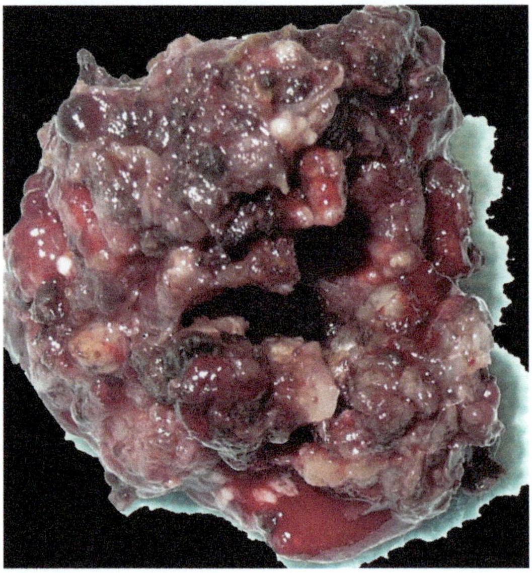

Fig. 13.15 Cavernous angioma removed

13.6.3.2 Case 2 (Fig.s. 13.16, 13.17, and 13.18)

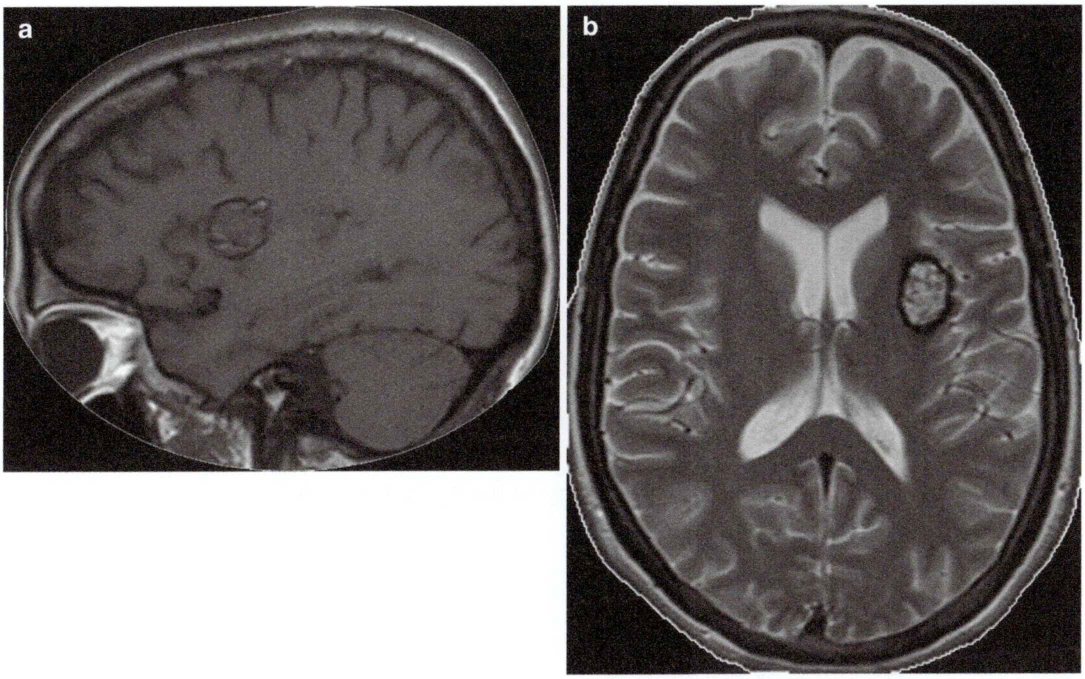

Fig. 13.16 (**a**, **b**) Putaminal cavernous angioma

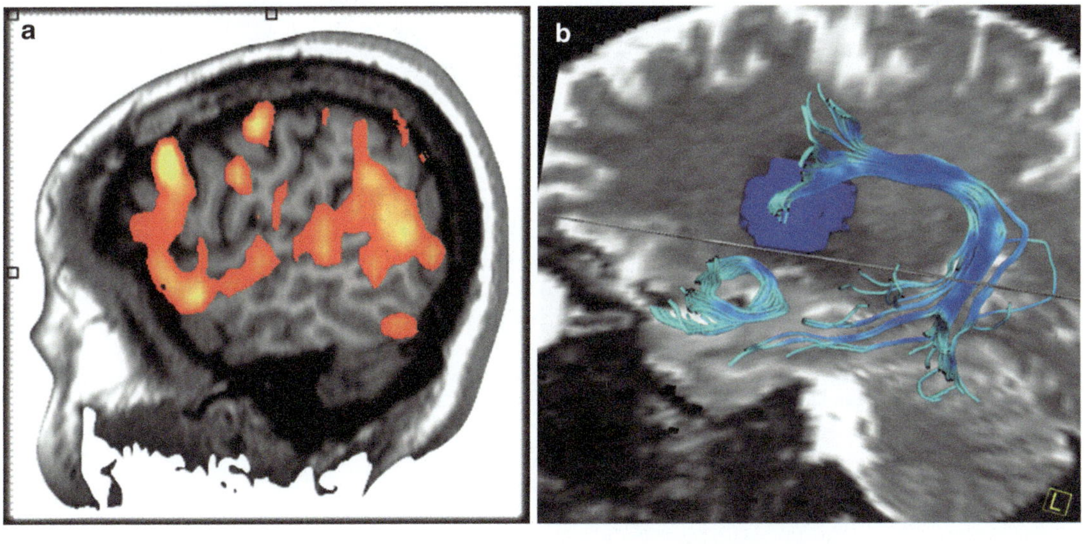

Fig. 13.17 (**a**) The distribution of speech areas over the cortex is demonstrated. In (**b**) it is possible to see the relations of the uncinate and arcuate fascicles to the cavernoma. The relationship with the corticospinal tract is shown in (**c**)

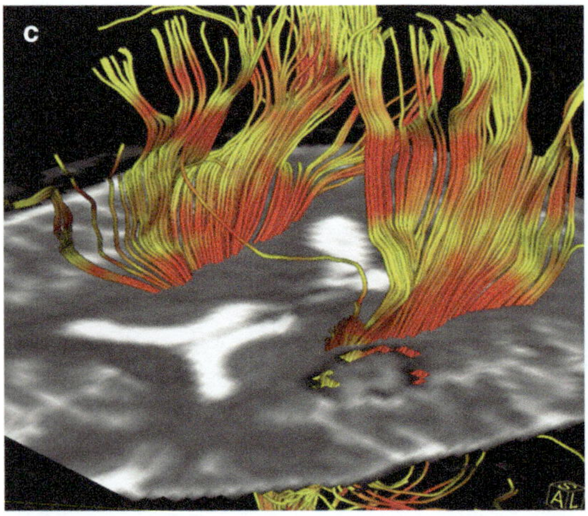

Fig. 13.17 (continued)

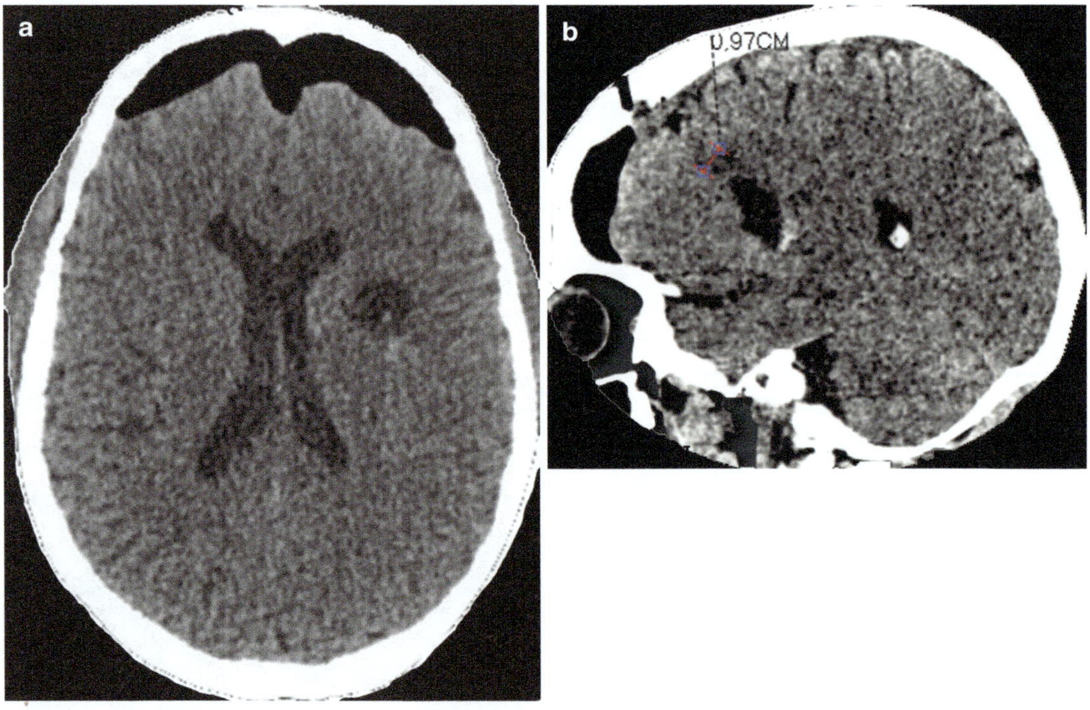

Fig. 13.18 (a, b) Immediate postop scan demonstrating complete resection of the cavernoma, the direction of the approach, and the bony opening (12 mm)

13.6.4 **Cerebellar Infarction** (Figs. 13.19 and 13.20)

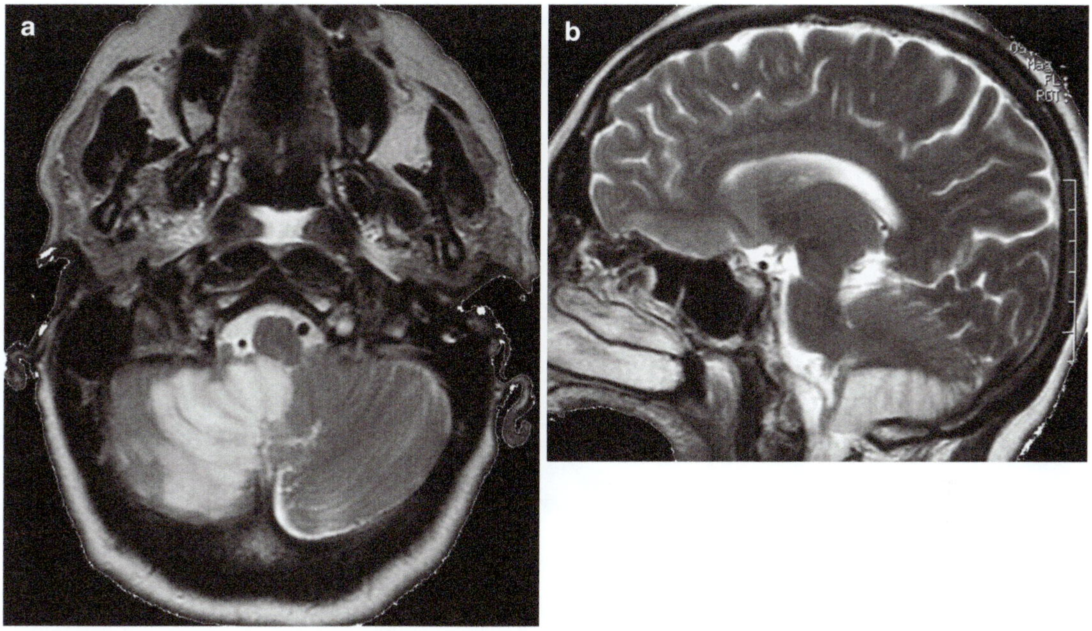

Fig. 13.19 (**a**, **b**) Images of cerebellar infarction compressing lower brainstem

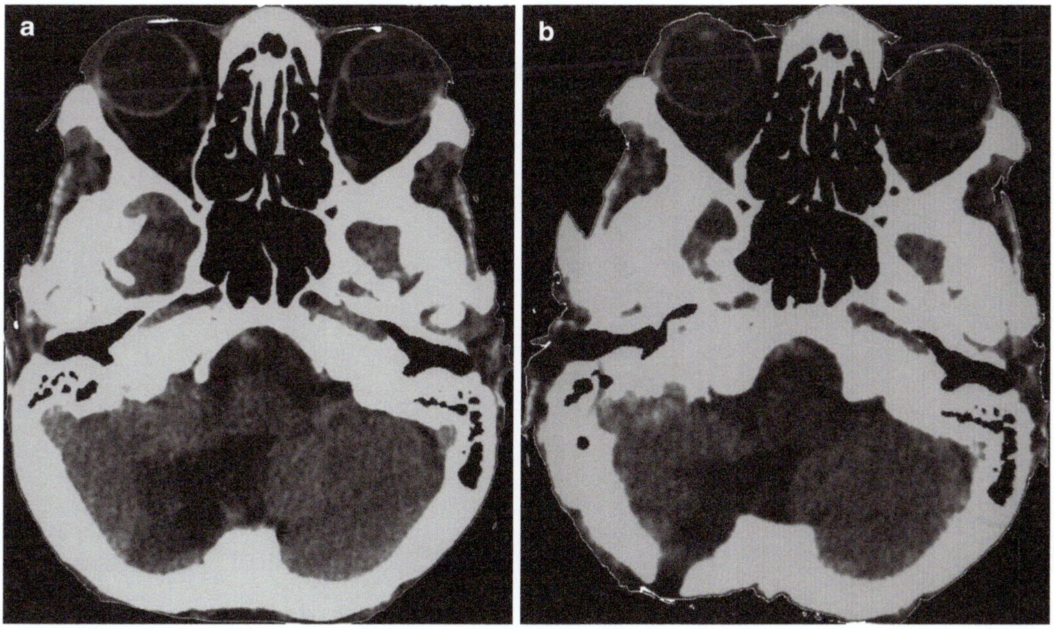

Fig. 13.20 (**a**, **b**) Postop CT control showing bone opening and bulbar decompression after endoscopic aspiration of ischemic tissue. Bimanual microsurgical technique was ensured

13.6.5 Brain Tumor (Fig. 13.21)

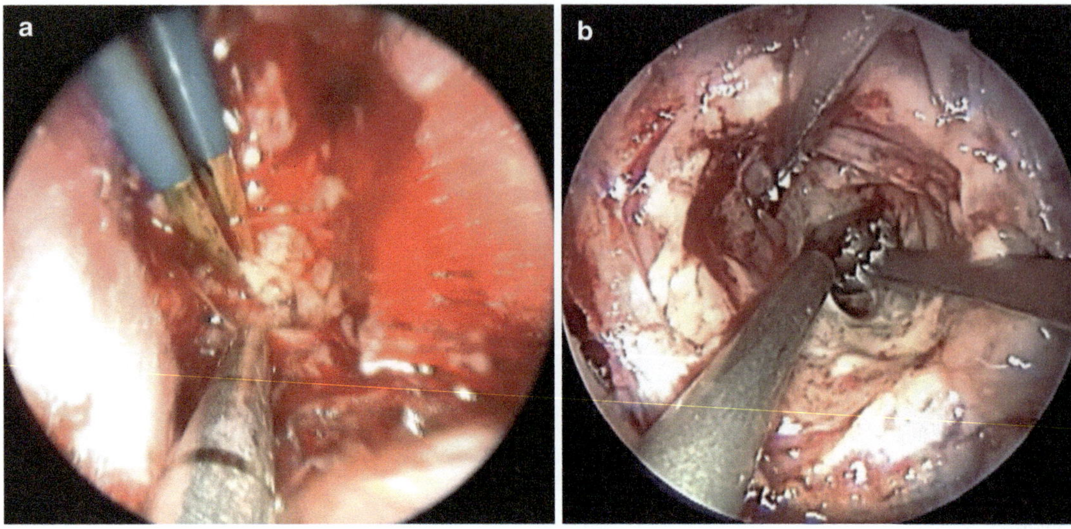

Fig. 13.21 (**a**, **b**) These images show endoscopic microsurgery of intraparenchymal gliomas. A small bone opening and a narrow tunnel through the cortex and subcortical tissue brought light and vision coupled to the suction tube, while the second hand controls the forceps. In this way, bimanual microdissection is achieved, obviating soft tissue, bone, and brain extensive damage

13.6.6 Hematoma (Fig. 13.22)

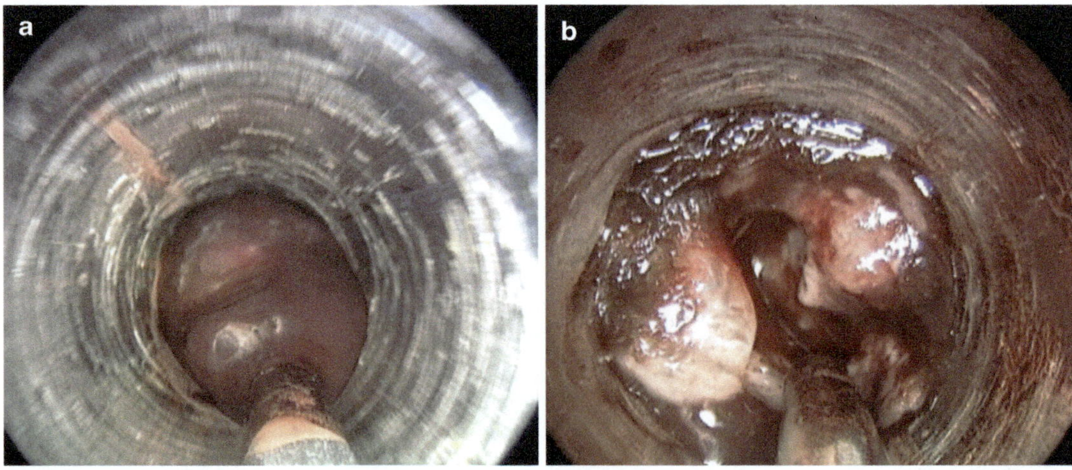

Fig. 13.22 (**a**) Aspiration of blood clot through a metallic cannula that is used to create a pathway along brain cortex and white matter to reach the hematoma. (**b**) The tip of the suction tube (which is coupled to the endoscope) inside the hematoma cavity after blood clot was removed

13.6.7 Sellar Tumor (Fig. 13.23)

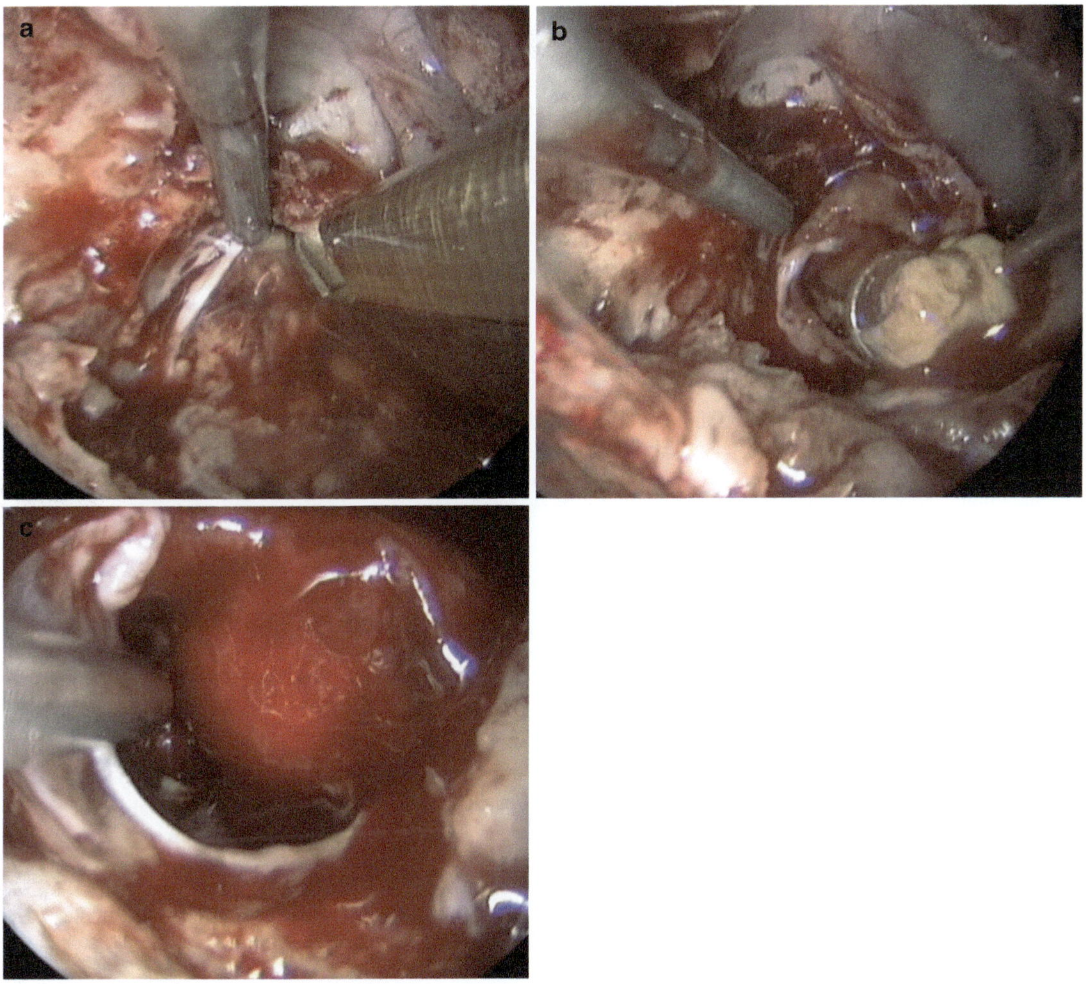

Fig. 13.23 (**a**, **b**) Endoscopic endonasal approach when the suction tube coupled to the endoscope is held in one hand, while different tools are used in the other hand. (**c**) The pituitary gland during removal of the tumor

Conclusion

Expanding possibilities in neurosurgical treatment of brain and skull base lesions with endoscopic techniques have been achieved in recent years. Microsurgical endoscopic approaches have added refinement in removal of tumors, cavernous angiomas, hematomas, abscesses, ischemic tissue, and sellar lesions. The application of the concept of Movement-Driven Vision has enhanced these possibilities, giving the neurosurgeon a technique and technology that ensures safety, time, and cost saving. It provides an opportunity to treat endoscopically lesions in solid organs.

References

1. Fries G, Perneczky A (1998) Endoscope-assisted brain surgery: part 2 – analysis of 380 procedures. Neurosurgery 42:226–231; discussion 231–232
2. Alencastro L (2012) Movement driven vision – a concept for endoscopic microsurgery. Endoworld 24
3. Andrews RJ, Bringas JR (1993) A review of brain retraction and recommendations for minimizing intraoperative brain injury. Neurosurgery 33:1052–1063; discussion 1063–1064
4. Ogura K, Tachibana E, Aoshima C, Sumitomo M (2006) New microsurgical technique for intraparenchymal lesions of the brain: transcylinder approach. Acta Neurochir (Wien) 148:779–785; discussion 785
5. Yokoh A, Sugita K, Kobayashi S (1983) Intermittent versus continuous brain retraction. An experimental study. J Neurosurg 58:918–923
6. Oi S (1999) Clinical application and future prospect of neuroendoscopic surgery. No To Hattatsu 31:299–304
7. Garrett M, Consiglieri G, Nakaji P (2010) Transcranial minimally invasive neurosurgery for tumors. Neurosurg Clin N Am 21:595–605, v
8. Kelly PJ, Ganslandt O, Fahlbusch R, Nimsky C, Stadlbauer A, Moser E (2004) Technology in the resection of gliomas and the definition of madness. Authors' reply. J Neurosurg 101:284–286
9. Hellwig D, Bauer BL (1991) Endoscopic procedures in stereotactic neurosurgery. Acta Neurochir Suppl 52:30–32
10. Hellwig D, Bauer BL (1992) Minimally invasive neurosurgery by means of ultrathin endoscopes. Acta Neurochir Suppl 54:63–68
11. Wan J, Jiang C (1998) Development and clinical application of a brain stereotactic endoscope. Zhonghua Wai Ke Za Zhi 36:536–538
12. Tirakotai W, Hellwig D, Bertalanffy H, Riegel T (2007) The role of neuroendoscopy in the management of solid or solid-cystic intra- and periventricular tumours. Childs Nerv Syst 23:653–658
13. Fiorindi A, Longatti P (2008) A restricted neuroendoscopic approach for pathological diagnosis of intraventricular and paraventricular tumours. Acta Neurochir (Wien) 150:1235–1239
14. Nakano T, Ohkuma H, Asano K, Ogasawara Y (2009) Endoscopic treatment for deep-seated or multiple intraparenchymal tumors: technical note. Minim Invasive Neurosurg 52:49–52
15. Nishihara T, Teraoka A, Morita A, Ueki K, Takai K, Kirino T (2000) A transparent sheath for endoscopic surgery and its application in surgical evacuation of spontaneous intracerebral hematomas. Technical note. J Neurosurg 92:1053–1055
16. Chen CC, Cho DY, Chang CS, Chen JT, Lee WY, Lee HC (2005) A stainless steel sheath for endoscopic surgery and its application in surgical evacuation of putaminal haemorrhage. J Clin Neurosci 12:937–940
17. Oi S, Samii A, Samii M (2005) Frameless free-hand maneuvering of a small-diameter rigid-rod neuroendoscope with a working channel used during high-resolution imaging. Technical note. J Neurosurg 102:113–118
18. Akai T, Shiraga S, Sasagawa Y, Okamoto K, Tachibana O, Lizuka H (2008) Intra-parenchymal tumor biopsy using neuroendoscopy with navigation. Minim Invasive Neurosurg 51:83–86
19. Kassam AB, Engh JA, Mintz AH, Prevedello DM (2009) Completely endoscopic resection of intraparenchymal brain tumors. J Neurosurg 110:116–123
20. Rohde V, Reinges MH, Krombach GA, Gilsbach JM (1998) The combined use of image-guided frameless stereotaxy and neuroendoscopy for the surgical management of occlusive hydrocephalus and intracranial cysts. Br J Neurosurg 12:531–538
21. Hopf NJ, Grunert P, Darabi K, Busert C, Bettag M (1999) Frameless neuronavigation applied to endoscopic neurosurgery. Minim Invasive Neurosurg 42:187–193
22. Schroeder HW, Wagner W, Tschiltschke W, Gaab MR (2001) Frameless neuronavigation in intracranial endoscopic neurosurgery. J Neurosurg 94:72–79
23. Alberti O, Riegel T, Hellwig D, Bertalanffy H (2001) Frameless navigation and endoscopy. J Neurosurg 95(3):541–543
24. Froelich J, Bien S, Hoppe M, Eggers F, Klose KJ (1996) An intracerebral sonographic catheter as an adjunct to stereotactic guided endoscopic procedures. Minim Invasive Neurosurg 39:93–96
25. Fernandez-Miranda JC, Engh JA, Pathak SK et al (2010) High-definition fiber tracking guidance for intraparenchymal endoscopic port surgery. J Neurosurg 113:990–999
26. Oka K, Go Y, Yamamoto M, Kumate S, Tomonaga M (1999) Experience with an ultrasonic aspirator in neuroendoscopy. Minim Invasive Neurosurg 42:32–34

Neuroendoscopic Techniques in the Management of Pineal Region Tumors

14

Tai-Tong Wong

14.1 Introduction

In recent years the use of the endoscope is a valid alternative to the classical microscopical approaches for the treatment of the pineal tumors. It can be used for endoscopic tumor biopsy (ETB) as well as endoscopic-assisted complete tumor removal in some cases [1, 2]. At the same time, if there is coexisting hydrocephalus, this can be treated endoscopically with endoscopic third ventriculostomy (ETV) [3].

The characteristics of the patient populations and as a consequence the therapeutic modalities differ between Japan and Korea on one hand and the rest of the world on the other [4, 5]. Our experience in Taipei is comparable to the Japan-Korea group (Table 14.1) [6].

Since 1970 we have treated 176 patients with germ cell tumors and from them 85 have been pineal (Table 14.2).

In the majority of patients, hydrocephalus has coexisted as shown on Table 14.3. The simultaneous presence of active hydrocephalus is well reported in the literature and needs to be treated.

At the pineal region a variety of lesions can occur, single or bifocal tumors, and with varying histology (pineoblastoma, pineocytoma, astrocytoma, meningioma, cyst, and also midbrain tumors) [7, 8] (Fig. 14.1).

14.2 Management of Pineal Region Tumors

The management of pineal region tumors can be summarized as follows:

1. In case of suspected germinoma or pineoblastoma with accompanying hydrocephalus and normal values of AFP and β-hCG, we propose endoscopic tumor biopsy and third ventriculostomy. At the same time an estimation of the tumor vascularity can be made as well as the presence of tumor seeding to the walls of the ventricles (Fig. 14.2). If the biopsy provides tumor-type diagnosis, further oncological management is pursued as the next step.
2. In case of suspected mature teratoma, nongerminomatous malignant germ cell tumor (NGMGCT), or other tumors, we propose radical excision of the tumor, endoscopically assisted when needed and navigation assisted if necessary (Figs. 14.3 and 14.4).
3. In case of midbrain tumors, we propose endoscopic third ventriculostomy combined with biopsy in selected cases. In some cases, an endoscopic removal of the tumor can be achieved [9–11] (Figs. 14.5, 14.6, and 14.7).

T.-T. Wong, MD
Department of Surgery, Cheng Hsin General Hospital, Taipei, Taiwan 112, China
e-mail: ttwong@vghtpe.gov.tw

S. Sgouros (ed.), *Neuroendoscopy*,
DOI 10.1007/978-3-642-39085-2_14, © Springer-Verlag Berlin Heidelberg 2014

Table 14.1 Confrontation of series

Types of tumors	Japan[a] N=118 1–25 years	Korea[a] N=125 1–12 years	TVGH[b] N=84 (8.5%) 1–18 years	Australia[c] N=37 1–16 years
Pineal tumors			74 (88.1 %)	
Suprasellar-pineal tumors			10 (11.9 %)	
Germ cell tumor	71.2 %	80.0 %	79.8 %	54.1 %
Germinoma	46.6 %	47.2 %	42.8 %	35.1 %
NGMGCT			26.2 %	16.2 %
MT			8.3 %	2.7 %
Neuroectodermal tumors/ pineoblastomas	15.2 %	16.8 %	9.5 %	16.2 %
Astrocytoma			2.4 %	8.1 %
No histological/ clinical Dx			5.9 %	16.2 %

[a]Oi et al. [12], multicenters
[b]Wong et al. [6], hospital series
[c]Drummond and Rosenfeld [13], hospital series

Table 14.2 Types of pineal GCTs in children series of Taipei Veterans General Hospital, 1970–2007

	Other sites GCTs	Pineal GCTs	Pineal GCTs seeding at Dx[a]
No. of patients	91	85	
Germinoma	*58.2 %*	*58.8 %*	*5.6 % (V 1, IS 1)*
Mature teratoma	1.1 %	8.2 %	
NGMGCT	35.2 %	31.2 %	0 %
Immature teratoma	13.2 %	8.2 %	
Mixed GCT	16.5 %	14.1 %	
Yolk sac tumor	6.6 %	4.7 %	
Dx by tumor marker	3.3 %	4.7 %	
Unclassified GCT	1.1 %	1.2 %	

V ventricular, *IS* intraspinal, *Dx* diagnosis
[a]Excluded double midline tumor

Table 14.3 Tumoral hydrocephalus with obstruction at posterior third ventricle, pineal, and midbrain tumors, 1970–2007

	No. of patients	Hydrocephalus (%)
	116	87.1
Pineal tumors	105	85.7
Germ cell tumors	85	83.5
Astrocytic tumors	2	100
Pineal parenchymal tumors	11	90.9
Embryonal tumors	2	100
No. of clinical/ histological Dx	6	83.3
Midbrain tumors	11	100

Excluding cases of questionable recording for hydrocephalus
Dx diagnosis

14.3 Endoscopic Techniques in the Management of Pineal Tumors

Our endoscopic technique includes one burr hole in case of only ETV (coronal suture burr hole) and two burr holes (coronal and behind hairline) in case of combined ETV and ETB (Fig. 14.8). We use rigid rod lens endoscope (0° and 30°), transparent sheath introducer, microforceps, and neuroballoon or angioplasty balloon catheter (Figs. 14.9 and 14.10). In Taipei VGH we use also the basket perforator for perforation and dilatation of the floor of the third ventricle [14, 15].

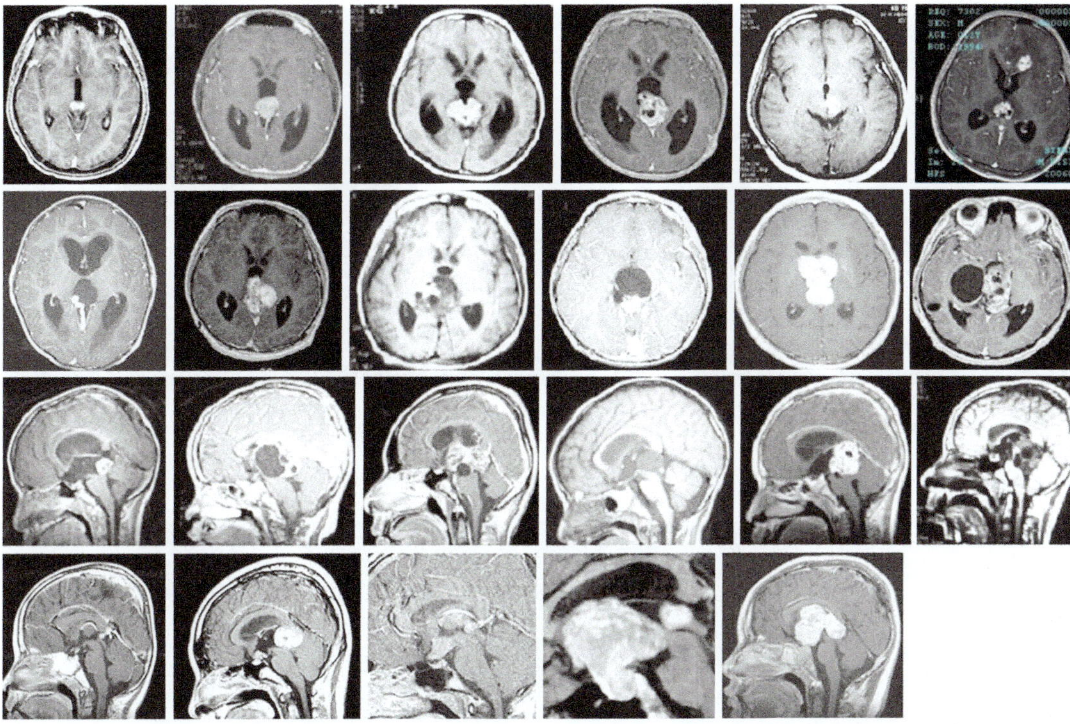

Fig. 14.1 MR scans with examples of pineal germinomas/NG-GCTs, single and bifocal tumors

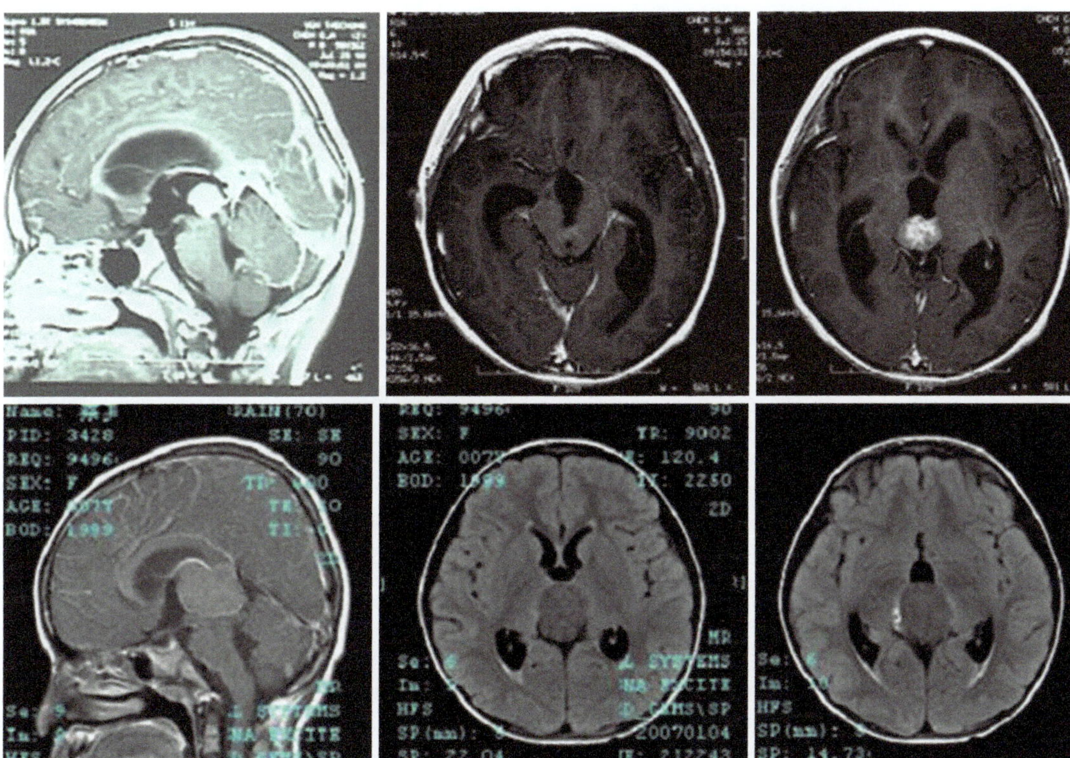

Fig. 14.2 MR scans with examples of pineoblastoma (2 *first rows*) and pineocytoma (*third row*)

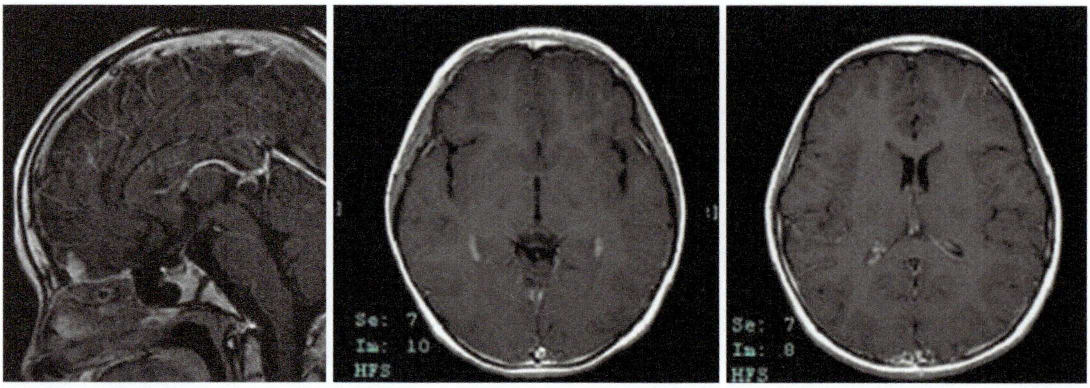

Fig. 14.2 (continued)

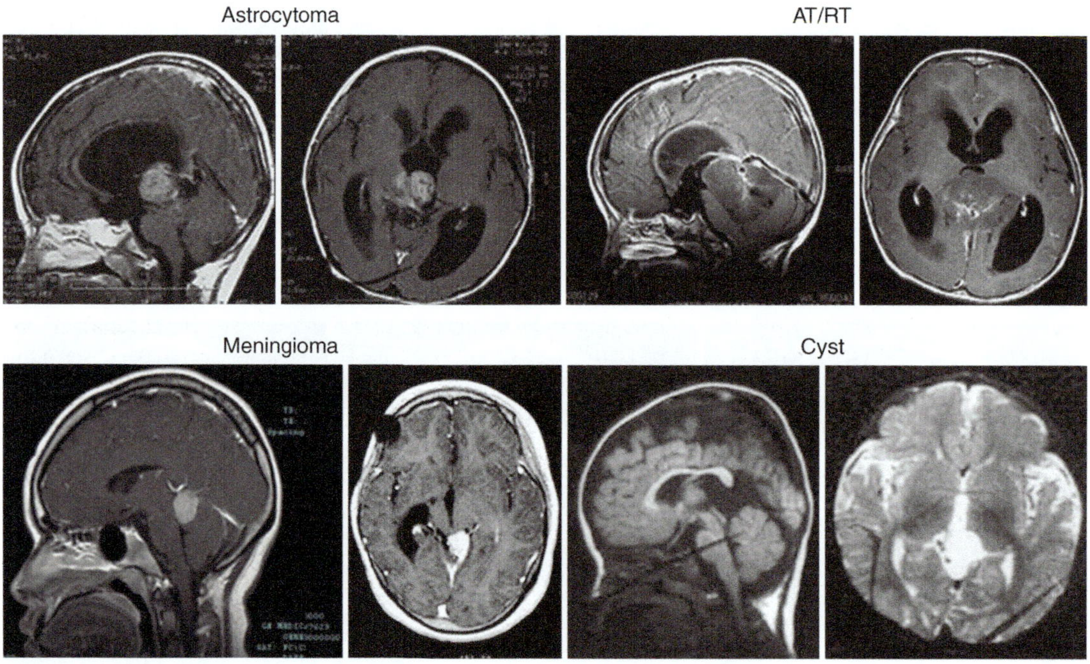

Fig. 14.3 MR scans with examples of other tumor types and cysts in the pineal/juxtapineal region

In case of small ventricles, we take some measures in order to avoid inadvertent penetration into the periventricular structures. For endoscopic third ventriculostomy (ETV), a precoronal burr hole is usually made in the midpupillary line. However, the entry point (burr hole), the trajectory of cannulation of the lateral ventricle, and the depth of the puncture with a peel-away sheath introducer can be planned by measurement of the preoperative MR image (Fig. 14.11). Stereotactic placement of the sheath introducer (Fig. 14.12) and endoscope is also safe and convenient. After the sheath is fixed in place, the stylet is removed. Thus, we can avoid inadvertent penetration into the periventricular structures such as the hypothalamus, internal capsule, basal ganglia, as well as the veins around the foramen of Monro [16].

The last years we have performed 44 ETV procedures (median age 9.8) for cases of obstructive hydrocephalus because of pineal and midbrain

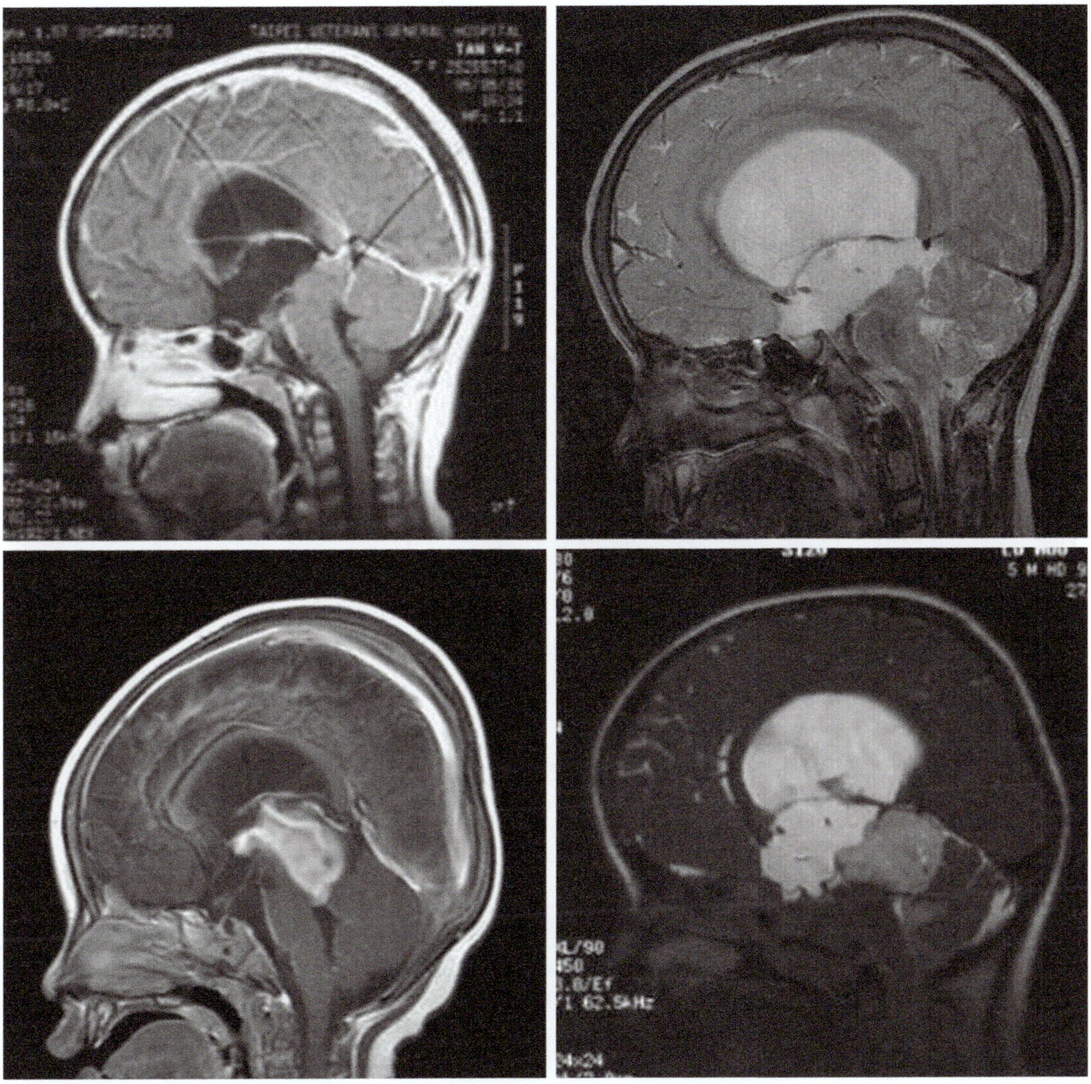

Fig. 14.4 MR scans with examples of Juxtapineal tumors – midbrain tumors

tumors (Table 14.4). We performed both ETB and ETV in 27 cases (31 ETBs in total). We have done a follow-up from 9 months to 12.4 years (mean 4.8). At the last follow-up we observed that 9 (20 %) procedures of ETV malfunctioned. At seven we performed ventriculoperitoneal shunt and two had to be revised again with ETV (median time to failure 4.6 months). However, the long-term success rate remains high 79.5 %. There was also a failure of 6 out of 31 ETB (20 %). Our results are comparable to the series of O'Brien DF et al. [17], but we achieved a better long-term success rate.

We have performed also 10 ETV for midbrain tumors, 6 of them with tumor biopsy (4 of them were diagnostic). The long-term functioning ETVs were only two with median follow-up of 4 years.

14.4 Complications

With respect to complications, we had 9 ETV malfunctions, 4 tumoral hemorrhages (2 catastrophic and 1 death of delayed hemorrhage),

4 subdural fluid collections (1 needed to be shunted), and no vascular injury (Fig. 14.13). Seeding of the tumor by the endoscopic procedures has been a matter of concern by some authors. However, for their series of 12 patients with intracranial germinomas, Shono et al. [2] reported that the risk of tumor dissemination due to neuroendoscopic procedures appears to be minimal when the appropriate chemotherapy and radiotherapy are provided postoperatively. Our opinion is that there is no correlation of endoscopic procedure and tumor dissemination/recurrence. In our series we had only two recurrences irrelevant to the use of endoscope (1 to a case with ETV performed but no ETB after 3.8 years and 1 thoracic spine dissemination to a case with ETV and ETB performed after 16 months) [18–20] (Fig. 14.14).

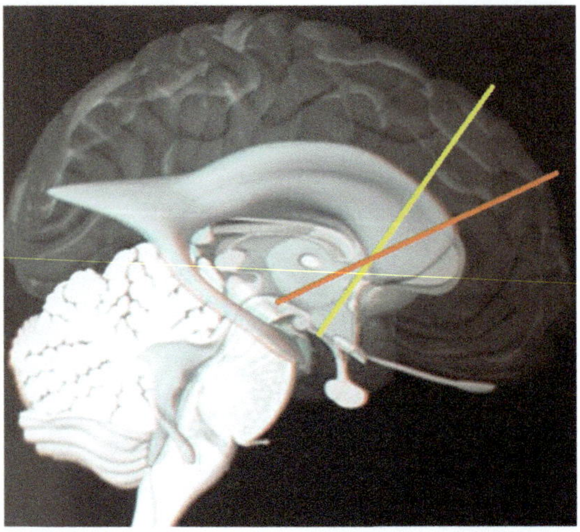

Fig. 14.5 Trajectories of coronal burr hole for ETV (*yellow line*) and behind hairline burr hole for ETB (*orange line*) (Drawings modified from Martin C. Hirsch, Thomas Kramer)

Conclusion

As a conclusion we can say that endoscopic tumor biopsy with third ventriculostomy is becoming an important alternative for the initial surgical management of pineal region tumors [21]. These procedures can be performed in a single step that achieves tumor biopsy for histological diagnosis, cerebrospinal fluid sampling for tumor markers and cytological diagnosis, and resolution of hydrocephalus. According to a multicenter study, the diagnostic

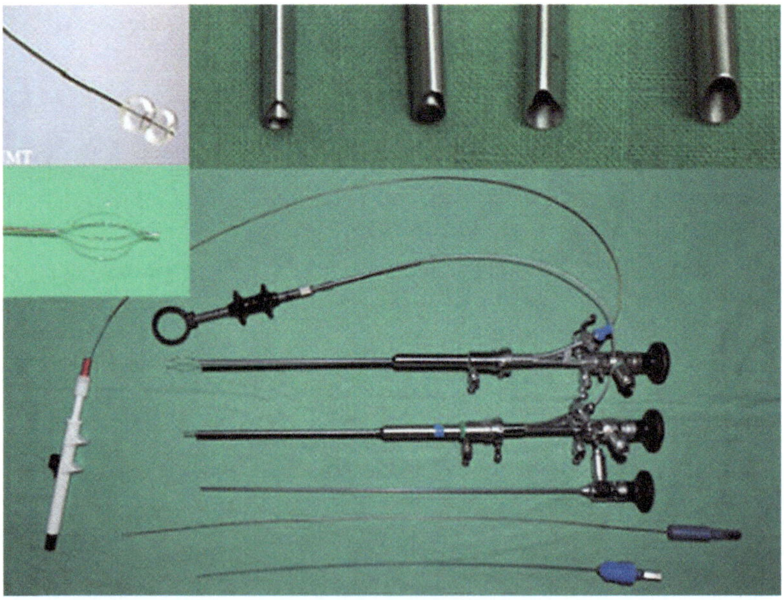

Fig. 14.6 Endoscopic instruments. The STORZ DECQ endoscope is used, with the 0° and 30° rod lenses. At the *upper left* the Integra neuroballoon and urological basket perforator (KARL STORZ GmbH & Co., Tuttlingen, Germany; Integra, Plainsboro, NJ, USA)

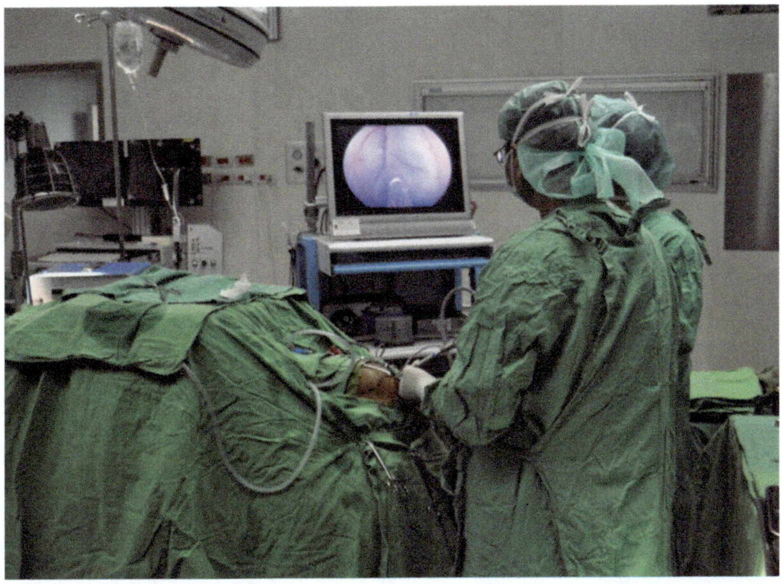

Fig. 14.7 View of the setup in the operating theater

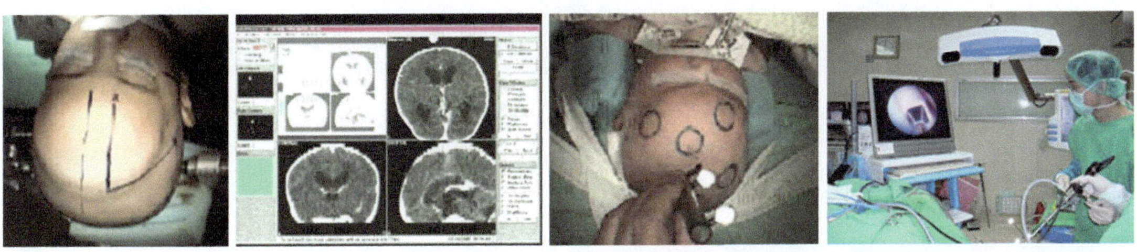

Fig. 14.8 Surgical incision and trajectory planning without (*left*) and with image guidance (*right*), insertion of the endoscope using image guided neuronavigation

capability and complication rate of neuroendoscopic biopsy and stereotactic needle biopsy are comparable [18]. For this reason, the ETB technique should be preferred especially for lesions within the ventricular walls [22]. The ETV technique has great results for the resolution of obstructive hydrocephalus due to lesions at the region of the posterior third ventricle, pineal, midbrain, and thalamus [23, 24]. At our hospital the trend of using ETV instead of VP shunt has changed the past decades and has turned to be the procedure of choice, and as a result fewer patients need a shunt (Table 14.5). ETV/ETB techniques are nowadays an important tool in the modern neurosurgeon's armamentarium and useful for the treatment of pineal lesions [25, 26].

Acknowledgment We would like to thank Dr C. Chamilos, of "Mitera" Children's Hospital, Athens, Greece, for the significant assistance in the writing of this manuscript.

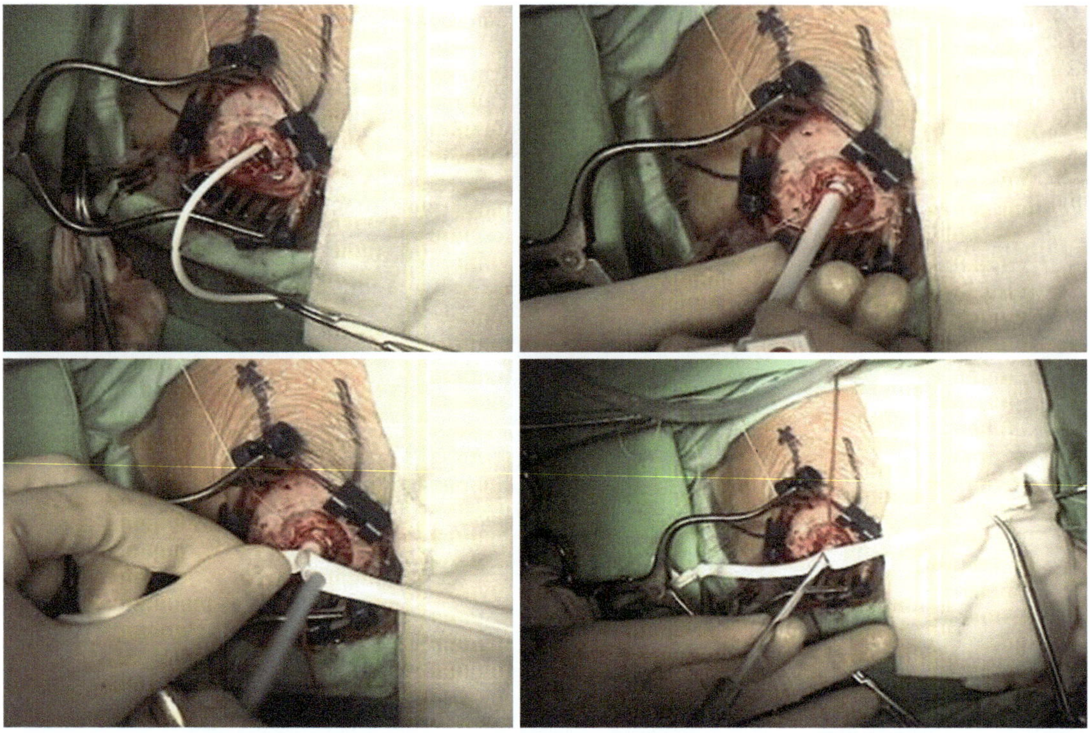

Fig. 14.9 Insertion and anchorage of peel-away transparent sheath trocar

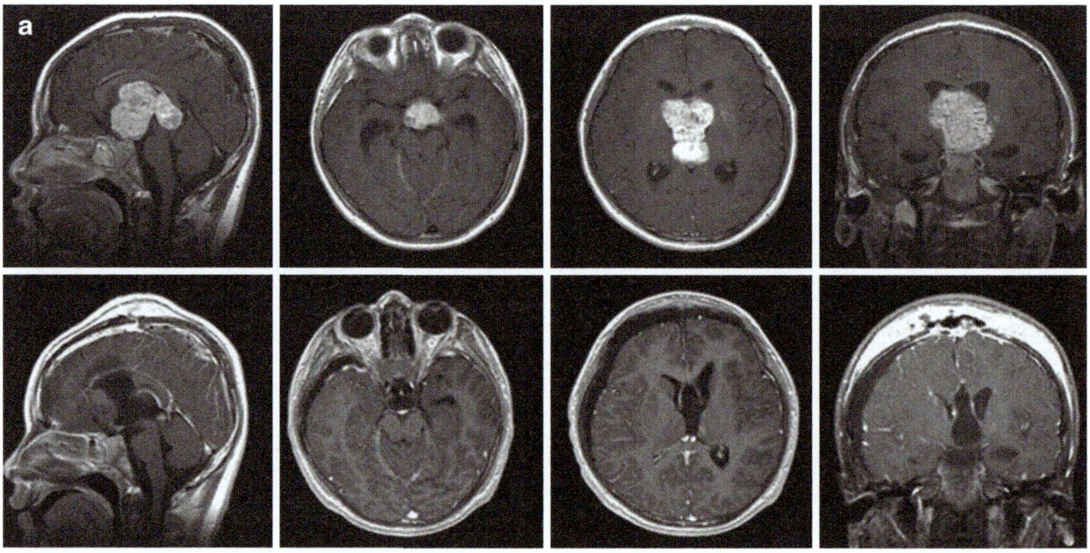

Fig. 14.10 Transcallosal interfoniceal approach for an 8-year-old boy with bifocal IT/YST/EC, ↑ serum AFP/HCG, endoscope-assisted gross total removal. (**a**) Preop (*upper row*), postop (*lower row*) MR images. (**b**) Intraoperative view of the tumor, seen through the endoscope

Fig. 14.10 (continued)

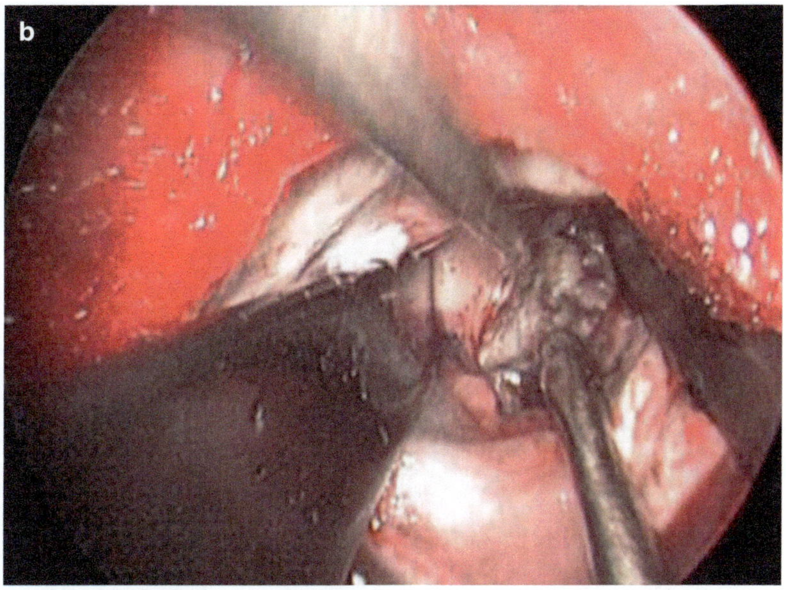

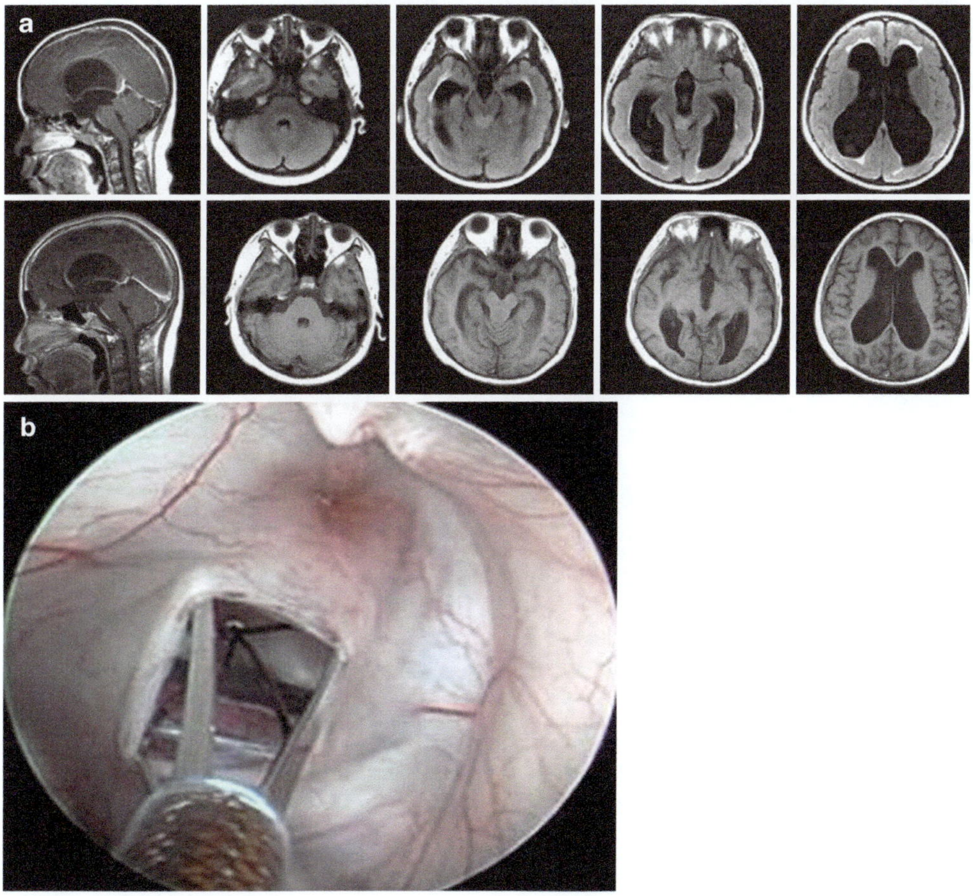

Fig. 14.11 Patient with midbrain tumor and hydrocephalus. (**a**) Preop (*upper row*) and postop images (*lower row*) after ETV. (**b**) Intraoperative during ETV. The basket perforator has created the stoma at the floor of the third ventricle and is dilating it

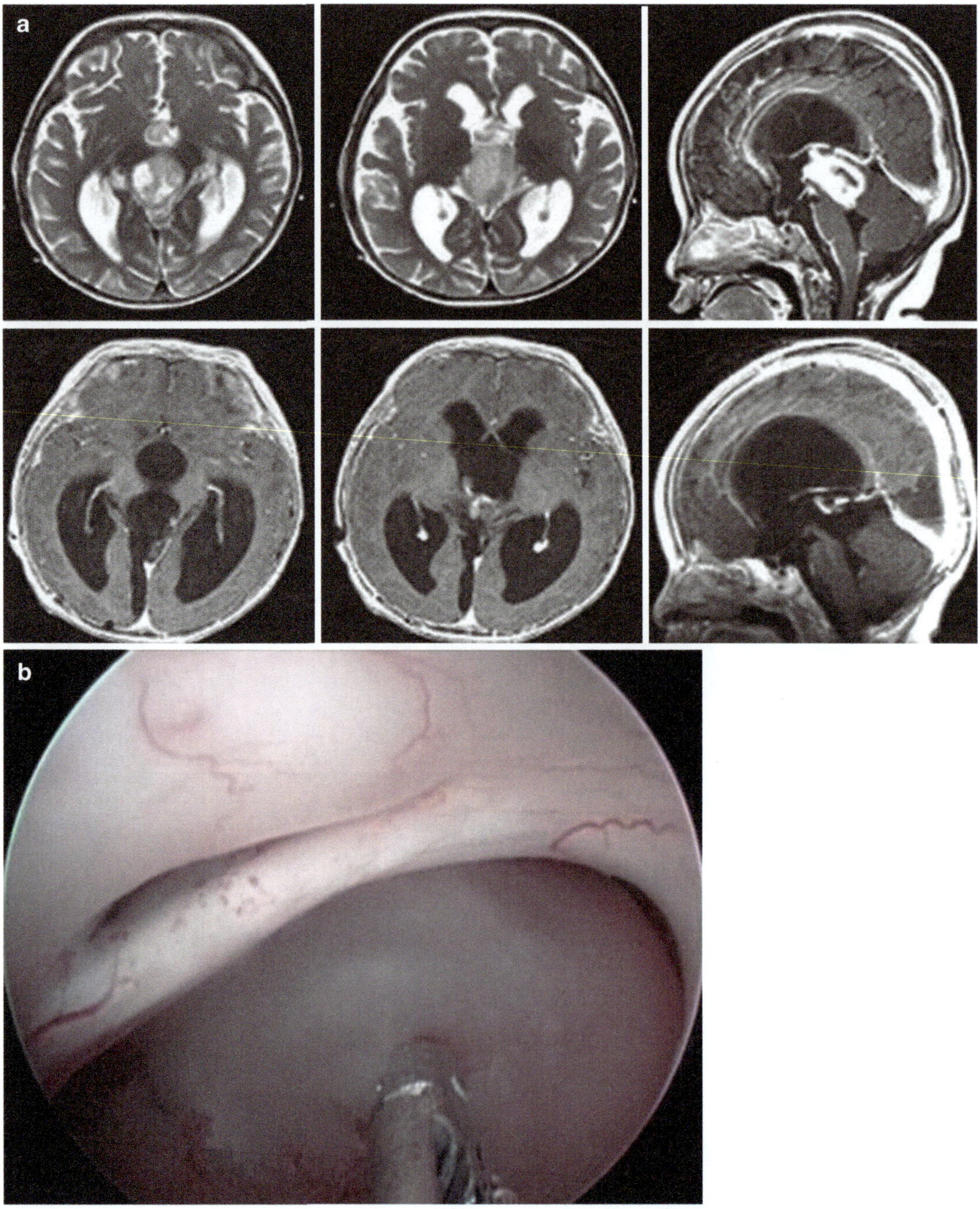

Fig. 14.12 An 11-month-old girl with midbrain anaplastic astrocytoma, hydrocephalus, s/p VP shunt at 7mos (referral hospital), ETV/ETB → NTR → SP shunt → VP shunt. (**a**) Preop (*upper row*) and postop (*lower row*) MR images. (**b**) Intraoperative view of endoscopic biopsy. (**c**) Intraoperative view of removal through occipital interhemispheric transtentorial approach

Fig. 14.12 (continued)

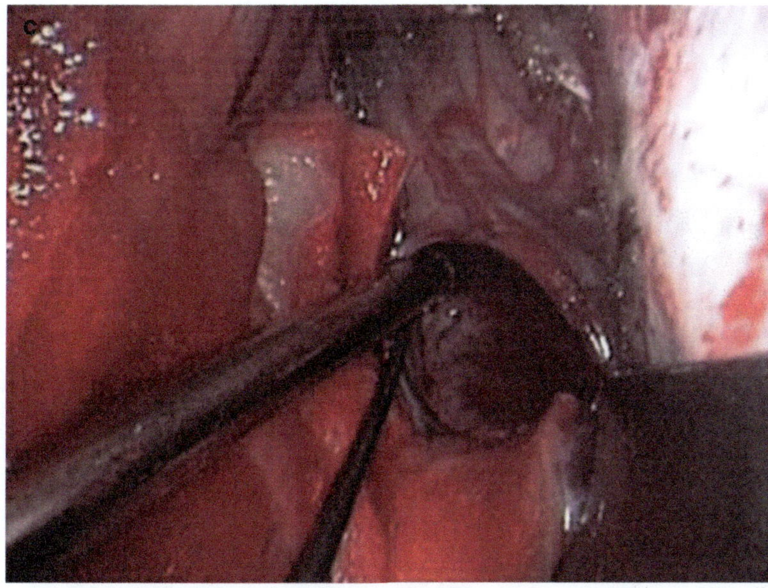

Table 14.4 ETV of 44 pineal and midbrain tumors at Taipei VGH

Location/no. of cases	NTV related to tumor resection			Histological Dx
	No./before	Along with	After	
	5/4	28	7	
Pineal 34	3/3	22	6	GCT 27
Sellar-pineal 5				G 11, MT 2
				NGMGCT 13
				Unclassified 2
				Pineoblastoma 6
				Ast. 1
Midbrain 10	*2/1*	*6*	1	Astrocytic T. 5
				PNET 1
				No hist. Dx 4

Dx diagnosis

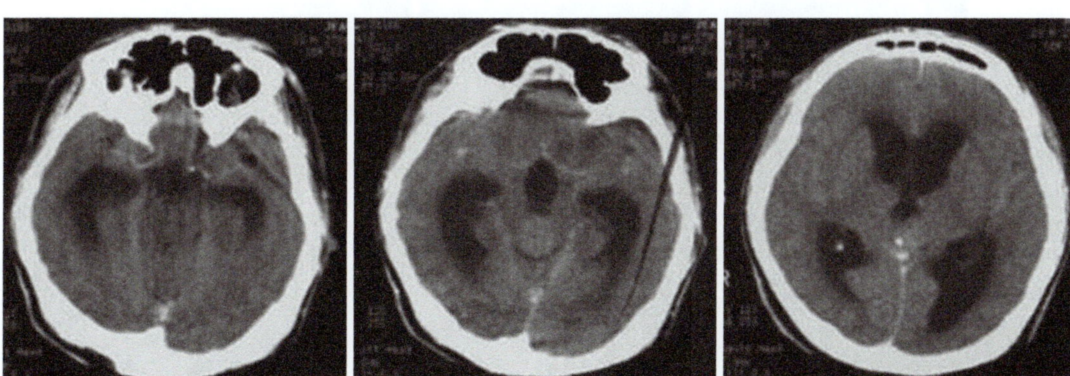

Fig. 14.13 A 21-year-old man with germinoma-YST. He died of delayed intratumoral hemorrhage 2 weeks after ETV and ETB

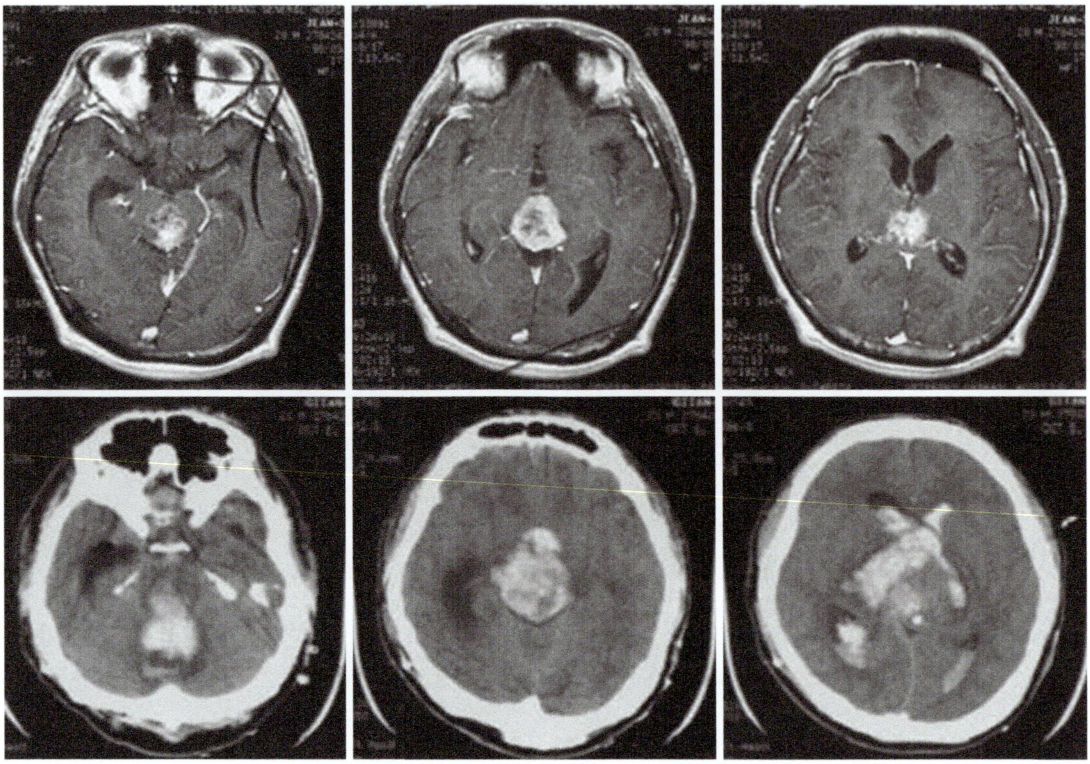

Fig. 14.13 (continued)

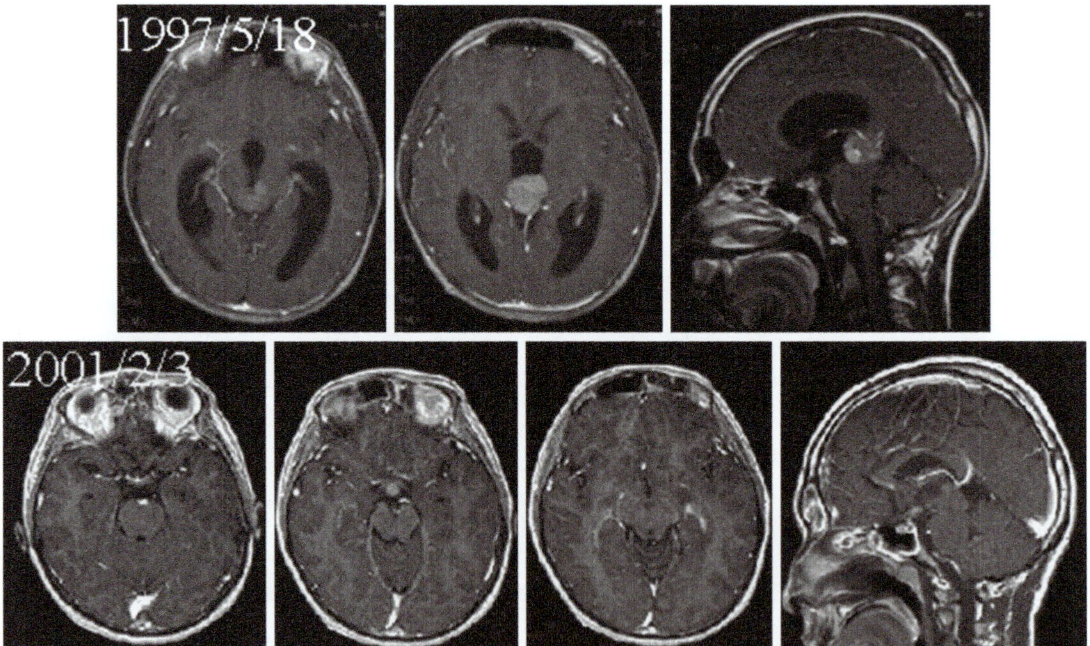

Fig. 14.14 A 15-year-old boy with normal serum tumor markers, ETV without tumor biopsy. He had chemotherapy with complete response (*upper row*). He developed recurrence 3.8 years later at the third ventricular floor (*lower row*)

Table 14.5 Changes of VP shunt insertion in different periods for posterior third ventricle, pineal, midbrain, and thalamus lesions at Taipei VGH, 1971–2008

Year period	No. of patients	No. (%) with hydrocephalus	No. (%) with VP shunt
1981–1990	28	24 (85.7 %)	24 (100 %)
1991–2000	50	45 (90.0 %)	41 (71.1 %)
2001–2008	54	46 (85.2 %)	11 (23.9 %)

References

1. Sood S, Hoeprich M, Ham SD (2011) Pure endoscopic removal of pineal region tumors. Childs Nerv Syst 27(9):1489–1492
2. Shono T, Natori Y, Morioka T, Torisu R, Mizoguchi M, Nagata S, Inamura T, Fukui M, Oka K, Sasaki T (2007) Results of a long-term follow-up after neuroendoscopic biopsy procedure and third ventriculostomy in patients with intracranial germinomas. J Neurosurg 107(Suppl 3):193–198
3. Morgenstern PF, Souweidane MM (2013) Pineal region tumors: simultaneous endoscopic third ventriculostomy and tumor biopsy. World Neurosurg 79(2):S18.e9–13
4. Oi S, Kamio M, Joki T, Abe T (2001) Neuroendoscopic anatomy and surgery in pineal region tumors: role of neuroendoscopic procedure in the 'minimally-invasive preferential management. J Neurooncol 54(3):277–286
5. The Committee of Brain Tumor Registry of Japan (2003) Brain tumor registry of Japan (1969–1996). Neurol Med Chir 43(Suppl):i–vii, 1–111
6. Wong TT, Ho DM, Chang KP, Yen SH, Guo WY, Chang FC, Liang ML, Pan HC, Chung WY (2005) Primary pediatric brain tumors: statistics of Taipei VGH, Taiwan (1975–2004). Cancer 104(10):2156–2167
7. Schmidek HH (2000) Management of pineal region neoplasms. In: Schmidek HH (ed) Operative neurosurgical techniques. Saunders, Philadelphia, pp 891–894
8. Fontana EJ, Garvin J, Feldstein N, Anderson RC (2011) Pediatric considerations for pineal tumor management. Neurosurg Clin N Am 22(3):395–402, ix
9. Blakeley JO, Grossman SA (2006) Management of pineal region tumors. Curr Treat Options Oncol 7(6):505–516
10. Kobayashi T, Lunsford LD (eds) (2009) Pineal region tumors, diagnosis and treatment options, Progress in neurological surgery. Karger, Basel. pp 26–43
11. Chen YW, Huang PI, Hu YW, Ho DM, Chang KP, Guo WY, Chang FC, Lee YY, Shiau CY, Wong TT, Yen SH (2012) Treatment strategies for initially disseminated intracranial germinomas: experiences at a single institute. Childs Nerv Syst 28(4):557–563
12. Oi S, Matsuzawa K, Choi JU, Kim DS, Kang JK, Cho BK (1998) Identical characteristics of the patient populations with pineal region tumours in Japan and Korea and therapeutic modalities. Childs Nerv Syst 14(1–2):36–40
13. Drummond KJ, Rosenfeld JV (1999) Pineal region tumours in childhood. A 30-year experience. Childs Nerv Syst 15(2–3):119–126
14. Wong TT, Liang ML, Chen HH, Chang FC (2011) Hydrocephalus with brain tumors in children. Childs Nerv Syst 27(10):1723–1734
15. Wong TT, Chen HH, Liang ML, Yen YS, Chang FC (2011) Neuroendoscopy in the management of pineal tumors. Childs Nerv Syst 27(6): 949–959
16. Naftel RP, Shannon CN, Reed GT, Martin R, Blount JP, Tubbs RS, Wellons JC 3rd (2011) Small-ventricle neuroendoscopy for pediatric brain tumor management. J Neurosurg Pediatr 7(1):104–110
17. O'Brien DF, Hayhurst C, Pizer B, Mallucci CL (2006) Outcomes in patients undergoing single-trajectory endoscopic third ventriculostomy and endoscopic biopsy for midline tumors presenting with obstructive hydrocephalus. J Neurosurg 105(3 Suppl):219–226
18. Costantini S, Sgouros S, Hellwig D, Veshchev I, Abbott R (2005) The International Neuroendoscopic Biopsy Study (INEBS): an ISGNE retrospective survey. Childs Nerv Syst 21:502
19. Lefranc M, Touzet G, Caron S, Maurage CA, Assaker R, Blond S (2011) Are stereotactic sample biopsies still of value in the modern management of pineal region tumours? Lessons from a single-department, retrospective series. Acta Neurochir (Wien) 153(5):1111–1121; discussion 1121–1122
20. Kombogiorgas D, Sgouros S (2006) Assessment of the influence of operative factors in the success of endoscopic third ventriculostomy in children. Childs Nerv Syst 22(10):1256–1262
21. Yamini B, Refai D, Rubin CM, Frim DM (2004) Initial endoscopic management of pineal region tumors and associated hydrocephalus: clinical series and literature review. J Neurosurg 100(5 Suppl Pediatrics):437–441
22. Ahn ES, Goumnerova L (2010) Endoscopic biopsy of brain tumors in children: diagnostic success and utility in guiding treatment strategies. J Neurosurg Pediatr 5(3):255–262
23. Ray P, Jallo GI, Kim RY, Kim BS, Wilson S, Kothbauer K, Abbott R (2005) Endoscopic third ventriculostomy for tumor-related hydrocephalus in a pediatric population. Neurosurg Focus 19(6):E8
24. Morgenstern PF, Osbun N, Schwartz TH, Greenfield JP, Tsiouris AJ, Souweidane MM (2011) Pineal region tumors: an optimal approach for simultaneous endoscopic third ventriculostomy and biopsy. Neurosurg Focus 30(4):E3
25. Al-Tamimi YZ, Bhargava D, Surash S, Ramirez RE, Novegno F, Crimmins DW, Tyagi AK, Chumas PD (2008) Endoscopic biopsy during third ventriculostomy in paediatric pineal region tumours. Childs Nerv Syst 24(11):1323–1326
26. Broggi M, Darbar A, Teo C (2010) The value of endoscopy in the total resection of pineocytomas. Neurosurgery 67(3 Suppl Operative):159–165

The "Complex" Management of Sylvian Fissure Arachnoid Cysts

15

Concezio Di Rocco, Federica Novegno, and Gianluca Trevisi

15.1 Introduction

Sylvian fissure arachnoid cysts are different from similar lesions localized in other intracranial regions. In fact, while the occurrence of chiasmatic, quadrigeminal, and, to a less extent, interhemispheric fissure cysts is nearly always recognized on the grounds of clinical manifestations of intracranial hypertension, a large proportion of the temporal region arachnoid cysts are detected incidentally in asymptomatic subjects undergoing neuroradiological examination for a variety of intercurrent causes (head injuries, psychomotor retardation, headache, and so on).

Furthermore, when "symptomatic," these cysts present with symptoms and signs so nonspecific to prevent any reliable surgical indication and, even more, to anticipate the surgical result. In spite of such significant limitations, the current debate among the neurosurgical community is mostly centered on the choice of the surgical procedure rather than aimed at evaluating the actual need to surgically treat all the subjects with Sylvian arachnoid cysts, including the asymptomatic ones.

C. Di Rocco, MD (✉) • G. Trevisi, MD
Department of Pediatric Neurosurgery,
Catholic University Medical School,
Largo Gemelli 8, 00168 Rome, Italy
e-mail: cdirocco@rm.unicatt.it

F. Novegno, MD
Department of Neurosurgery,
Tor Vergata University Medical School, Rome, Italy

15.2 The Limits of Surgical Indications

The surgical indication in cases of Sylvian fissure cysts is a challenging decision-making process. It can be easy in patients with symptoms or signs of increased intracranial pressure (Fig. 15.1) or in the presence of clear-cut focal neurological deficits attributable to a mass effect of the lesion. Unfortunately, in the great majority of the so-called symptomatic patients, the clinical manifestations referred to the cyst tend to be relatively nonspecific so as to make their causative relationships with the lesion disputable. In fact, Sylvian arachnoid cysts have been reported in association with a variety of conditions which include headache, epilepsy, psychomotor retardation, attention deficit, hyperactivity, manic depression, schizophrenia-like symptoms, paranoia, psychoses, anosmia, Ménière's disease, and hearing loss, just to quote the most frequently described [5].

Among the clinical manifestations of Sylvian fissure arachnoid cysts, three are considered to be particularly relevant for the surgical indication: headache, epilepsy, and psychomotor retardation.

Actually, about 70 % of "symptomatic" subjects complain of headache, which is often of a chronic type. Unfortunately the characteristics of this symptom are nearly always nonspecific and not easily attributable to the presence of the cyst. The headache, in fact, does not appear to correlate with the size of the cyst or to phenomena of compression/distortion over the neighboring vascular or meningeal structures. However, if not

S. Sgouros (ed.), *Neuroendoscopy*,
DOI 10.1007/978-3-642-39085-2_15, © Springer-Verlag Berlin Heidelberg 2014

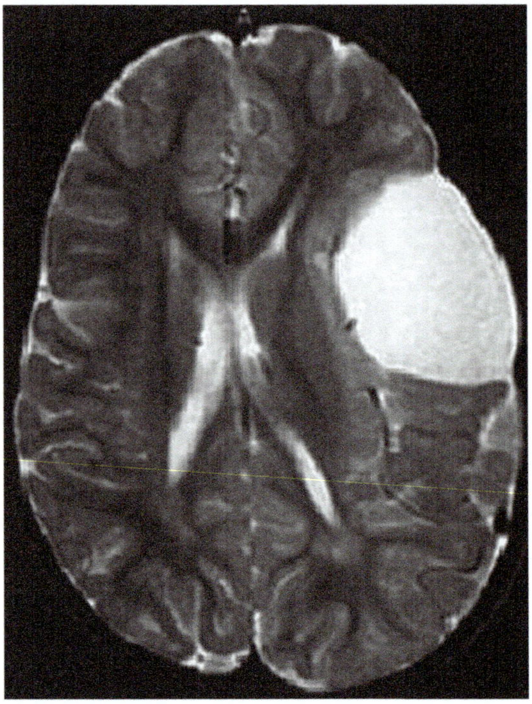

Fig. 15.1 Axial T2w MRI of left medium-size Sylvian cyst inducing a shift of midline cerebral structures with compression and distortion of the ipsilateral ventricle. CSF spaces of the convexity are reduced on the left side compared to the contralateral side. The volume of the left hemicranium is slightly bigger than the right one. The association of the abovementioned signs suggests a mass effect of the lesion

interpreted differently, headache may be considered at least for justification of further diagnostic work-up and even invasive intracranial pressure recordings [23].

Prolonged ICP recordings may actually reveal an abnormally high mean CSF pressure or point out the occurrence of abnormally high pressure waves during physiological sleep as well as arterial pulses of excessively large amplitude. On this ground, the results of a study we carried out on a series of pediatric patients with temporal cysts who underwent prolonged ICP recordings demonstrated that Galassi type I cysts were almost always associated with a normal ICP, whereas abnormally high ICP pressure values were found in all the Galassi type III cysts [4]. Both normal and abnormally high intracranial pressures could be detected in children with Galassi type II cysts, so making impossible to predict the values of intracranial pressure on the basis of neuroradiological investigations in this specific subgroup of patients, that is, in a significant percentage of cases.

Epilepsy is a common cause for performing neuroradiological exams; consequently it is possible that in some subjects these investigations may reveal the presence of temporal arachnoid cysts. However, a strict correlation of seizure disorder with the presence of the lesion is still lacking in the literature. First of all, in the majority of cases, there is no direct concordance of the seizures semeiology and the location of the cyst. Furthermore, in many children the electrophysiological exams often reveal contralateral anomalies, suggesting a high probability of associated diffuse developmental cortical anomalies involving also the opposite hemisphere. Finally, the surgical excision of the cyst or its marsupialization is not necessarily followed by seizure disappearance or reduction, even when the volume of the cyst is significantly reduced postoperatively.

Mental retardation and behavior problems are also described frequently in association with Sylvian fissure arachnoid cysts. With regard to epilepsy, the relationships between the cognitive and behavioral anomalies and the presence of the cyst are far to be demonstrated. In the same way, the benefit of surgical treatment over these symptoms is yet to be confirmed. Only a single group of scientists reported an improvement of the cognitive disorders on a series of adult patients [24]. In children, the majority of authors experienced different results: indeed, no significant psychomotor improvement has been reported regardless of the surgical modality and, above all, the entity of cysts size reduction in more recent series [1, 20, 23]. In fact, a primary developmental hypoplasia of the temporal lobe rather than an atrophy or compression exerted by the lesion may be taken into account for the interpretation of the clinical manifestations. In favor of such a hypothesis is also the common observation of absent neuropsychological impairment even in children with large cysts and those located into the dominant hemisphere.

Large percentages of patients having arachnoid cysts in the middle cranial fossa identified by radiological means develop no symptoms at all

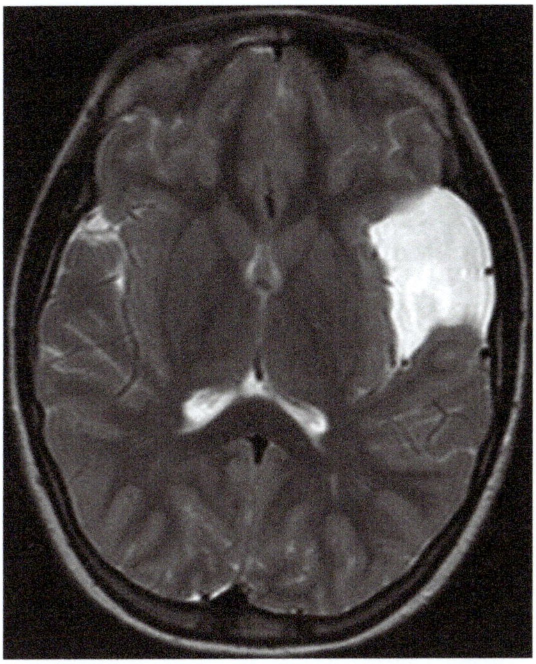

Fig. 15.2 Axial T2w MRI of left medium-size Sylvian cyst showing no mass effect on the adjacent cerebral parenchyma. This patient was followed for 4 years after diagnosis, and neither symptoms nor signs which could be referred to the lesion were exhibited by the patient during that period

(Fig. 15.2) [21]. Indeed, as was pointed out from an international survey [23], most pediatric neurosurgeons (more than 60 %) would adopt a "wait and see" policy in cases of incidental diagnosis or at least would suggest further diagnostic examinations, such as functional MRI, cine-MRI, SPECT, PET neuropsychological evaluations, and EEG to confirm the pathological role of the lesion.

No doubts concerning surgical indication arise when symptoms or signs due to increased intracranial pressure are detected, namely, focal neurological deficit or decreased consciousness, often related to a hemorrhagic complication; however these are, actually, rare events. However, in the absence of specific symptoms related to a localized or diffused increasing intracranial pressure, several authors advocate the use of a "prophylactic" operation in order to prevent the risk of intracranial bleeding due to spontaneous or traumatic tearing of the cyst linings and their fragile vessels, resulting in intracranial hemorrhage and subdural fluid accumulation. The actual incidence of spontaneous rupture of middle cranial fossa arachnoid cysts is still unknown: Bilginer et al. found a 2.27 % incidence of subdural hematoma requiring surgical therapy over a series of 132 pediatric patients [3]. In a retrospective review of 343 patients affected by Sylvian fissure arachnoid cysts, Sprung et al. found a series of 60 cases (17.4 %) admitted for subdural and/or intracystic effusions, among whom 54 (15.7 % of the entire series of 343 patients) required surgical intervention [21]; they found also that most of the cysts (41/60) fulfilled the criteria for type II cysts, that subdural effusions were mostly ipsilateral located and occurred after traumatic events, and that almost half of the patients were younger than 19 years of age. This occurrence rate of subdural collections is significantly higher than those reported by other authors [25] and was interpreted as due to the large number of cases who were referred to the center as well as to the common availability of a CT scan examination.

Overall, according to the available data from the literature, the incidence of subdural fluid collections in the set of untreated temporal arachnoid cysts may be estimated from about 2–17.4 % of cases, which does not differ significantly from the occurrence rate described in most series after surgical operation, challenging so far the prophylactic value of the surgical treatment of temporal arachnoid cysts for such type of risk [5]. In particular, in the series by Spacca et al., four patients suffered a head injury 3–60 months after successful surgery resulting in hemorrhagic complications [20]. Moreover, spontaneous disappearance of even large middle cranial fossa cysts has been described [2, 18, 26].

15.3 The Choice of Surgical Technique

The main goals of the surgical treatment of Sylvian fissure arachnoid cysts are the elimination of the mass effect of the lesion and the prevention of its recurrence in order to improve or normalize the CSF dynamics. These goals can be pursued with a variety of surgical procedures: extra-thecal shunts from the cyst to the peritoneal cavity, shunting of the cyst content into the ventricular system, microsurgical opening (marsupialization) of the cyst linings into the adjacent arachnoid spaces and cisterns, cyst lining excision, and endoscopic opening of the cyst into the basal cisterns.

According to a recent international survey among pediatric neurosurgeons [23], craniotomy and cyst wall marsupialization/removal was considered the primary surgical treatment in 66 % of the obtained responses; 28.8 % of the neurosurgeons interviewed would prefer an endoscopic approach (pure 15.5 % and assisted 13.3 %, respectively). Only 6.6 % would consider, nowadays, cysto-peritoneal shunt as the first-line treatment in Sylvian fissure arachnoid cysts.

In recent years, the cysto-peritoneal shunt, once regarded the most simple and effective procedure to treat Sylvian fissure arachnoid cysts, has been progressively abandoned because of the known complications of shunt surgery (shunt malfunction, occlusion, infection) [1, 11, 19] and, in particular, the late development of shunt dependency and acquired Chiari type I malformation, even though the procedure is associated with the higher evidence of objective results, that is, the cerebral parenchyma re-expansion.

Consequently, cyst lining excision and cyst membrane marsupialization have become the most utilized techniques worldwide. Unfortunately, the degree of cerebral parenchymal re-expansion associated with these types of surgical procedure as shown by computed tomographic (CT) scan or magnetic resonance imaging (MRI) is not so obvious as in cases managed by cysto-peritoneal shunt. As a result, the "success" of the surgical treatment is more difficult to establish when using these techniques.

Paradoxically, the comparative analysis of series focusing on the surgical outcomes may only define the percentage of "failure," that is, a cyst whose size remains unchanged after the surgical treatment with certainty. On the other hand, successes are considerably more difficult to be assessed in the large majority of patients, that is, in cases where the cyst decreases in size only partially.

Indeed, some authors simply report "satisfactory" reduction of the cyst without referring to the relative decrease in size of the lesion or to absolute numeric values defining the entity of the surgical "success." Others group into the category of good outcome all the cases in which the size of the lesion appears to be diminished after the operation using, however, adjectives such as "minimal," "partial," "moderate," and "incomplete" which obviously do not allow a reliable evaluation or comparative analysis. Actually, the "complete" resolution of the cyst is rarely reported. Furthermore, only exceptionally the postoperative modifications of the cyst volume, which define the surgical outcome, have been associated with the effects of the treatment on the clinical manifestations. It is evident how, in the absence of objective evaluation criteria, the definition of outcomes might be biased by the subjective judgment of the neurosurgeon. The neuroradiologist could contribute to alleviate such a limitation not only by measuring the degree of the cyst reduction objectively but by furnishing also additional data with regard to the cerebrovascular compression, stretching, and distortion. Unfortunately, even though the introduction of progressively more effective neuroimaging tools to calculate the volume of the cyst might provide more sound figures in the future, until now no objective measurements are available to relate the "success" of the surgical treatment based on the variations of specific pre- and postoperative parameters.

Historically, the principal debate over temporal arachnoid cysts management has focused on the comparison of microsurgical techniques and shunt implantation [1, 8, 14, 16, 19, 28], endoscopic procedure being applied increasingly on temporal arachnoid cysts cases "only" in the last 10 years [6, 7, 9, 10, 13, 15, 20].

The implantation of a cysto-peritoneal shunt has been considered for long time the less invasive surgical procedure to treat temporal arachnoid cysts in terms of perioperative morbidity with a higher success rate of significant decrease in size or complete obliteration of the cyst [19].

Cysto-peritoneal shunts, however, are weighted by the constant risk of shunt infections/malfunctions, occlusions, as well as shunt dependency [1, 11, 19]. Later on, the occurrence of hindbrain caudal and upward herniation may be observed due to a progressive craniocerebral disproportion, especially in subjects operated on in early age [5]. Differently from a ventriculoperitoneal CSF shunt, the cysto-peritoneal shunt should, at least theoretically, drain from a close cavity, consequently making difficult to understand why the induced change in size of the lesion may differ in the various patients, without considering a coexisting primary hypoplasia of the temporal lobe. Some attempts have been made to investigate the action of this type of shunt. Arai et al. in a series of 77 subjects with temporal arachnoid cyst who had undergone the implantation of a cysto-peritoneal shunt device monitored the intracystic pulse wave by puncturing the shunt system [1]. They found that the intracystic pressure and the amplitude of the intracystic pulse wave increased when the shunt was closed to subsequently decrease when it was open. The authors concluded that the action of the shunt in decreasing the cyst volume was not limited to the fluid subtraction but also at diminishing a possible pathogenetic factor for cyst enlargement, namely, the intracystic pressure pulsations. They also proposed the removal of the outer membrane of the cysts wall to avoid shunt malfunction, considering that the outer membrane detaches easily from the dura mater after the shunt procedure, causing plugging of the shunt tube.

On the other hand, open craniotomy and cyst fenestration with or without cyst wall removal are considered an aggressive approach, being weighted by major complications, namely, subdural hematomas or hygromas, oculomotor palsy, meningitis, hemiparesis, seizures, and even death [22]; however, this type of procedures allows marsupialization of the cyst under direct microscopic vision, avoiding stripping of the arachnoid membrane so reducing the risk of bleeding [9]. Actually, in recent reports, perioperative mortality and morbidity are similar in comparison with shunting procedures [23]. According to some authors [19], the complete removal of the cyst wall is neither possible nor necessary to obtain an effective decompression of the cyst. However, despite anecdotal reports suggesting that a limited partial excision of the cyst wall might be an effective and sufficient treatment, fenestration of the cyst into the basilar cisterns has widely proved to offer a greater chance of successfully dealing with the condition and restoring normal CSF dynamics, resulting in the elimination of the need of a shunt in many cases [16].

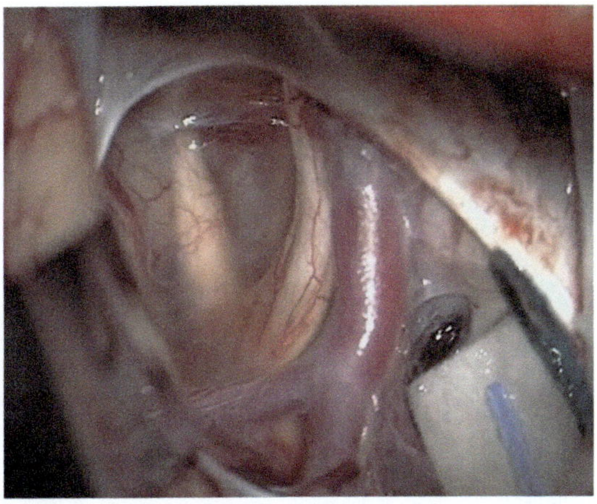

Fig. 15.3 Microscopic visualization during the opening of the basal cyst's membrane into the basal cisterns

The keyhole microsurgical approach performing a minicraniotomy has proved to be effective in treating temporal arachnoid cysts with a success rate over 80 % [17] (Fig. 15.3).

With the advent of neuroendoscopy and the progressive improvement of neurosurgeons' expertise in approaching intracranial pathologies endoscopically, the debate has been extended, further focusing on the possible advantage of the technique in creating alternative CSF pathways. However, the results reported in the literature are still controversial [6, 7, 10, 13, 15, 19, 20].

The main criticisms to the endoscopic management of temporal arachnoid cysts address its technical limitations mainly. The available instrumentation allows the use of only an instrument at the time in the working channel or two instruments, in the case of larger diameter endoscopes, working in the same axis of the endoscope, so that the control of hemostasis (bleeding may reduce the vision,

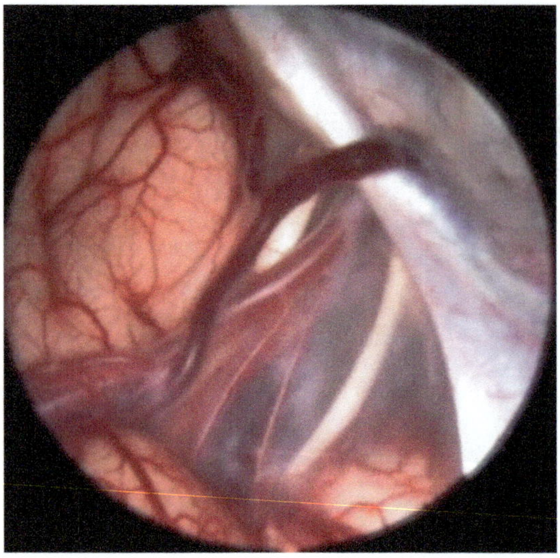

Fig. 15.4 Endoscopic view during the fenestration of the basal membrane of a Sylvian fissure arachnoid cyst showing similar visualization to that provided by the microscopic approach. The fine delineation of the third cranial nerve and the perforating branches of the internal carotid artery is noted

imposing the interruption of the procedure) or the action of pulling gently the thick arachnoidal membranes may be difficult [6]. Another issue is related to the possibility of losing the orientation especially within large and dark cavities, whose topographic anatomy may be rather disorienting. Neuronavigation may be useful in this context in order to plan the best trajectory and to provide real-time control of the endoscope position, with the limit of possible modifications of landmarks due to intraoperative CSF loss [20, 23]. However, type II cysts may be challenging for the endoscopic approach because the temporal lobe may constitute an obstacle along the ideal trajectory line toward the basal cistern [19].

If the endoscope bears the significant limitation of monocular vision compared to the microscope, it has the advantage of allowing a better visualization of the different membranes in cases of loculated cysts that have to be opened to ensure a sufficient flow (Fig. 15.4) [6]. When flexible endoscopes are utilized, a further advantage is the possible shifting in the line of action according to the specific morphology of the lesion.

Johnson et al. reported the results of a series of 91 reviewed cases from the literature, treated using endoscopic techniques with a 95 % successful clinical improvement (74 % cyst reduction) [13]. Most recent series showed a satisfactory clinical outcome in 90–92.5 % of cases, with a significant cyst reduction in the range of 55–75 % of the cases [10, 15, 20].

According to the review of 304 cases affected by temporal arachnoid cysts by Gangemi et al. over a cohort of 160 patients treated by craniotomy and cyst excision, 141 (88 %) had a complete or partial clinical remission; among 94 patients treated with cysto-peritoneal shunt, 91 (96.8 %) had "good" clinical outcome, and among 50 cases of endoscopic treatment, 35 (70 %) showed clinical improvement [9].

If the aim of the surgical treatment is obtaining cyst size reduction, some authors [1, 19] showed that CP shunt was the best option for the complete obliteration of large cyst in infants or young children, although with a high shunt-related complications.

From a retrospective review of the last 34 consecutive cases of middle cranial fossa cysts randomly selected to be treated microscopically or endoscopically in a 6-year period at our institution (unpublished data), we observed that patients younger than 3 years of age at treatment presented a variable reduction of the cyst size (from a mild, less than 25 %, to a noticeable, more than 75 %, decrease in volume). None of the cysts of these very young children resulted unmodified or increased in size at radiological follow-up after the operation. In particular, about one fourth of them (26.7 %) were noticeably reduced in size (more of 75 % of the preoperative volume) (Fig. 15.5) and a further fourth were minimally decreased (less than 25 % of the preoperative volume). The degree of reduction of the remaining cysts (46.6 %) ranged among these two extremes. On the other hand, about 1/3 (31.6 %) of the children older than 3 years did not show any modification in their volume after the operation (Fig. 15.6). Among this age group only 10.5 % of the children showed a more than 75 % cyst volume reduction. Another 31.6 % had a mild reduction (less than 25 %) and 26.3 % of the cysts had a volume reduction between 25 and 75 %.

The two age groups, comparable for Galassi classification, also showed a different rate of

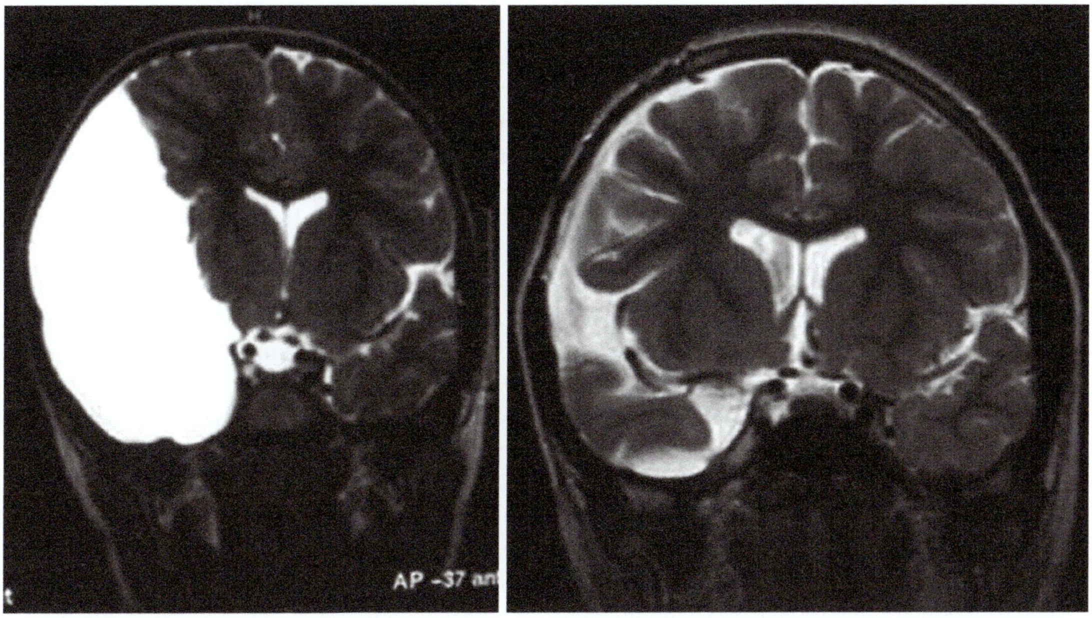

Fig. 15.5 Preoperative (*left*) and postoperative (*right*) coronal T2w MRI images of right Sylvian arachnoid cyst. Brain re-expansion and cyst's volume reduction after marsupialization of cyst membrane. CSF is normally distributed within peripheral subarachnoid spaces and the midline shift is resolved

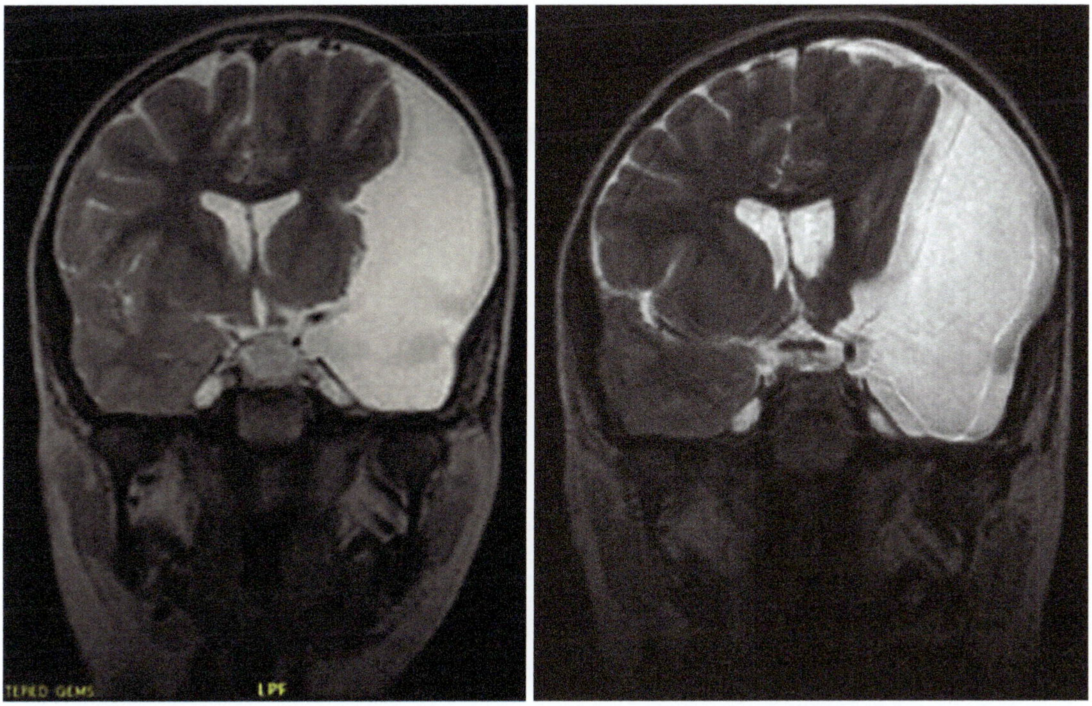

Fig. 15.6 Preoperative (*left*) and postoperative (*right*) coronal T2w MRI images of left Sylvian arachnoid cyst. Marsupialization of the cyst linings resulted in minimal re-expansion of the left lateral ventricle without significant changes of the cyst volume. An associated minimal subdural fluid collection is noted

long-term complications. Out of the older group, 10.5 % of the children, two out of six of patients who had no cyst reduction, finally needed a cysto-peritoneal shunt insertion. Another 15.8 % of the patients older than 3 years of age developed a postoperative hygroma that needed a permanent subdural-peritoneal shunt. In contrast, only 1 out of 15 (6.7 %) patients in the younger age group (less than 3 years old) needed the insertion of a permanent subdural-peritoneal shunt because of postoperative subdural hygroma. These data seem to indicate that patients younger than 3 years of age have a higher chance of brain re-expansion and lower rate of long-term complications. In other words, age more than the type of surgical treatment influenced the results in the population considered.

Our data further support what was observed by Di Rocco et al. [6] who stated that among their series of 17 patients who underwent endoscopic procedure for fenestration of Sylvian fissure arachnoid cysts, children operated on before age 1 had a complete reduction in volume of the cysts and an expansion of the temporal lobe at last neuroimaging follow-up.

An interesting hypothesis concerning the age factor is that by Zada et al. [27]. The authors observed that patients under 2 years of age affected by temporal arachnoid cysts are more prone to present with nonspecific macrocephaly, in some cases associated to mild ventriculomegaly, confirming previous observation by Levy et al. [17]. In a retrospective series of 22 patients under 2 years of age at diagnosis affected by temporal arachnoid cysts, they found that these are more likely to become shunt dependent and propounded a direct relationship between the development of an arachnoid cyst and an abnormal CSF dynamics, suggesting that the development and expansion of arachnoid cyst may be considered a form *frusta* of hydrocephalus.

Actually, most of the postoperative complications of the treatment of Sylvian arachnoid cysts appear to depend on the complex relationships of these cysts and CSF pathways, rather than on surgical modality chosen [5]. In fact, even with comparable results in terms of clinical outcome, what endoscopy has not yet eliminated in comparison with microsurgical approach is the occurrence of postoperative subdural hygromas, reported in 5–23.5 % of cases, which may end in the necessary placement of a permanent subdural-peritoneal shunt in a significant proportion of the operated-on subjects (4–6 % of the cases) [6, 7, 10, 12, 15, 20, 22]. It is worth noting that these figures are two- to threefold higher than the incidence of the same complication occurring in the natural history of the condition (following the spontaneous or posttraumatic rupture of the cyst). On the base of this high incidence of postoperative subdural hygroma, Elhammady et al. proposed a transcortical approach to minimize the risk of cerebrospinal fluid diversion into the subdural space, with the aim of avoiding extra-axial fluid collections in the postoperative phase [7]. The effectiveness of the technique has not been confirmed yet.

Conclusion

Temporal arachnoid cysts continue to represent a challenging lesion for the neurosurgeon faced with a difficult surgical indication in cases of incidental discovery in asymptomatic subjects or recognition in patients presenting with nonspecific clinical manifestations, whose relationships to the presence of the cyst is questionable. In symptomatic subjects for whom surgical treatment is advised, further difficulties arise in the choice of the surgical option. Cysto-peritoneal shunting, once considered the most reliable and safe procedure, has been practically abandoned nowadays due to unacceptable rates of short-term and late complications. Consequently the current debate is about the comparison of microscopic and endoscopic techniques to be utilized in the fenestration of the cyst and the creation of alternative communication for the fluid content to drain within the subarachnoid spaces of the cranial base. Both techniques have the same limitations and are associated with the same complications, in particular postoperative subdural fluid accumulation, which may require further surgical treatment in a significant percentage of the cases. It is apparent that more than a technical advance the management of Sylvian fissure arachnoid cyst needs more reliable ways to identify the candidates for the surgical treatment, better understanding of the surgical goals, and more objective evaluation tools to assess successes as well as failures.

References

1. Arai H, Sato K, Wachi A, Okuda O, Takeda N (1996) Arachnoid cysts of the middle cranial fossa: experience with 77 patients who were treated with cystoperitoneal shunting. Neurosurgery 39(6):1108–1112
2. Beltramello A, Mazza C (1985) Spontaneous disappearance of a large middle fossa arachnoid cyst. Surg Neurol 24(2):181–183
3. Bilginer B, Onal MB, Oguz KK, Akalan N (2009) Arachnoid cyst associated with subdural hematoma: report of three cases and review of the literature. Childs Nerv Syst 25(1):119–124
4. Di Rocco C, Tamburrini G, Caldarelli M, Velardi F, Santini P (2003) Prolonged ICP monitoring in Sylvian arachnoid cysts. Surg Neurol 60(3):211–218
5. Di Rocco C (2010) Sylvian fissure arachnoid cysts: we do operate on them but should it be done? Childs Nerv Syst 26(2):173–175
6. Di Rocco F, R James S, Roujeau T, Puget S, Sainte-Rose C, Zerah M (2010) Limits of endoscopic treatment of Sylvian arachnoid cysts in children. Childs Nerv Syst 26(2):155–162
7. Elhammady MS, Bhatia S, Ragheb J (2007) Endoscopic fenestration of middle fossa arachnoid cysts: a technical description and case series. Pediatr Neurosurg 43(3):209–215
8. Fewel ME, Levy ML, McComb JG (1996) Surgical treatment of 95 children with 102 intracranial arachnoid cysts. Pediatr Neurosurg 25(4):165–173
9. Gangemi M, Seneca V, Colella G, Cioffi V, Imperato A, Maiuri F (2011) Endoscopy versus microsurgical cyst excision and shunting for treating intracranial arachnoid cysts. J Neurosurg Pediatr 8(2):158–164
10. Gui SB, Wang XS, Zong XY, Li CZ, Li B, Zhang YZ (2011) Assessment of endoscopic treatment for middle cranial fossa arachnoid cysts. Childs Nerv Syst 27(7):1121–1128
11. Hamid NA, Sgouros S (2005) The use of an adjustable valve to treat over-drainage of a cyst-peritoneal shunt in a child with a large sylvian fissure arachnoid cyst. Childs Nerv Syst 21:991–994
12. Hopf NJ, Perneczky A (1998) Endoscopic neurosurgery and endoscope-assisted microneurosurgery for the treatment of intracranial cysts. Neurosurgery 43(6):1330–1336
13. Johnson RD, Chapman S, Bojanic S (2011) Endoscopic fenestration of middle cranial fossa arachnoid cysts: does size matter? J Clin Neurosci 18(5):607–612
14. Kang JK, Lee KS, Lee IW, Jeun SS, Son BC, Jung CK, Park YS, Lee SW (2000) Shunt-independent surgical treatment of middle cranial fossa arachnoid cysts in children. Childs Nerv Syst 16(2):111–116
15. Karabagli H, Etus V (2012) Success of pure neuroendoscopic technique in the treatment of Sylvian arachnoid cysts in children. Childs Nerv Syst 28(3):445–452
16. Levy ML, Wang M, Aryan HE, Yoo K, Meltzer H (2003) Microsurgical keyhole approach for middle fossa arachnoid cyst fenestration. Neurosurgery 53(5):1138–1144
17. Levy ML, Meltzer HS, Hughes S, Aryan HE, Yoo K, Amar AP (2004) Hydrocephalus in children with middle fossa arachnoid cysts. J Neurosurg 101(Suppl 1):25–31
18. McDonald PJ, Rutka JT (1997) Middle cranial fossa arachnoid cysts that come and go. Report of two cases and review of the literature. Pediatr Neurosurg 26(1):48–52
19. Shim KW, Lee YH, Park EK, Park YS, Choi JU, Kim DS (2009) Treatment option for arachnoid cysts. Childs Nerv Syst 25(11):1459–1466
20. Spacca B, Kandasamy J, Mallucci CL, Genitori L (2010) Endoscopic treatment of middle fossa arachnoid cysts: a series of 40 patients treated endoscopically in two centres. Childs Nerv Syst 26(2):163–172
21. Sprung C, Armbruster B, Koeppen D, Cabraja M (2011) Arachnoid cysts of the middle cranial fossa accompanied by subdural effusions–experience with 60 consecutive cases. Acta Neurochir (Wien) 153(1):75–84
22. Tamburrini G, Caldarelli M, Massimi L, Santini P, Di Rocco C (2003) Subdural hygroma: an unwanted result of Sylvian arachnoid cyst marsupialization. Childs Nerv Syst 19(3):159–165
23. Tamburrini G, Dal Fabbro M, Di Rocco C (2008) Sylvian fissure arachnoid cysts: a survey on their diagnostic workout and practical management. Childs Nerv Syst 24(5):593–604
24. Wester K, Hugdhal K (1995) Arachnoid cysts of the temporal fossa: impaired preoperative cognition and postoperative improvement. J Neurol Neurosurg Psychiatry 59:293–298
25. Wester K, Helland CA (2008) How often do chronic extra-cerebral haematomas occur in patients with intracranial arachnoid cysts? J Neurol Neurosurg Psychiatry 79(1):72–75
26. Yamauchi T, Saeki N, Yamaura A (1999) Spontaneous disappearance of temporo-frontal arachnoid cyst in a child. Acta Neurochir (Wien) 141(5):537–540
27. Zada G, Krieger MD, McNatt SA, Bowen I, McComb JG (2007) Pathogenesis and treatment of intracranial arachnoid cysts in pediatric patients younger than 2 years of age. Neurosurg Focus 22(2):E1
28. Zeng L, Feng L, Wang J, Li J, Wang Y, Chen J, Chen J, Lei T, Li L (2008) Comparative study on two surgical procedures for middle cranial fossa arachnoid cysts. J Huazhong Univ Sci Technolog Med Sci 28(4):431–434

Neuroendoscopy in Spinal Pathology: Our Experience, New Trends, and Developments

16

Alvaro Cordoba

16.1 Introduction

Current trends in surgical disciplines have been directed toward the use of minimally invasive, effective forms of diagnosis and treatment. Endoscopy represents one such modality in the spectrum of minimally invasive techniques. Although current interest in endoscopy is great, the application of endoscopic surgery for the treatment of neurosurgical disorders is not new.

The general components of instruments for neurosurgical endoscopy are identical to those of the instrumentation used in other surgical disciplines, except for the small size of the neurosurgical endoscope. Presently, two general types of endoscopes are available: rigid lens scopes and fiberscopes. Rigid endoscopes transmit images through a series of lenses, whereas fiberscopes transmit images through carefully arranged optic fibers. Rigid systems give clearer images than fiberscopes, but fiberscopes can be bent or maneuvered without image distortion. In addition to the basic elements for viewing, other ports or working channels may be available for the insertion of instruments, including energy delivery systems (i.e., laser fibers or electrocautery systems) and irrigation apparatuses (with or without suction). The diameter of the working channel is the factor limiting the type of endoscopic instrumentation that can be developed. Rigid scopes that offer an assortment of different viewing angles are available but are useful only for viewing. Preoperative planning determines the appropriate endoscope for a particular procedure. Although a procedure may be viewed directly through the endoscope, most surgeons (the author included) prefer to operate with the aid of a viewing system that comprises of a camera, a monitor, and a light source. The light source is connected to the endoscope via a fiberoptic cable and must be bright enough to illuminate the operative field without transmitting excessive heat to the scope tip. Halogen, mercury vapor, and xenon light sources are available. The camera, which is connected to the endoscope via an adaptor, transmits the image to a video monitor for viewing by the surgical team. Irrigation is essential during the operative procedure to clear the lens of debris, clear the operative field of any blood, and help prevent collapse of the CSF spaces; care must be taken in the amount of irrigation.

Spinal endoscopic procedures were performed in cadavers by Burman in 1931 and Stern in 1936 and were first performed in patients by Pool in 1938. Pool's primitive instrumentation enabled the visualization of the intradural contents and the diagnosis of arachnoiditis and spinal neoplasms. Despite significant advances in endoscope technology, few references exist between these early reports and recent ones that describe the application of endoscopy to the examination

A. Cordoba, MD
Minimal Invasive Neurosurgery,
British Hospital, Montevideo, Uruguay
e-mail: alvarocordoba61@gmail.com

Tribute to Prof. Dr. Roberto De Bellis – In Memoriam

S. Sgouros (ed.), *Neuroendoscopy*,
DOI 10.1007/978-3-642-39085-2_16, © Springer-Verlag Berlin Heidelberg 2014

of the various compartments of the spinal axis [11, 12, 15, 18]. Perhaps the greatest challenge to endoscopic applications for neurosurgery is presented by the extradural space.

16.2 Endoscopic Applications in the Intradural Compartment

16.2.1 Cyst Fenestration

The spinal axis can be divided into the intradural and extradural compartments. The intradural compartment can be divided further into the intramedullary and extramedullary components. Endoscopic applications in the intradural compartment include fenestration of both the extramedullary cysts and the intramedullary cavities commonly seen in hydrosyringomyelia.

Huewel and colleagues described the use of a fiberscope to inspect intramedullary cavities in syringomyelia [6]. After a myelotomy has been performed, a small-diameter fiberscope inserted into the spinal cord syrinx is used to visualize the many septations traversing the cavity and, in rare instances, the compartmentalization of the syrinx. Fenestration of the membranes permits communication throughout the syrinx and facilitates its complete collapse. Biopsy of an intramedullary tumor associated with a syrinx has also been performed, but complete resection of spinal cord neoplasms has not been reported.

For extramedullary applications, the subarachnoid space permits introduction of small fiberscopes into the spinal canal. Potential applications include fenestration of either arachnoid cysts or postoperative cysts that originate from previous spinal procedures [2, 4, 8, 11–13, 18].

16.3 Endoscopic Applications in the Extradural Compartment

16.3.1 Endoscopic Discectomy

Within the extradural compartment, efforts have been directed at endoscopic discectomy, including cervical discectomies, thoracoscopic removal of thoracic discs, posterolateral approaches for removal of L4–L5 discs, and laparoscopic approaches for removal of L5–S1 discs (Fig. 16.1). Paraspinal tumors in the thoracic and lumbar regions may also be approached with thoracoscopic and laparoscopic techniques, respectively. The current surgical management for lumbar disc disease is microsurgical discectomy, a safe and effective procedure that requires a short hospital stay. Although percutaneous lumbar discectomy encompasses many techniques, its goal is to remove herniated nucleus pulposus in the dorsal portion of the disc space. However, if an endoscope is not used, most percutaneous techniques are limited to removal of the central disc contents. If subligamentous prolapse is included in the spectrum of indications, then endoscopic control is necessary. Single and biportal approaches as well as transforaminal discectomy with small fiberscopes have been described. The indications for these approaches at present are few, the essential instrumentation for surgery has not yet been perfected, and extensive comparisons for their role as alternatives to microdiscectomy are not available. Despite these limitations, efforts to perfect percutaneous dorsolateral discectomy, laparoscopic lumbar discectomy with fusion, and thoracoscopic discectomy are continuing. Certainly, these procedures will evolve to become the techniques of choice for spinal surgery in various clinical situations.

16.3.2 Epiduroscopy

The usefulness and effectiveness of this technique is a matter of discussion. It is most commonly applied in post-laminectomy peridural fibrosis [5, 14–17]. Via the hiatus sacralis and with the use of intraoperative radiology, a 0.9–2.5-mm 0° semiflexible or flexible neuroendoscope is introduced through a sheath (Fig. 16.2). Adhesiolysis is performed with a balloon catheter and cauterization. No more than 120 ml of irrigation is recommended. Our series includes 26 patients with confirmed peridural fibrosis on epiduroscopy despite negative MRI scans. Targeted adhesiolysis was performed in half of the patients, whereas the other half underwent nontargeted adhesiolysis. Epidural

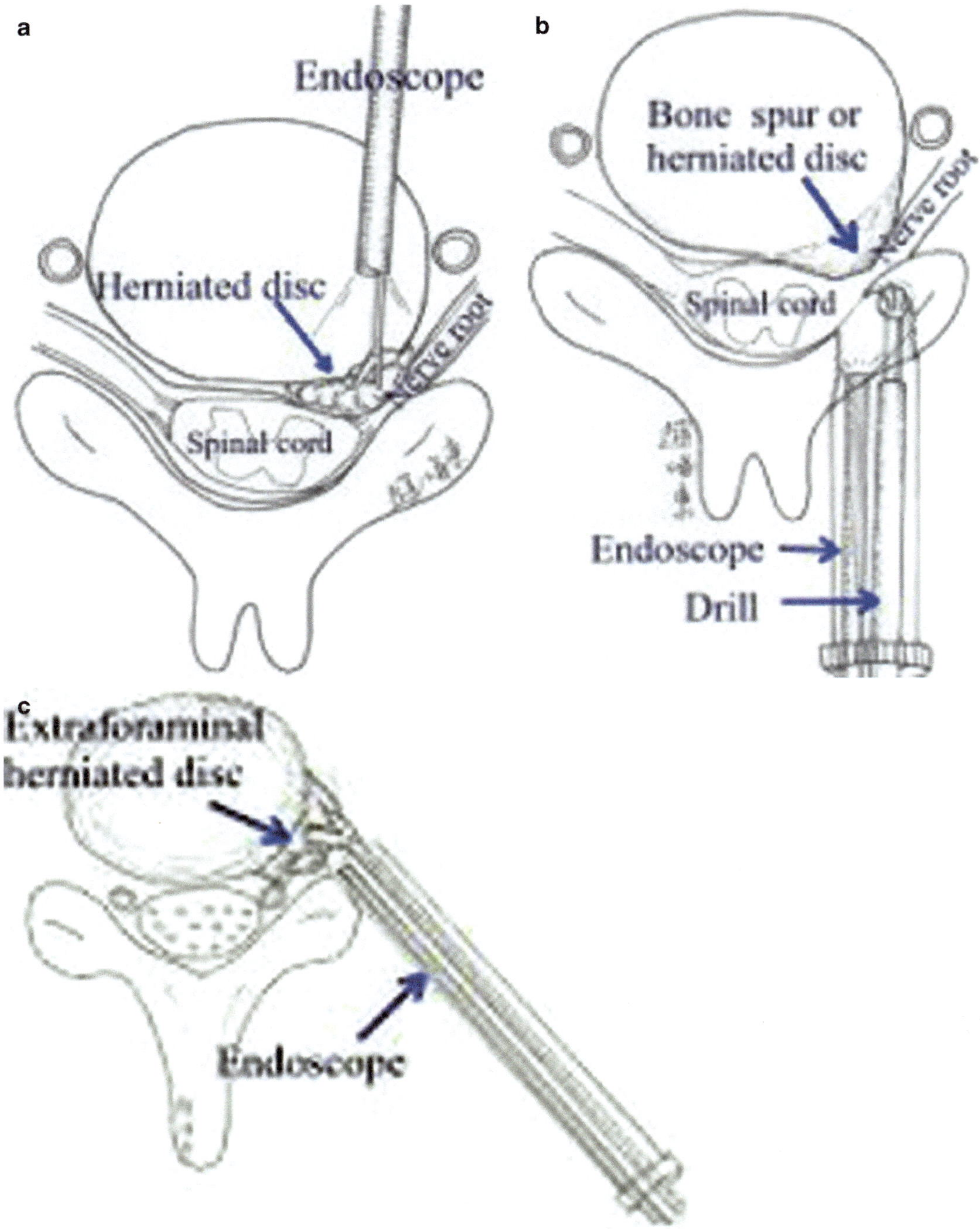

Fig. 16.1 Diagrams showing the possible endoscopic approaches that can be employed in the removal of cervical, thoracic, and lumbar herniated discs. (**a**) Anterior, to remove the herniated part of the disc. (**b**) Posterior, to decompress the spinal root canal as well, in the presence of a lateral osteophyte. (**c**) Lateral, to remove extraforaminal disc herniation

adhesiolysis was followed by the injection of steroids (triamcinolone) and local anesthetic (lidocaine) during epiduroscopy. In one patient, the procedure was repeated 6 months later, and an epidural catheter was left in place for 3 days postoperatively.

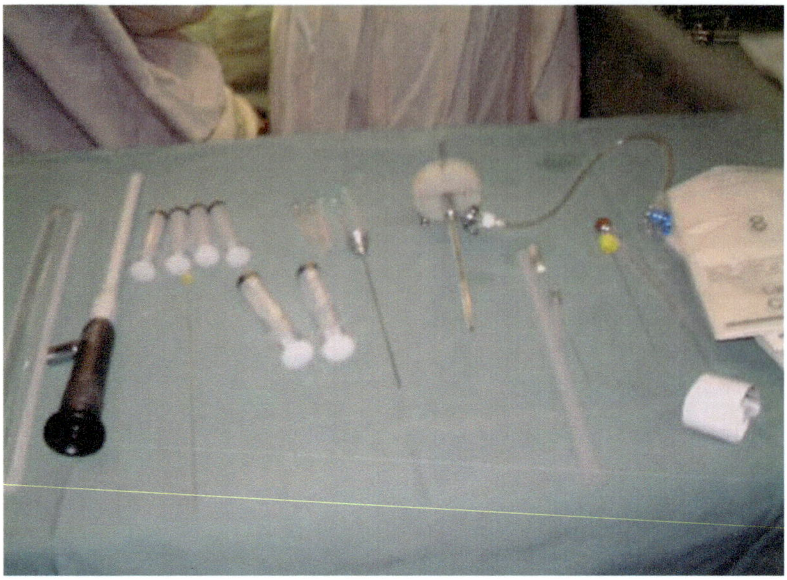

Fig. 16.2 Semiflexible and flexible spinal 0.9-mm 0° neuroendoscopy equipment used for epiduroscopy

After treatment, sciatic pain improved in all patients; however, low back pain was persistent, a finding that is concordant to previous literature reports. Based on the findings during epiduroscopy, 83.3 % of all patients with persistent pain after back surgery had severe (grade 3 or 4) epidural fibrosis, while 91.0 % had significant (grade 2, 3, or 4) fibrosis. In patients who had undergone more extensive surgery, severe fibrosis was present in 91.1 % and significant fibrosis in 95.6 %. Using MRI, epidural fibrosis was diagnosed only in 16.1 % of these patients. All patients with severe epidural fibrosis had a filling defect on epidurography. Concordant pain was present in 84.3 % of patients and was dependent on the severity of fibrosis. Epiduroscopy demonstrates that the prevalence of severe epidural fibrosis after back surgery syndrome is substantially higher than is generally reported in MRI evaluations. Severe epidural fibrosis is the underlying pathology in most patients with failed back surgery syndrome. Epidural adhesiolysis followed by the injection of steroids and local anesthetic during epiduroscopy alleviates pain and functional disability and reduces dysfunction of A-β and A-δ fibers in patients with chronic sciatica. Complication rate was about 2–7 % and included bleeding, visual loss and retinal hemorrhages, root injury, and infection. There are still some problems to be solved in the epiduroscope development, but its dramatic effect in pain reduction has been recognized, and it is considered as an attractive diagnostic and therapeutic tool.

16.3.3 Spinaloscopy

The lumbar and lower thoracic subarachnoid space of 26 human autopsy subjects was studied using rigid endoscopy by Blomberg in 1994 [1] with the aim to detect fibrous structures. This procedure is known as spinaloscopy. Fibrous attachments were found between nerve roots and/or nerve roots and the arachnoid membrane at least at one spinal level in 16 subjects. The appearance and density of the structures varied and caused restriction of nerve root mobility in nine subjects. In three of them, the impeded mobility prevented the nerve root from yielding to the contact and pressure exerted either by the tip of the endoscope or by a spinal needle introduced into the subarachnoid space. In another three subjects, a distinct membranous structure was identified in the posterior midline of the subarachnoid space in the lower thoracic and upper lumbar regions. These findings may be possibly associated with the variation in the extent of subarachnoid block and to the development of isolated nerve root trauma in connection with this procedure. The learning curve for spinal endoscopy is steep, and the procedure should not be attempted alone by a novice surgeon. Nevertheless, with training and experience, the spine surgeon can achieve better outcomes and reduced morbidity with spinal endoscopy, and the operating times are comparable to open procedures. As technology evolves and more experience is obtained, neuroendoscopy will likely achieve a more central role in spine surgery. In our clinical series we used flexible and semiflexible 0.9-mm 0° neuroendoscope, in a minimal approach (small laminectomy) or percutaneous procedure in lumbosacral and dorsal lesion like tumor biopsy. We closed with fibrin glue. Different kinds of pathologies were approached by this technique.

Our clinical series consists of 30 cases within a 9-year period (2002–2010). We used a flexible and semiflexible 0.9-mm 0° neuroendoscope either through a minimal surgical approach (small laminectomy) or as a percutaneous procedure in the management of dorsal lumbosacral lesions. Fibrin glue was utilized during closure. Overall, there was no associated intra- or postoperative mortality or morbidity. Infection rate was 1.6 %. Mean follow-up period was 48 months. Our total list of patients includes diverse pathologies:

- 13 arachnoid cysts, of which 8 are subdural and 5 are extradural. All of the arachnoid cysts were seen in pediatric patients (age range 2–14 years) and 50 % in patients with MMC and secondary tethered cord. Only 2 patients demonstrated radiological improvement. Clinical and/or EMG improvement after endoscopy for arachnoid cyst varied from 53.5 % in patients with previous MMC to 87.4 % in patients without MMC.
- 6 spinal tumors, of which 3 are less than 2 cm, 1 extended dorsal tumor which was biopsied, 1 meningioma, and 1 non-Hodgkin lymphoma. There are no previous reports of gross total resections of spinal tumors endoscopically. Published papers mention partial resections and biopsies.
- 14 patients with syringomyelia (7 posttraumatic, 2 in the cervical region, 5 dorsolumbar). Success rate was 82 % in the management of posttraumatic syringomyelia. Sometimes a septated syringomyelia is treated with endoscopic fenestrations in order to achieve free communication of fluid between the cavities and subsequent collapse with clinical improvement. However, despite the fenestrations, very often the cavity remains unchanged in size. In a second operation under endoscopic view, a small tube can be inserted into the cystic cavity to drain the fluid. Its efficacy is a matter of discussion and controversy.

16.4 The Future: Stem Cell Implants Through Neuroendoscopy (Restorative Neurosurgery)

Experimental and clinical research [7, 9, 10, 20] has shown the plasticity of the multipotent adult progenitor cell (MAPC) in various conditions of tissue damage. It was observed that in some neuromuscular disorders, clinical improvement of the pathological condition can be reached after the transplantation of MAPCs.

Amyotrophic lateral sclerosis (ALS) is a degenerative disorder characterized by loss of upper and lower motor neurons resulting in progressive muscle weakness, respiratory insufficiency, and ultimately death. Up to now, there are no effective treatments to reverse the natural course of the disease that is fatal. Considering the devastating effects of the ALS, we have designed a trial in which stem cells were implanted in the spinal cord and in the CSF of patients with ALS through a minimally invasive neuroendoscopic procedure. We also utilized stem cell implants in 7 patients with traumatic spinal cord injury and 1 patient with Alzheimer's disease.

16.5 Our Experience in Patients with Amyotrophic Lateral Sclerosis (ALS)

16.5.1 Materials and Methods

Twenty-four patients with ALS met the inclusion criteria for this study. Spirometry with a forced expiratory volume (FEV) and forced vital capacity (FVC) ratio not inferior to 60 % was required.

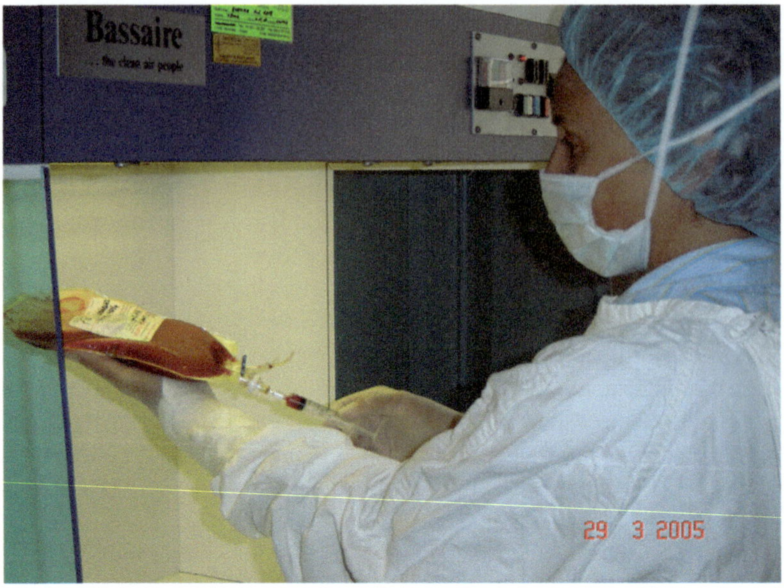

Fig. 16.3 Processing of peripheral blood stem cells

All patients were measured with an ALS function scale to set an individual initial score. Based on this scale, all our patients with ALS were graded from a minimum of 0 to a maximum of 40 points. A minimum score of 17 points was a prerequisite for inclusion in the study.

Bone marrow was stimulated with filgrastim 10 mg/kg 1 day before admission. Peripheral blood stem cells were collected from the patient through a central venous catheter by a continuous-flow apheresis equipment (Fig. 16.3). A buffy coat was separated from plasma, and CD34+ cells were tested and selected.

Laboratory manipulation of peripheral stem cells was done immediately before neuroendoscopy to preserve cell viability. Under general anesthesia, the first step was to insert a spinal needle in the intervertebral space between L4–L5 to obtain 4 ml of cerebrospinal fluid (CSF) (Fig. 16.4). Two milliliter of stem cells was then suspended in the CSF sample, and the mixture was injected back into the subarachnoid space (Fig. 16.5). The second step is to locate the intervertebral space between T8–T9 and to introduce percutaneously a semiflexible 0.9-mm 0° neuroendoscope. Once 1 mm deep in the posterior part of the spinal cord, 1 ml of concentrated stem cells is transplanted. Two milliliter of concentrated stem cells is then injected in the perispinal space before BioGlue is used to seal the dura mater (Fig. 16.6). The whole procedure lasted for about 45 min. The remaining stem cells were injected through the central venous catheter which is then removed at the end of the procedure.

16.5.2 Results

Stimulation during 6 days with filgrastim increased the white cell count to an average of 33.200/ml (range 24–55.000/ml). Mononuclear cells obtained were 8.13 × 10~8 per kg (range 5.3–12). After purification, CD34+ cells employed were 7.6 × 10~6 per kg (3.3–17.8).

No complications were observed during the stimulation period, the peripheral progenitor cell harvest, or the neuroendoscopic procedure.

Discharge from the hospital was 48 h after the transplantation with follow-up in the outpatient clinic. Periodic assessment of patients with the ALS function scale revealed that, at 6 months, 15 patients improved their initial scores while 9 patients remained stable with no progressive deterioration of their neurological performance. In all cases a remarkable decrease of the muscular fasciculations was observed.

The mortality rate of the treated group at 2 years follow-up was 20.8 %. This compares

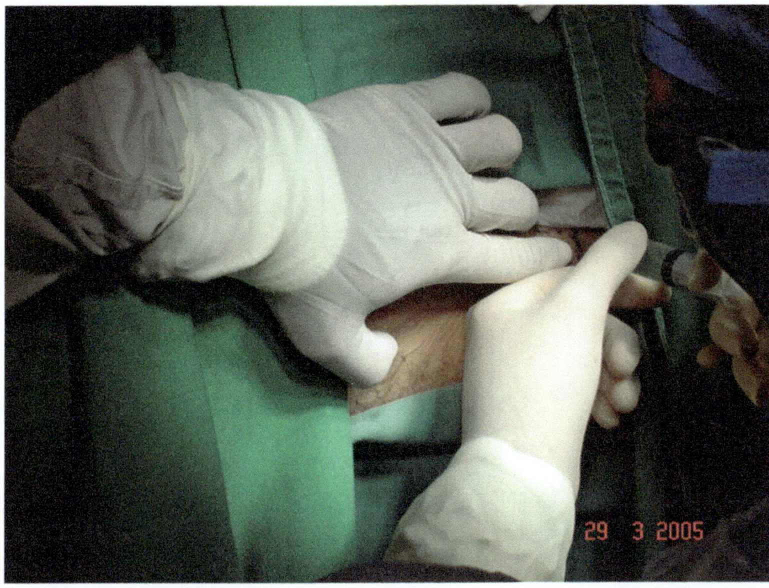

Fig. 16.4 Through a lumbar puncture, CSF is removed and used to suspend the stem cells

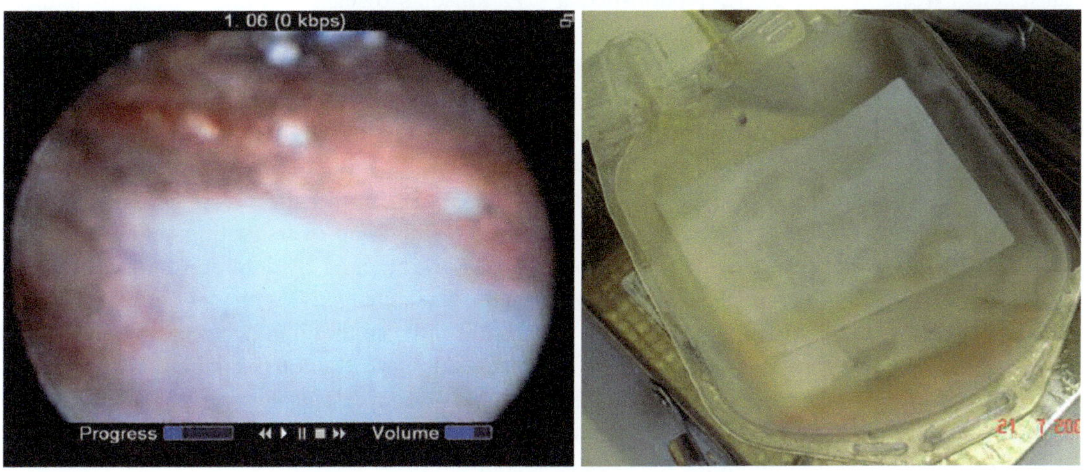

Fig. 16.5 The mixture of CSF and suspended stem cells is injected back into the subarachnoid space

favorably with the reported 36.1–53.6 % in the control group. Three patients died with pulmonary insufficiency in the first 18 months after the treatment.

16.5.3 Discussion

Since the introduction of stem cells as a potential therapeutic tool, their potential role in the treatment of various clinical entities has been studied including neurodegenerative diseases, e.g., Alzheimer's and Parkinson's [19], cerebrovascular diseases, cerebral tumors, and traumatic spine injury. Different kinds of stem cells have been utilized like olfactory and mesenchymal stem cells. Other study employed neural stem cells in culture for 15 days which were implanted through neuroendoscopy.

The discovery of stem cells in the adult human brain and developing stem cell technology opens a possible future scenario of autotransplantation, where stem cells are harvested from the patient and propagated in vitro before they are used as

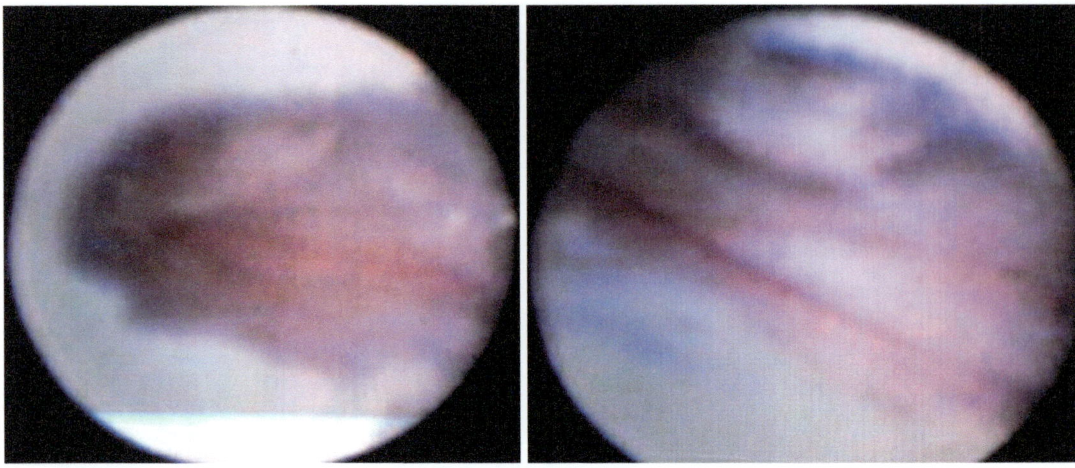

Fig. 16.6 Using the 0.9-mm 0° endoscope, concentrated stem cells are transplanted in the posterior part of the spinal cord and the perispinal space

transplants. Westerlund et al. [21] published a study in 2005 with the following objectives: (1) to investigate the feasibility of harvesting tissue containing neural stem cells by endoscopy, (2) to study the possibility of propagating and multiplying stem cells from this tissue efficiently in vitro, and (3) to examine whether the stem cells differentiate into functional neurons. In 13 patients undergoing routine neurosurgical endoscopy procedures for hydrocephalus, the authors used an endoscope and a 3-mm biopsy forceps to harvest the small piece of the ventricular wall that was detached by the introduction of the endoscope. Cells were cultured as neurospheres and after induced differentiation, they were investigated with immunocytochemistry and whole-cell patch-clamp recordings. All cells characterized were propagated under strict clonal conditions. There were no complications in harvesting the part of the lateral ventricular wall that was penetrated with the inner lumen of the endoscope. Single cells, isolated and cultivated in vitro, multiplied to form neurospheres in a serum-free environment. Only 7 % of cells generated a new neurosphere. A single stem cell had the potential to give rise to approximately 63,000 new cells after two passages. The total number of cells produced from a single biopsy was already, after the second passage, far beyond the number required for clinical effect in, for instance, Parkinson's disease. Within 1 week of induced differentiation, cells expressing markers for neurons (β-III-tubulin or NeuN), oligodendrocytes (RIP or 04), and astrocytes (glial fibrillary acidic protein) appeared. After 3 weeks, cells with a neuronal phenotype showed a firing pattern distinctive of mature neurons, including repetitive, short-lasting, and overshooting action potentials that were blocked by inhibiting voltage-dependent Na+ channels with tetrodotoxin. These results indicate that it may be feasible to produce neural tissue for autotransplantation from endoscopically harvested stem cells [3], but further work is needed in refining culture protocols to control phenotype fate.

In Latin America, we are developing an Iberamerican stem cells working group with a common protocol with the cooperation of scientists from Chile, Brazil, Uruguay, and Spain for the next 5 years. Our results in prognosis of ALS are similar in comparison to other methodologies.

Conclusion

The procedure is safe, feasible, and easy to reproduce. No complications or morbidity were observed. Improvement of neurological condition was registered in 15 patients and stabilization of the progressive disease in the other 9, not responding to the previous treatments. We considered the possibility of repeating stem cell implantation several times in order to increase the stem cells' population and to improve the results. In spite of the short follow-up, we think it is an encouraging new approach for an, up to now, always fatal disease.

References

1. Blomberg RG (1995) Fibrous structures in subarachnoid space: a study with spinaloscopy in autopsy subjects. Anest Analg 80(5):875–879
2. Bosscher HA, Heavner JE (2010) Incidence and severity of epidural fibrosis after back surgery: an endoscopic study. Pain Pract 10(1):18–24
3. De Bellis R, Cordoba A, Bello L (2006) Treatment of 12 patients with ALS, grafting cells through neuroendoscopy. Bone Marrow Transplant 37(Suppl 1):S133
4. Eguchi T, Tamaki N, Kurata H (1999) Endoscopy of the spinal cord: cadaveric study and clinical experience. Minim Invasiv Neurosurg 42:146–151
5. Fukushima T, Schramm J (1975) Klinischer: Versuch der Endoskopie des Spinalkanals: Krzmitteilung. Neurochirurgie 18:199–203
6. Huewel N, Perneczky A, Urban V et al (1992) Neuroendoscopic technique for the operative treatment of septated syringomyelia. Acta Neurochir (Wien) 54(Suppl):59–62
7. Janson CG, Ramesh TM, During MJ, Leone P, Heywood J (2001) Human intrathecal transplantation of peripheral blood stem cells in amyotrophic lateral sclerosis. J Hematother Stem Cell Res 10: 913–915
8. Karakhan VB et al (1994) Operative spinal endoscopy. Acta Neurochir 68(Suppl):108–114
9. Mazzini L, Fagioli F, Boccaletti R, Mareschi K, Oliveri G, Olivieri C et al (2003) Stem cell therapy in amyotrophic lateral sclerosis: a methodological approach in humans. Amyotroph Lateral Scler Other Motor Neuron Disord 4:158–161
10. Mazzini L, Fagioli F, Boccaletti R (2004) Stem-cell therapy in amyotrophic lateral sclerosis. Lancet 364:1936–1937
11. Ooi Y, Satoh Y, Inoue K, Mikanagi K, Morisaki N (1978) Myeloscopy. Acta Orthopedics Belgium 44:881–894
12. Ooi Y, Satoh Y, Sugawara S, Mikanagi K, Morisaki N (1977) Myeloscopy. Int Orthopedics 1:107–111
13. Perneczky A, Tschabischter M, Resch KDM (1993) Spinal subarachnoidal space in Atlas of Endoscopy. Thieme Medical Publishers, New York, p 263–267
14. Pheasant HC (1975) Sources of failure in laminectomies; symposium on the lumbar spine. Orthop Clin North Am 6(1):319–329
15. Saberski L, Kitahata L (1995) Direct visualisation of the lumbosacral epidural space through the sacral hiatus. Anesth Analg 80:839–840
16. Saitoh K (2001) Epiduroscopy in patients with chronic low back pain without remarkable findings on MRI. Masui 50(11):1257–1259
17. Sakai T, Aoki H, Hojo M, Takada M, Murata H, Sumikawa K (2008) Adhesiolysis and targeted steroid/local anesthetic injection during epiduroscopy alleviates pain and reduces sensory nerve dysfunction in patients with chronic sciatica. J Anesth 22(3): 242–247
18. Schutze G, Kurtze H (1995) Direct observation of the epidural space with a flexible catheter. Regional Anaesth 19(2):85–89
19. Svendsen CN, Langston JW (2004) Stem cells for Parkinson disease and ALS: replacement or protection? Nat Med 10:224–225
20. Vastag B (2001) Stem cells step closer to the clinic: paralysis partially reversed in rats with ALS-like disease. JAMA 285:1691–1693
21. Westerlund U, Svensonn M, Moe MC, Varghese M, Gustavsson B, Wallsted L, Bergjohnsen J, Langmoen IA, Hodge CJ, Boulis NM (2005) Endoscopically harvested stem cells: a putative method in future autotransplantation. Neurosurgery 57(4):779–784

17 Endoscopy-Assisted Craniosynostosis Surgery

Erik J. van Lindert, Anke M. Ettema, and Wilfred A. Borstlap

17.1 Introduction

The surgical methods to treat craniosynostosis have evolved from a relatively simple strip craniectomy to a diverse spectrum of partial or complete cranial vault remodeling [1, 3, 9, 16, 18]. More complex procedures, such as the biparietal craniectomy [8], pi procedure [14], and partial or complete cranial vault remodeling [6] have shown excellent results but often with high comorbidity [13]. There is general agreement that the younger a child is, the less extensive a craniofacial procedure should be. This is especially true in case of scaphocephaly [1, 15].

Recently, there is a renewed interest in early management for the correction of craniosynostosis, now revitalized by means of an endoscopy-assisted strip craniectomy before the sixth month of age, and combined with postoperative helmet molding therapy [2, 4, 7, 9, 10, 12, 13, 17]. The philosophy underlying this technique is the possibility to perform extensive surgical procedures through minimal incisions, decreasing blood loss, decreasing operative times, and shortening the hospitalization period, thus rendering not only good cosmetic results but also limit peri- and postoperative morbidity [5, 9].

17.2 General Principles and Surgical Technique

The main principle of endoscopy-assisted craniosynostosis surgery (EACS) is the suturectomy of the affected suture (Fig. 17.1). Since this was the primary treatment in the past for craniosynostosis with dissatisfying results overall, the suturectomy now relies on two additional conditions: early surgery (age below 6 months, but preferably earlier) and additional skull molding by a helmet. Early intervention not only halts a progressive deformity but may also reverse a deformity [11]. EACS does not claim to reach better results than conventional surgical methods but intends to reach comparable results with less morbidity and fewer complications than other extensive surgeries.

To perform endoscopy and thus claim a "minimally invasive technique" is not a goal in itself. The use of the endoscope must be regarded as an additional tool that improves illumination and visibility, thus allowing small skin incisions without compromising optical control. The endoscope is used for dural dissection and relieving the dura from the bone and synostotic suture. This is usually easily done, since dura is hardly attached to a synostotic suture, which is in strong contrast to dura that is firmly attached to intact

E.J. van Lindert, MD, PhD (✉)
Department of Neurosurgery, Radboud University Nijmegen Medical Centre, Nijmegen, The Netherlands
e-mail: e.vanlindert@nch.umcn.nl

A.M. Ettema, MD, PhD • W.A. Borstlap, MD, PhD
Department of Oromaxillofacial Surgery, Radboud University Nijmegen Medical Centre, Nijmegen, The Netherlands

S. Sgouros (ed.), *Neuroendoscopy*,
DOI 10.1007/978-3-642-39085-2_17, © Springer-Verlag Berlin Heidelberg 2014

a

b

c

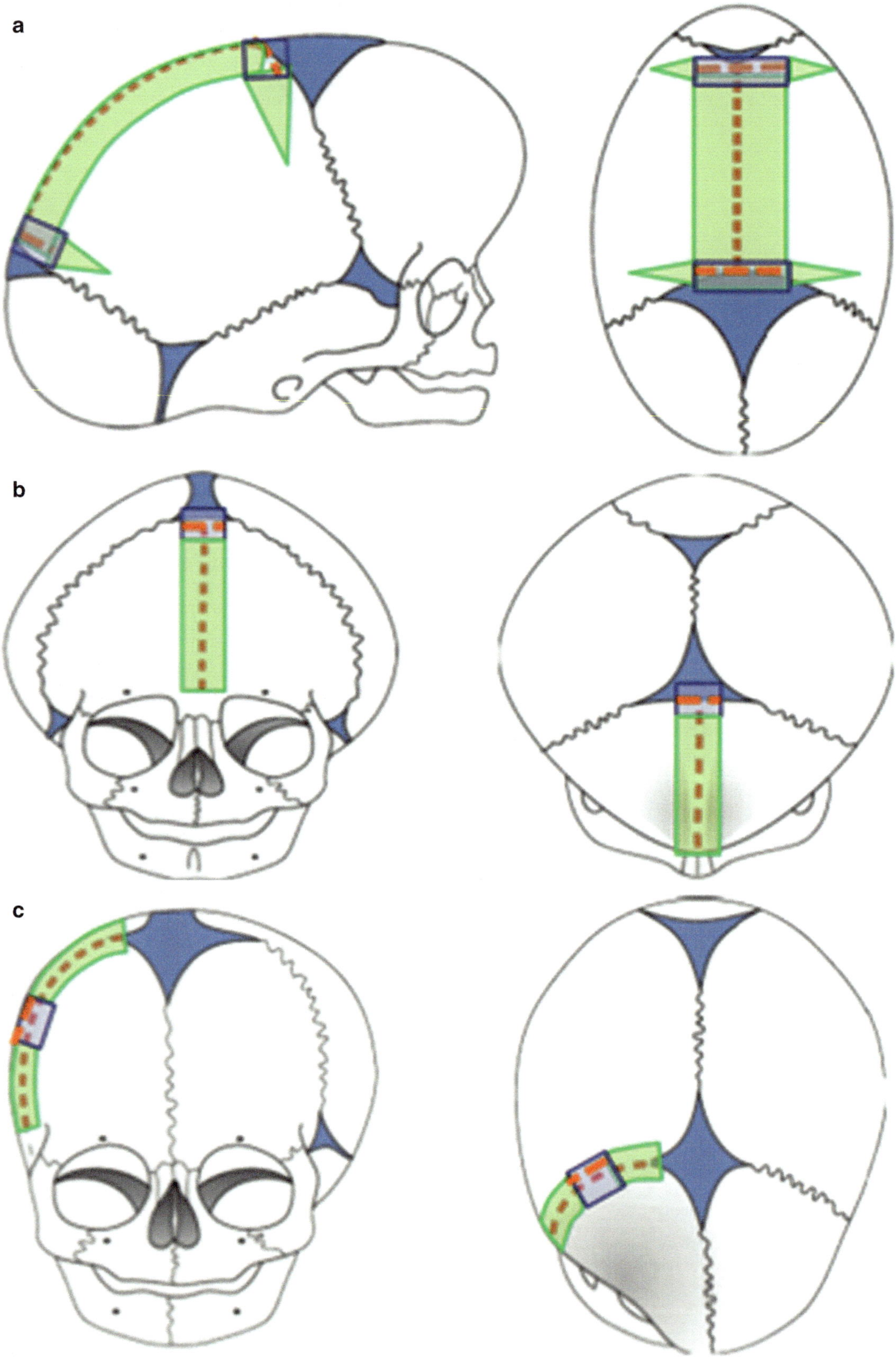

Fig. 17.1 Extent of suturectomy in (**a**) scaphocephaly, (**b**) trigonocephaly, and (**c**) frontal plagiocephaly

cranial sutures. The endoscopic control allows early optical control of emissary veins that then can be coagulated and cut.

EACS should be considered simple and easy surgery if it is well performed.

17.2.1 Diagnostics

Craniosynostosis requires neurological, ophthalmological, radiological, and human genetics diagnostic evaluation, but these are nonspecific and independent of the type of surgery chosen. A skull X-ray does not contribute to the diagnostics, but we consider a 3D CT scan of the skull obligatory. Not as much as to establish a diagnosis, since the diagnosis can be obtained by simply observing and investigating the patient, but to acquire as much information as possible to be optimally prepared for surgery. Attention should be paid to opacities in the bone that can be present in the small baby so that inadvertent breaking or perforating of the skull can be prevented. Sometimes the affected suture is not completely synostotic. The open part of an otherwise synostotic suture does not necessarily have to be removed. Also, since the dura is more firmly attached to the open suture as compared to the synostotic suture, this should be known to prevent the risk of dural laceration. The thickness of the skull that can be irregular should be addressed also, as usually a pair of scissors is used to cut the skull under endoscopic view. The skin incision should be determined paying attention to all these factors.

For evaluation of the surgical result, we do not want to rely on radiological examinations because of the irradiation. Therefore, we prefer 3D stereophotogrammetry in the preoperative setting that can be repeated unrestrictedly during many years of follow-up.

17.2.2 Timing of Surgery

Jimenez and Barone already found that the critical age for EACS seems to be 6 months. After that age the cosmetic results become worse, and insufficient correction of skull shape is reached. However, one should not wait until the infant reaches the age of 5 or 6 months. The earlier an EACS is performed, the better the result. This is of even more importance in case of plagiocephaly and trigonocephaly. Therefore, below the age of 4 months, we always offer EACS as the treatment of choice, but, for infants of 5 or 6 months, we restrict EACS for mild and moderate cases and consider open remodeling procedures for severe cases. An optimal age for EACS is in our opinion 3 months. The child has grown after birth and acquired some weight, can tolerate some moderate blood loss, and is able to tolerate the molding helmet. Unfortunately, there is quite often a significant diagnostic delay with general practitioners and pediatricians, because of which many patients are seen in a later phase and this goal of surgery at 3 months cannot be reached.

In syndromic cases diagnosis is usually obtained early after birth. This offers a window of opportunity for early treatment. We prefer to operate these children at an age of 4–8 weeks. The idea is not to offer a definitive treatment of for instance the brachycephaly but to reduce a progressive deformity and prevent increased intracranial pressure. Parents are informed that cranial vault expansion and bifrontoorbital advancement procedures may still be required at a later stage. Because of the very young age and additional problems, such as sleep apnea, redression helmet therapy is not added in these cases. At this moment, however, the experience in syndromic cases of craniosynostosis is evolving, which may change our policy in the future.

17.2.3 Anesthesia, Monitoring, and Postoperative Care

Standard anesthetic monitoring techniques are used, including electrocardiography, noninvasive blood pressure monitoring, pulse oximetry, temperature monitoring, and blood loss monitoring. EACS on the metopic and coronal sutures is performed with the patient in a supine position. The sagittal suture is best operated upon with the

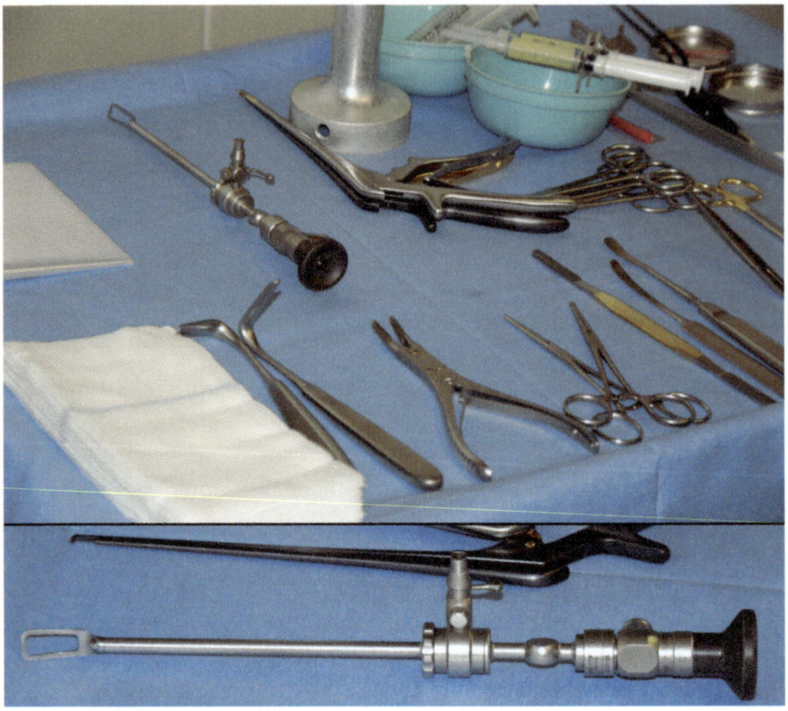

Fig. 17.2 Endoscope, endoscope shaft, and instruments used in EACS

patient in a sphinx position (see Fig. 17.4a), while the lambdoid sutures are reached with the patient in a prone position.

Since blood loss is usually minimal and OR times limited to 45–75 min, a central venous line is not required nor an arterial line. Two peripheral venous lines suffice in all cases. Antibiotic prophylaxis consists of 25 mg/kg cefazolin i.v. given 20 min before skin incision in all cases. All patients are monitored postoperatively in pediatric high dependency unit, and hemoglobin/hematocrit is controlled at the end of surgery and 6 h later. ICU monitoring is never needed. Postoperative pain is treated with prophylactic paracetamol and low-dose i.v. morphine until the first day after surgery. The patient is usually dismissed from the hospital on the first or second postoperative day.

In our series postoperative blood transfusion was required in 15 % of cases, while intraoperative blood transfusion was never required. The only postoperative complication was a Norovirus infection in one case. We have not encountered infection, air embolus, hyponatremia, hypotension, injury to the sagittal sinus, dural tear, postoperative hematoma, seizure, coagulopathies, or mortality in 40 successive cases of EACS.

17.2.4 Instrumentation and Surgical Hemostasis

EACS can be performed with a standard armamentarium. To limit blood loss, we use monopolar cutting for galea and periosteum. The endoscope is a Storz 0° lens scope with a working shaft used for endoscopic facial lift surgery without irrigation or suction (Fig. 17.2). A separate aspirator parallel to the endoscope performs blood aspiration. Craniectomy is performed with a high-speed drill initially and continued with different rongeurs and Kerrisons. In scaphocephaly, a pair of strong scissors is used to cut the bone from one craniectomy site to the other in order to remove a piece of bone of 11 × 4 cm (see Fig. 17.4c, f).

Bleeding during surgery from the epidural space and bone edges is easily controlled with FloSeal® Matrix Hemostatic Sealant (Baxter Healthcare Corporation, Fremont, CA, USA).

17.2.5 Helmet Molding Therapy

Within 2 weeks after surgery, a plaster imprint of the skull is taken, which serves as an initial template for the fabrication of the custom-made helmet.

The children are wearing the helmet within 3 weeks postoperatively. During follow-up special attention is paid concerning the development of pressure ulceration areas and/or other complications due to the wear of the helmet.

Changes in cranial shape occur immediately after initiation of the surgery and are noted especially postoperatively. The helmet corrects the calvarial growth pattern and, subsequently, the direction of growth. The plasticity of the infant cranial vault, along with rapid brain growth during the first months of life, permits skull remodeling in the postoperative time. Whereas, our data also confirmed that after approximately 6 months, the helmet is used to maintain the cephalic index and prevent or reduce a relapse of the deformity [13].

There are different types of molding helmets on the market for positional occipital plagiocephaly. However, they may not all be suitable for treatment of craniosynostosis. We experienced an improvement of our results, especially in case of scaphocephaly, after we changed from a one-piece helmet to a two-piece helmet (Fig. 17.3). The advantage of the two-piece helmet is that these are thinner and lighter, better aerated, easier to put on and off, more stable on

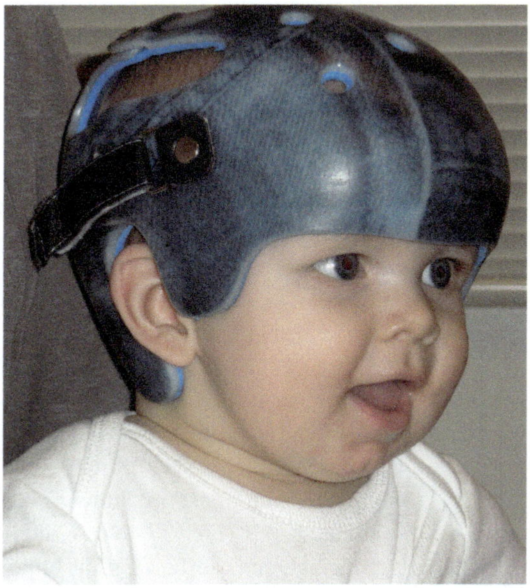

Fig. 17.3 Two-piece molding helmet

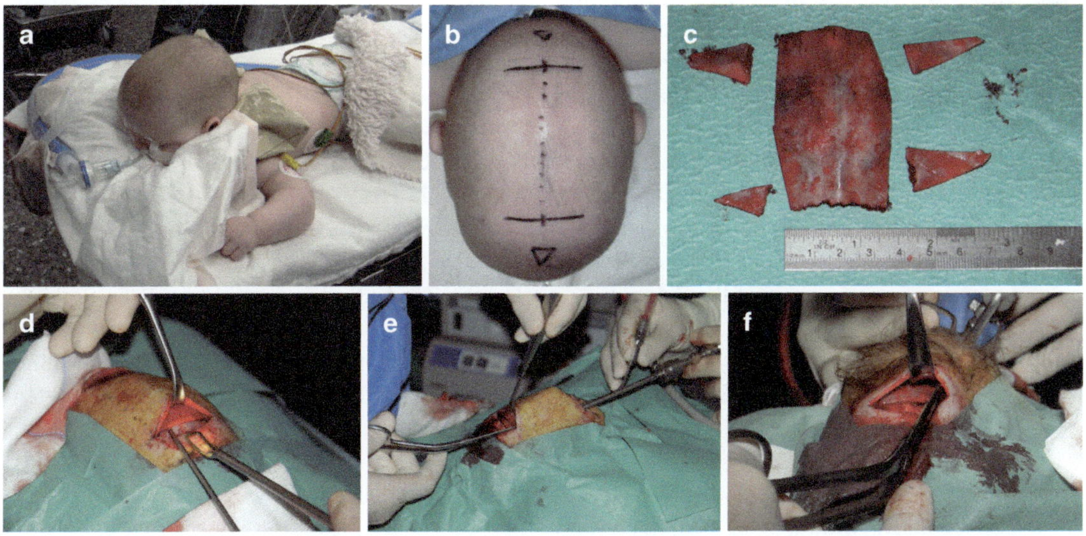

Fig. 17.4 (**a**) Sphinx positioning for scaphocephaly surgery, (**b**) position and extent of skin incisions, (**c**) extent of bone removal in scaphocephaly, (**d**) epidural insertion of the endoscope and dural dissection, and (**e**, **f**) epidural placement of the endoscope from one incision site and bone cutting with scissors from the other incision

the head (less "sliding" of the helmet), and easily adjustable shaping by heating the helmet.

In our series the helmet is worn for 10 months (range 6–16 months) on average. None of the patients developed pressure ulcer, whereas dry skin or development of eczema under the helmet was documented in two patients. These dermal problems were resolved after finishing the helmet therapy.

17.3 Scaphocephaly

Scaphocephalic patients are positioned in a modified prone sphinx position bringing the synostotic sagittal suture in a horizontal plane (Fig. 17.4). The craniectomy is performed from the anterior to the posterior fontanelle but may be adapted in case a part of the suture is still open and patent. The removed strip should be 4–5 cm wide. Lateral barrel stave osteotomies or wedge-shaped osteotomies behind the coronal sutures and in front of the lambdoid sutures should assist in allowing an increased biparietal width (Fig. 17.4c). A video demonstrating this surgery can be seen on http://www.youtube.com/watch?v=oUIEhPsKT3E.

Already in the first days and weeks after surgery and before administration of the helmet, the head shape is changing. Most prominent is the rounding of the occiput which is first noticed by the parents. Later, the biparietal width increases. In contrast to these early changes, the correction of the frontal bossing is relatively delayed and more influenced by the redression helmet, than by surgery itself. As with classical surgical techniques, a slight relapse may occur after some time with a mild decrease of the cephalic index. The redression helmet seems to assist in limiting this relapse.

17.4 Trigonocephaly, Plagiocephaly, and Brachycephaly

In trigonocephaly, frontal plagiocephaly, and brachycephaly, the patients are in a supine position, stabilized in a vacuum mattress, with the head contralaterally rotated (in plagiocephaly and brachycephaly cases) or in a neutral position (in trigonocephaly cases). For both indications a single 2–3 cm-wide skin incision within the hairline is made (Fig. 17.5). In trigonocephaly the skin incision is positioned close and anterior to the anterior fontanelle, and in plagiocephaly and brachycephaly the skin incision is made halfway between the anterior fontanelle and the pterion. A small craniectomy is performed with a high-speed drill. Subsequently, at the upper surface the periosteal layer is lifted from the bone and at the undersurface the dura is dissected from the synostotic suture under endoscopic guidance. The synostotic suture is removed with a width of 1–1.5 cm from the anterior fontanel to the nasion (in trigonocephaly) or the pterion (in plagiocephaly and brachycephaly) in an osteoclastic fashion using rongeurs. If a partially patent suture is encountered, further removal of the suture is stopped.

At the pterion or at the nasion, some thick cancellous bone can be encountered which may be responsible for some venous bleeding. This, however, is easily controlled by FloSeal®. In trigonocephaly one or two bridging veins can be encountered when nearing the skull base. This may need sometimes bipolar electrocoagulation. After surgery a head bandage for 1 day is applied to prevent postoperative subcutaneous hematoma development. Facial and periorbital swelling is usually mild.

17.5 Syndromic and Nonsyndromic Multisutural Craniosynostosis

Jimenez and Barone have shown that nonsyndromic multisutural craniosynostosis can be treated successfully in the same fashion as monosutural synostosis with excellent results and reversal of the deformities [11]. They had no serious morbidity and only very few postoperative blood transfusions. However, there are hardly any other significant surgical series confirming these results yet.

We have little experience with multisutural craniosynostosis, but our initial results are

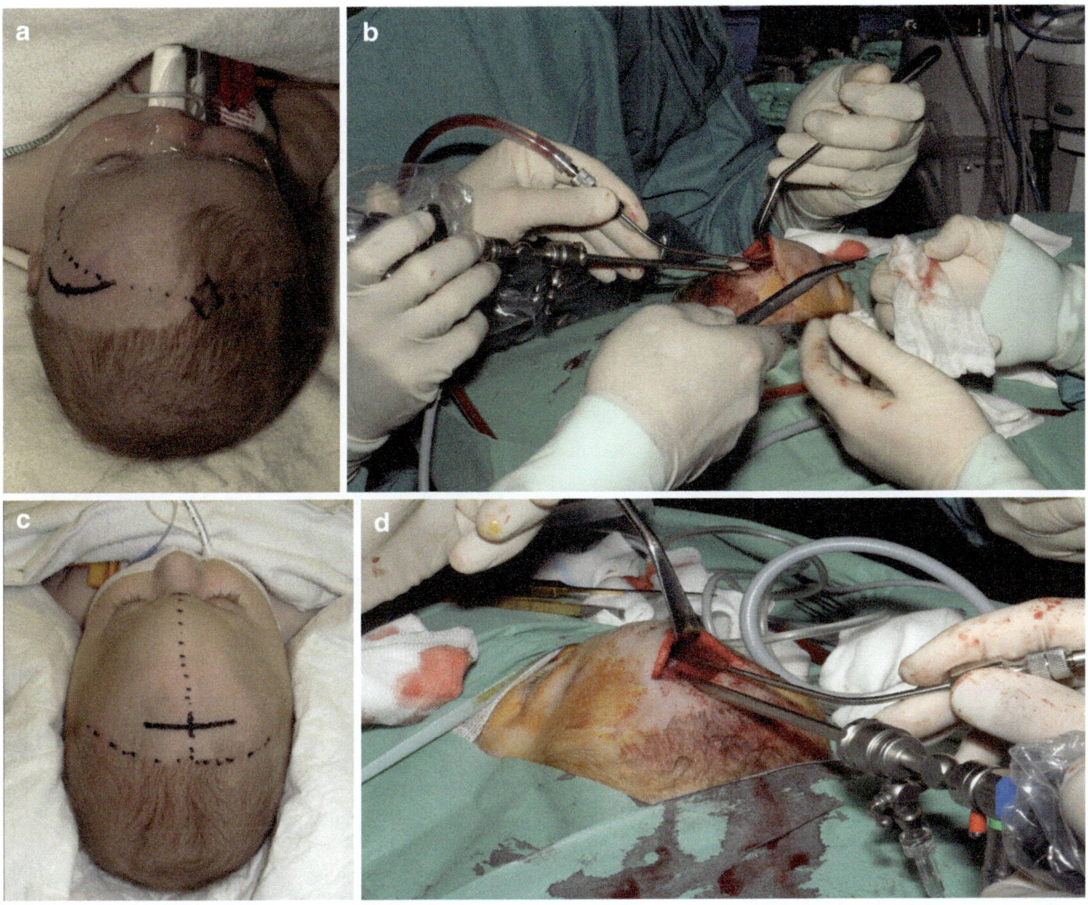

Fig. 17.5 (**a**) Positioning and skin incision for left frontal plagiocephaly, (**b**) positioning and skin incision for trigonocephaly, and (**c**, **d**) skin lifting and endoscope introduction in EACS for trigonocephaly

gratifying. In one patient with a severe brachyplagiocephaly caused by bilateral lambdoid and unilateral coronal suture synostosis, a simple suturectomy followed by helmet molding therapy was sufficient for a good cosmetic result, even though the initial goal for surgery was to halt a progressive deformity with the intention for definitive reconstructive surgery at a later stage. This, however, was not necessary anymore.

We are not aware of reports of EACS in syndromic multisutural craniosynostosis. Nevertheless, we started to perform EACS in those cases. In syndromic craniosynostosis, surgery is usually postponed to a later stage in which the children are 9–12 months old. The reason is that early surgery goes with a higher incidence of relapse and consequently repeat surgery. However, this means that the deformity will be progressive in the meantime and also may lead to an increased intracranial pressure. Some groups started to perform posterior cranial vault expansion as an intermediate solution before performing frontoorbital advancement later on.

It is our goal to try to halt the progressive deformity, prevent intracranial hypertension, and simplify reconstructive surgery at a later stage by performing EACS in a very early stage (6–8 weeks of age) but without helmet molding. The idea is that this is very easy and simple surgery with very low morbidity. It is, however, not meant to be a replacement for conventional surgical techniques but a supplement treatment. Initial results in three Apert syndrome and one Muenke syndrome cases are promising, but we do not have long-term results yet.

17.6 Future Developments

Although EACS already exists over 15 years, it is still a relatively new technique. Comparison of the technique and the results of treatment with classical techniques should not only be performed with regard to the perioperative phase and results after 1 year but also be evaluated after 10–15 years. Also, it should be evaluated whether EACS is ideal for all syndromic and nonsyndromic cases or only for special subgroups.

Probably the easiest way of improving results is to get the patient as soon as possible under the attention of the surgeon and the surgery scheduled before 3 months of age. Therefore, information and education of general practitioners and pediatricians as well as training of all those paramedic professionals who are working with children with an "abnormal" head shape (pediatric physiotherapists, manual therapists, etc.) should be actively looked for if one intends to perform this kind of surgery.

3D CAD should enhance the making of the molding helmet, making it a more reliable tool, allowing easier adaptations, and giving the opportunity to the surgeon to interfere with the making process of the helmet. The technique is already available but at the moment is more expensive than handmade customized helmets.

Although custom available surgical instruments are good enough to perform EACS safely and with success, there is also room for refinement and development of dedicated instruments for this specific type of surgery. One can think of new endoscope shaft, dedicated instruments for surgical hemostasis, but especially of a craniotome that can be used below the skin under endoscopic guidance. At the moment, however, these instruments are not available.

Last but not least, EACS may become combined with other surgical techniques as well. Spring expansion, internal and external distraction, and orbitofrontal advancement may all be combined with EACS, in which the combination of two techniques allows further improvement of the result.

This, however, requires the surgeon to refrain from dogmas and teaching schools and therefore will be a long way out.

References

1. Alvarez-Garijo JA, Cavadas PC, Vila MM, Alvarez-Llanas A (2001) Sagittal synostosis: results of surgical treatment in 210 patients. Childs Nerv Syst 17: 64–68
2. Barone CM, Jimenez DF (1999) Endoscopic craniectomy for early correction of craniosynostosis. Plast Reconstr Surg 104:1965–1973; discussion 1974–1975
3. Boulos PT, Lin KY, Jane JAJ, Jane JAS (2004) Correction of sagittal synostosis using a modified Pi method. Clin Plast Surg 31:489–498, vii
4. Clayman MA, Murad GJ, Steele MH, Seagle MB, Pincus DW (2007) History of craniosynostosis surgery and the evolution of minimally invasive endoscopic techniques: the University of Florida experience. Ann Plast Surg 58:285–287
5. Di Rocco C (2003) How to decrease the impact of surgical scar in the correction of sagittal synostosis. Childs Nerv Syst 19:42–45
6. Epstein N, Epstein F, Newman G (1982) Total vertex craniectomy for the treatment of scaphocephaly. Childs Brain 9:309–316
7. Esparza J, Hinojosa J (2008) Complications in the surgical treatment of craniosynostosis and craniofacial syndromes: apropos of 306 transcranial procedures. Childs Nerv Syst 24:1421–1430
8. Greene CSJ, Winston KR (1988) Treatment of scaphocephaly with sagittal craniectomy and biparietal morcellation. Neurosurgery 23:196–202
9. Hinojosa J, Esparza J, Munoz MJ (2007) Endoscopic-assisted osteotomies for the treatment of craniosynostosis. Childs Nerv Syst 23:1421–1430
10. Jimenez DF, Barone CM (1998) Endoscopic craniectomy for early surgical correction of sagittal craniosynostosis. J Neurosurg 88:77–81
11. Jimenez DF, Barone CM (2010) Multiple-suture nonsyndromic craniosynostosis: early and effective management using endoscopic techniques. J Neurosurg Pediatr 5:223–231
12. Jimenez DF, Barone CM, Cartwright CC, Baker L (2002) Early management of craniosynostosis using endoscopic-assisted strip craniectomies and cranial orthotic molding therapy. Pediatrics 110:97–104

13. Jimenez DF, Barone CM, McGee ME, Cartwright CC, Baker CL (2004) Endoscopy-assisted wide-vertex craniectomy, barrel stave osteotomies, and postoperative helmet molding therapy in the management of sagittal suture craniosynostosis. J Neurosurg 100:407–417
14. Kanev PM, Lo AK (1995) Surgical correction of sagittal craniosynostosis: complications of the pi procedure. J Craniofac Surg 6:98–102
15. Marchac D, Renier D, Broumand S (1994) Timing of treatment for craniosynostosis and facio-craniosynostosis: a 20-year experience. Br J Plast Surg 47:211–222
16. McCarthy JG, Glasberg SB, Cutting CB, Epstein FJ, Grayson BH, Ruff G, Thorne CH, Wisoff J, Zide BM (1995) Twenty-year experience with early surgery for craniosynostosis: I. Isolated craniofacial synostosis–results and unsolved problems. Plast Reconstr Surg 96:272–283
17. Persing JA, Nichter LS, Jane JA, Edgerton MTJ (1986) External cranial vault molding after craniofacial surgery. Ann Plast Surg 17:274–283
18. Shillito JJ, Matson DD (1968) Craniosynostosis: a review of 519 surgical patients. Pediatrics 41: 829–853

Endoscopic Endonasal Repair of CSF Leak

18

Yaron A. Moshel, Madeleine R. Schaberg, Vijay K. Anand, and Theodore H. Schwartz

18.1 Background

Cerebrospinal (CSF) rhinorrhea most commonly occurs as a result of trauma and iatrogenic disruption of the skull base and leptomeningeal membranes and secondary to skull base erosion from inflammatory, neoplastic, and pseudotumor syndromes. Spontaneous lesions, as seen in cases of pseudotumor, are exceedingly rare and have been theorized to result from either increased ICP or preformed developmental pathways [2, 13, 40]. Progressive erosion of the skull base in patients with increased ICP and well-pneumatized sphenoid sinuses may result in focal areas of dehiscence and herniation of intracranial contents. This is often associated with primary empty sella in which the suprasellar arachnoid cistern is prolapsed inside the sellar cavity [27, 35]. Errors in the embryological development of the sphenoid bone may result also in congenital defects of the skull base and may present in adulthood as an incidental neuroimaging finding of meningoencephalocele or symptomatically with CSF rhinorrhea and meningitis. The development of the sphenoid bone is complex and involves the fusion of multiple cartilaginous precursors into a single osseous structure. Incomplete fusion of the precursor of the greater wing of the sphenoid with the presphenoid and basisphenoid areas can result in a persistent channel termed the lateral craniopharyngeal (Sternberg) canal [32, 36].

Cerebrospinal fluid leaks can be divided into post-traumatic, iatrogenic, and spontaneous, the first of which generally resolve without surgical intervention. The latter two categories can be particularly challenging to repair due to their high volume of flow, the difficulty in identifying the precise location of the leak, the potential for unrecognized mild increases in intracranial pressure, or congenital thinning of the skull base. Surgical repair of encephaloceles and CSF rhinorrhea is recommended to prevent meningitis, intracranial abscess, and pneumocephalus. Traditionally, CSF leaks have been managed via a craniotomy with a 70–80 % successful closure rate [15]. Advantages of the transcranial approach include direct visualization of the dural defect, the ability to address associated brain injury, and the potential to use a large vascularized pericranial flap. However, many studies have reported a 40 % recurrence rate with this approach and significant patient morbidity including anosmia,

Y.A. Moshel, MD, PhD
Division of Neuro-Oncology,
Department of Neurosurgery, Thomas Jefferson University, Philadelphia, PA, USA

M.R. Schaberg, MD, MPH
Department of Otolaryngology Head and Neck Surgery, The New York Eye and Ear Infirmary, New York, NY, USA

V.K. Anand, MD, FACS
Department of Otolaryngology and Head and Neck Surgery, Weill Cornell Medical College, New York, NY, USA

T.H. Schwartz, MD (✉)
Department of Neurological Surgery, Weill Cornell Medical College – New York Presbyterian Hospital, New York, NY, USA
e-mail: schwarh@med.cornell.edu

S. Sgouros (ed.), *Neuroendoscopy*,
DOI 10.1007/978-3-642-39085-2_18, © Springer-Verlag Berlin Heidelberg 2014

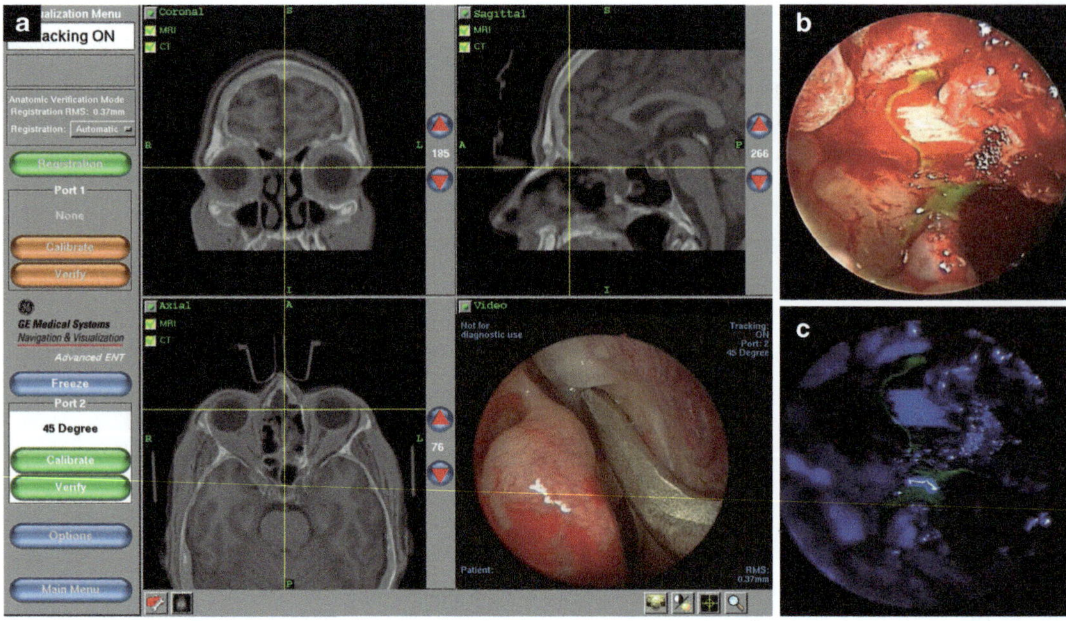

Fig. 18.1 (**a**) Representative figure demonstrating an intraoperative stereotactic system that displays the standard orthogonal views based on the preoperative MRI scan. A trajectory view or the intraoperative endoscopic high-definition video feed can be displayed also to cross correlate the anatomy. (**b**, **c**) Intraoperative view in a patient that received intrathecal fluorescein prior to the start of surgery. The green-tinged cerebrospinal fluid demonstrates the location of the arachnoid defect and the need for a watertight closure. The fluorescein-stained cerebrospinal fluid can be visualized with white light (**a**) or with a blue light filter with a blocking filter

frontal lobe retraction, seizures, memory deficits, and intracranial hemorrhage [1, 30, 31]. In attempt to avoid these complications and improve closure rates, the endonasal endoscopic approach has evolved to address CSF leaks and encephaloceles of the anterior skull base involving pathology along the cribriform plate, fovea ethmoidalis, sphenoid bone, or temporal bone (Fig. 18.1). The endoscope not only provides excellent visualization, but outcome studies have demonstrated decreased morbidity and improved closure rates [4, 12, 30, 38]. The approach also allows for close postoperative surveillance of the wound site and the ability to identify recurrences. The endoscopic repair of CSF leaks is quickly becoming the most favored method for closure of anterior skull base CSF leaks. We have performed over 43 endoscopic endonasal procedures for repair of CSF leaks and encephaloceles since 2004 with a 94 % successful closure rate. The particular approach depended on the individual anatomy and location of the skull base defect.

18.2 Surgical Techniques

18.2.1 Use of Intrathecal Fluorescein

The presence and site of a CSF leak can be verified using a combination of diagnostic methods including β-2 transferrin testing, nuclear pledget scan, rigid nasal endoscopy, CT imaging, MR imaging, cisternography, and intraoperative intrathecal fluorescein. The intrathecal administration of fluorescein to stain CSF has been described for over 40 years and is an important adjunct to endoscopic repair of CSF rhinorrhea [33, 34, 37]. Intrathecal fluorescein is helpful in localizing the CSF leak, determine the extent of the defect, and ensure a watertight closure. It is equally of great value in facilitating closure of large defects following endoscopic skull base surgery. The green color is easily distinguished from the surrounding blood and secretions in the operative field that may otherwise obscure the naturally clear, translucent CSF. Although the use of intrathecal fluorescein is generally considered safe [25], older reports have described complications, including seizures, radicular symptoms, and transient paraparesis or hemiparesis [22, 25, 26, 28]. The dosages of fluorescein varied in these reports, and patients were not always premedicated to avoid a reaction to the drug. With use of low-dose intrathecal fluorescein with premedication, these complications have been avoided [24, 37, 38]. We have used low-dose intrathecal fluorescein in over 300 endoscopic endonasal procedures without any adverse-effect incident.

Patients are generally premedicated with 50 mg of diphenhydramine and 10 mg of dexamethasone following induction of general anesthesia. Prior to the procedure, a lumbar puncture is performed to enter the intrathecal space and withdraw 10 mL of CSF. This is mixed with 25 mg of fluorescein (0.25 mL of injectable 10 % solution, Akorn Inc., Buffalo Grove, IL) and is slowly reinjected into the intrathecal space. In patients undergoing planned lumbar drainage, the CSF is obtained following drain placement, and the lumbar drain is clamped following fluorescein injection. The intrathecal injection stains the CSF that is already in circulation.

Endoscopic visualization of the fluorescein-stained CSF is performed throughout the surgery with either a white light or a blue light filter (465–495 nm) with a blocking filter (515–555 nm). The operative field is inspected at the time of the surgical approach to confirm the location and volume of any CSF leak in patients with suspected preoperative CSF leak or encephalocele. In patients undergoing endoscopic tumor resection, the operative field is inspected for CSF leak following complete tumor removal and following reconstruction [24, 37, 38].

18.2.2 Endoscopic Repair of Skull Base Defects

The principles of endoscopic reconstruction of skull base defects are similar to those of traditional open craniotomy approaches, that is, to completely separate the cranial cavity from the sinonasal cavity and eliminate dead space. This closure, especially for large defects with high flow of CSF output, relies on a multilayered reconstruction to reestablish tissue barriers as is true in traditional open craniotomy techniques. The closure is achieved using a variety of techniques based on the severity of the intraoperative leak as well as the location and size of the cranial base defect [29, 39]. The first step of the surgery is to adequately expose the entire defect. The meningocele or encephalocele is resected, and the bony edges of the defect are defined circumferentially. The herniated dura should be resected or reduced into the intracranial cavity. Brain that has herniated into the nasal cavity is rarely functional and considered a potential source of intracranial infection if not resected. However, in certain rare instances of very large encephaloceles, the preoperative imaging must be carefully scrutinized to ensure that important vascular structures, such as the anterior cerebral arteries, have not herniated through the large defect. Another important step is to remove the mucosa surrounding the defect to allow the graft to adhere firmly to the skull base. These maneuvers will often worsen the CSF leak but is critical to obtain an eventual watertight seal and to define the bony defect.

Small isolated CSF leak/encephaloceles with a small bony defect can be closed with a single layer of autologous fat or fascia placed through the defect as an inlay, followed by application of tissue sealant. We also like to use Duraguard (Biovascular, Inc., St. Paul, MN) since it is more rigid than fascia lata. In some situations we have placed Medpor (Porex Surgical, Inc., Newnan, GA) as an inlay to cover the defect with a fascia lata onlay. A final layer of DuraSeal (Covidien, Hazelwood, MO) is helpful to maintain a watertight closure until a fibrotic seal can be obtained. Sellar lesions involving a bony skull base defect without arachnoid violation or intraoperative CSF leak can be closed by packing the cavity with Gelfoam and reconstructing the bony sella with vomer or Medpor graft. Reconstruction is achieved by placing the graft, which has been trimmed to size, as either an underlay or, more commonly, an onlay graft. Sellar reconstruction in the presence of intraoperative CSF leak is achieved by packing the tumor cavity

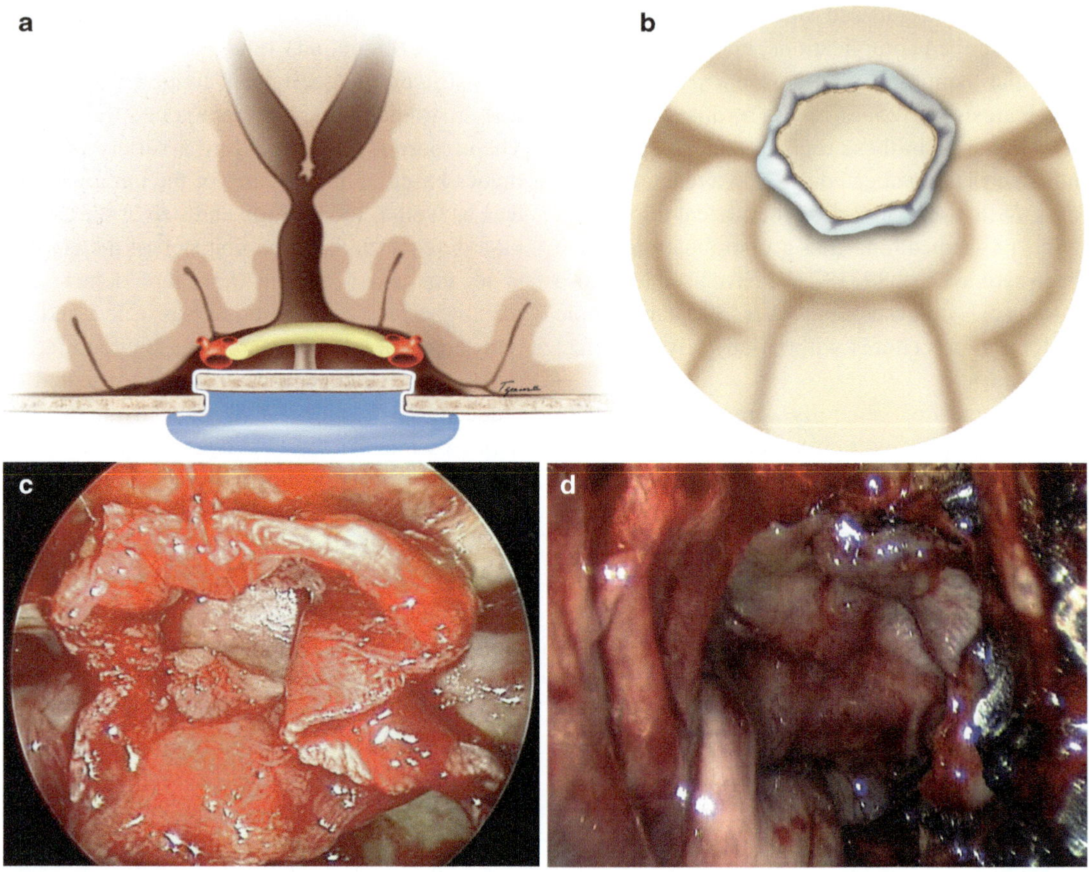

Fig. 18.2 (**a**) Diagrammatic demonstration with a coronal view of the suprasellar contents and closure of the skull base defect with a gasket seal. The countersunk rigid buttress is cut to the same size as the skull base defect and countersunk with overlying fascia lata for a watertight seal. (**b**) Diagrammatic demonstration of the intraoperative view of a gasket seal closure similar to (c). (**c**) Intraoperative image of a gasket seal reconstruction of the skull base. Note the large margin of overhanging fascia lata and the countersunk bone. (**d**) Intraoperative view demonstrating the nasoseptal flap secured in place

with autologous abdominal fat followed by reconstruction of the bony sella (with vomer or Medpor) and application of tissue sealant [24, 37].

Patients with larger skull base defects after endoscopic endonasal surgery for sellar and anterior skull base tumors (suprasellar, fovea ethmoidalis, cribriform plate) with a high-volume intraoperative CSF leak require multilayered closure [3, 5–10, 14, 16–20, 23]. This can be achieved often with an autologous fat graft in the tumor cavity followed by inlay placement of a fascial layer (harvested autologous fascia lata) and onlay placement of a bony buttress and application of tissue sealant. In cases involving direct communication between the ventricular spaces and the tumor cavity, packing of fat into the tumor cavity is avoided to minimize the risk of iatrogenic hydrocephalus [24, 37].

18.2.3 Gasket Seal Closure

These larger skull base defects usually created after endoscopic endonasal transphenoidal, transethmoidal, transcribriform, transclival, or transpterygoidal approaches to skull base tumors can be supplemented often with a gasket seal closure [24, 37] (Fig. 18.2). Gasket seal closure begins with elimination of any dead space with autologous fat to prevent pooling of CSF over the closure. A gasket seal closure is favored when the defect is >1 cm in diameter and consists of a soft tissue graft (generally fascia lata) centered over the defect with the edges of the graft exceeding the bony defect circumferentially. The radius of the graft must exceed the bone defect by at least 1 cm. If fascia lata is not available, we use bovine pericardium or AlloDerm (LifeCell Corp., Branchburg, NJ). These substances are sufficiently thick to create the gasket seal. Next, a piece of rigid material such as vomer or Medpor (Porex Surgical, Inc., Newnan, GA) is fashioned to be roughly the size of the bony defect and is centered over the soft tissue graft so that there is at least 1 cm of tissue graft extending circumferentially around the rigid graft and gently countersunk into the bony defect, forming a watertight gasket seal around the rigid graft [24]. Bioabsorbable plates and cartilage are not recommended; the former may not last long enough to ensure stable closure, and the latter is not sufficiently rigid. The closure is inspected to make sure there is no leakage of fluorescein-tinged CSF, which would indicate inadequate closure. If CSF is still leaking, either the closure is redone or a lumbar drain is placed. These types of large defects are then further covered with a vascularized nasoseptal flap followed by a final layer of DuraSeal to keep the flap in place.

18.2.4 Vascularized Nasoseptal Flap

The use of a pedicled nasoseptal vascular flap of the nasal septum mucoperiosteum based on the nasoseptal artery has become an important adjunct in the endoscopic reconstruction of large skull base defects. The nasoseptal flap is generally harvested at the beginning of the operation, before tumor removal and before the posterior septectomy is performed. The vascular supply of the nasoseptal flap is derived from the posterior septal artery, a terminal branch of the internal maxillary artery [11, 21]. The flap is raised by placing two parallel incisions within the septal mucosa, one along the nasal floor and the other just inferior to the most superior aspect of the septum. These incisions are joined anteriorly to create the flap, and posteriorly these incisions are extended over the rostrum of the sphenoid superiorly and to the choana inferiorly. The flap is elevated anterior to posterior and lateral with a dissector and tucked out of the way of the surgeon into the nasopharynx.

During skull base reconstruction, the nasoseptal flap is incorporated as a final layer of closure in addition to the previously placed gasket seal or bony buttress and inlay or inlay graft. The flap is secured in position with fibrin glue or DuraSeal ensuring that it is not twisted along its pedicle and that the mucosal surface is facing the nasal cavity. It is important that the flap abuts the skull base defect and surrounding bone and mucosa directly without any interposing hemostatic material. Furthermore it is important that the flap is planned large enough to cover all the edges of the skull base defect. After reconstruction and securing of the flap in position, Floseal (Baxter Inc., Vienna, Austria) is routinely placed into the sinonasal cavity, and small folds of Telfa are placed into the anterior nasal cavity and removed on the first postoperative day.

18.2.5 Ventriculoperitoneal Shunt and Lumbar Drain

A lumbar drain can be placed preoperatively in patients considered at high risk for failure of the endonasal skull base repair. Routine use of a lumbar drain is a widely debated subject. Patients considered at higher risk for failure of the skull base reconstruction include those that have failed prior attempts at encephalocele or CSF fistula repair, a BMI >30, a particularly large defect, an empty sella syndrome or hydrocephalus identified radiographically, a history of pseudotumor, or had entry into the ventricular system during suprasellar tumor resection [4]. By diverting the cerebrospinal fluid and maintaining a lower intracranial pressure, the lumbar drain can facilitate the initial healing process where the graft material and nasoseptal flap are incorporated into the skull base. This is particularly helpful during patient extubation after the surgery where coughing and bucking will transiently increase the intracranial pressure and push the graft or CSF out through the skull base defect and jeopardize the repair. However, there is a significant risk of developing pneumocephalus secondary to overdrainage in patients with anterior cranial fossa skull base defects. These patients must be monitored during this period for any change in neurological condition and should undergo a postoperative CT or MRI scan. To minimize these risks lumbar drains, when placed, are opened at a low rate of approximately 5 mL/h and are generally removed at the end of the first or second postoperative day. Patients noted to have pseudotumor, hydrocephalus, or empty sella before surgery are at high risk for failure of the skull base repair and may ultimately need placement of VP shunt in addition to the skull base repair to eliminate CSF rhinorrhea. We had to place a VP shunt for recurrent CSF fluid rhinorrhea in less than 5 % of cases after endoscopic endonasal repair of the skull base defect.

References

1. Aarabi B, Leibrock LG (1992) Neurosurgical approaches to cerebrospinal fluid rhinorrhea. Ear Nose Throat J 71:300–305
2. Abiko S, Aoki H, Fudaba H (1988) Intrasphenoidal encephalocele: report of a case. Neurosurgery 22: 933–936
3. Brown SM, Tabaee A, Singh A, Schwartz TH, Anand VK (2008) Three-dimensional endoscopic sinus surgery: feasibility and technical aspects. Otolaryngol Head Neck Surg 138:400–402
4. Carrau RL, Snyderman CH, Kassam AB (2005) The management of cerebrospinal fluid leaks in patients at risk for high-pressure hydrocephalus. Laryngoscope 115:205–212
5. Cavallo LM, Messina A, Cappabianca P, Esposito F, de Divitiis E, Gardner P, Tschabitscher M (2005) Endoscopic endonasal surgery of the midline skull base: anatomical study and clinical considerations. Neurosurg Focus 19:E2
6. Couldwell WT, Weiss MH, Rabb C, Liu JK, Apfelbaum RI, Fukushima T (2004) Variations on the standard transsphenoidal approach to the sellar region, with emphasis on the extended approaches and parasellar approaches: surgical experience in 105 cases. Neurosurgery 55:539–547; discussion 547–550
7. de Divitiis E, Cappabianca P, Cavallo LM (2002) Endoscopic transsphenoidal approach: adaptability of the procedure to different sellar lesions. Neurosurgery 51:699–705; discussion 705–697
8. de Divitiis E, Cavallo LM, Cappabianca P, Esposito F (2007) Extended endoscopic endonasal transsphenoidal approach for the removal of suprasellar tumors: Part 2. Neurosurgery 60:46–58; discussion 58–59
9. Dusick JR, Esposito F, Kelly DF, Cohan P, DeSalles A, Becker DP, Martin NA (2005) The extended direct endonasal transsphenoidal approach for nonadenomatous suprasellar tumors. J Neurosurg 102:832–841
10. Fraser JF, Nyquist GG, Moore N, Anand VK, Schwartz TH (2010) Endoscopic endonasal transclival resection of chordomas: operative technique, clinical outcome, and review of the literature. J Neurosurg 112:1061–1069
11. Hadad G, Bassagasteguy L, Carrau RL, Mataza JC, Kassam A, Snyderman CH, Mintz A (2006) A novel reconstructive technique after endoscopic expanded endonasal approaches: vascular pedicle nasoseptal flap. Laryngoscope 116:1882–1886
12. Hegazy HM, Carrau RL, Snyderman CH, Kassam A, Zweig J (2000) Transnasal endoscopic repair of cerebrospinal fluid rhinorrhea: a meta-analysis. Laryngoscope 110:1166–1172
13. Herman P, Sauvaget E, Guichard JP, Tran Ba Huy P (2003) Intrasphenoidal transsellar encephalocele repaired by endoscopic approach. Ann Otol Rhinol Laryngol 112:890–893
14. Hofstetter CP, Singh A, Anand VK, Kacker A, Schwartz TH (2010) The endoscopic, endonasal, transmaxillary transpterygoid approach to the pterygopalatine fossa, infratemporal fossa, petrous apex, and the Meckel cave. J Neurosurg 113:967–974
15. Hubbard JL, McDonald TJ, Pearson BW, Laws ER Jr (1985) Spontaneous cerebrospinal fluid rhinorrhea: evolving concepts in diagnosis and surgical management based on the Mayo Clinic experience from 1970 through 1981. Neurosurgery 16:314–321
16. Jho HD, Ha HG (2004) Endoscopic endonasal skull base surgery: part 1–the midline anterior fossa skull base. Minim Invasive Neurosurg 47:1–8
17. Jho HD, Ha HG (2004) Endoscopic endonasal skull base surgery: part 2–the cavernous sinus. Minim Invasive Neurosurg 47:9–15
18. Jho HD, Ha HG (2004) Endoscopic endonasal skull base surgery: part 3–the clivus and posterior fossa. Minim Invasive Neurosurg 47:16–23
19. Kassam A, Carrau RL, Snyderman CH, Gardner P, Mintz A (2005) Evolution of reconstructive techniques following endoscopic expanded endonasal approaches. Neurosurg Focus 19:E8
20. Kassam AB, Gardner P, Snyderman C, Mintz A, Carrau R (2005) Expanded endonasal approach: fully endoscopic, completely transnasal approach to the middle third of the clivus, petrous bone, middle cranial fossa, and infratemporal fossa. Neurosurg Focus 19:E6

21. Kassam AB, Thomas A, Carrau RL, Snyderman CH, Vescan A, Prevedello D, Mintz A, Gardner P (2008) Endoscopic reconstruction of the cranial base using a pedicled nasoseptal flap. Neurosurgery 63:ONS44–ONS52; discussion ONS52–ONS53
22. Keerl R, Weber RK, Draf W, Wienke A, Schaefer SD (2004) Use of sodium fluorescein solution for detection of cerebrospinal fluid fistulas: an analysis of 420 administrations and reported complications in Europe and the United States. Laryngoscope 114:266–272
23. Laufer I, Anand VK, Schwartz TH (2007) Endoscopic, endonasal extended transsphenoidal, transplanum transtuberculum approach for resection of suprasellar lesions. J Neurosurg 106:400–406
24. Leng LZ, Brown S, Anand VK, Schwartz TH (2008) "Gasket-seal" watertight closure in minimal-access endoscopic cranial base surgery. Neurosurgery 62:ONSE342–ONSE343; discussion ONSE343
25. Locatelli D, Rampa F, Acchiardi I, Bignami M, De Bernardi F, Castelnuovo P (2006) Endoscopic endonasal approaches for repair of cerebrospinal fluid leaks: nine-year experience. Neurosurgery 58:ONS-246–ONS-256; discussion ONS-256–ONS-257
26. Mahaley MS Jr, Odom GL (1966) Complication following intrathecal injection of fluorescein. J Neurosurg 25:298–299
27. Maira G, Anile C, Mangiola A (2005) Primary empty sella syndrome in a series of 142 patients. J Neurosurg 103:831–836
28. Moseley JI, Carton CA, Stern WE (1978) Spectrum of complications in the use of intrathecal fluorescein. J Neurosurg 48:765–767
29. Nyquist GG, Anand VK, Mehra S, Kacker A, Schwartz TH (2010) Endoscopic endonasal repair of anterior skull base non-traumatic cerebrospinal fluid leaks, meningoceles, and encephaloceles. J Neurosurg 113:961–966
30. Park JI, Strelzow VV, Friedman WH (1983) Current management of cerebrospinal fluid rhinorrhea. Laryngoscope 93:1294–1300
31. Ray BS, Bergland RM (1969) Cerebrospinal fluid fistula: clinical aspects, techniques of localization, and methods of closure. J Neurosurg 30:399–405
32. Schick B, Brors D, Prescher A (2000) Sternberg's canal–cause of congenital sphenoidal meningocele. Eur Arch Otorhinolaryngol 257:430–432
33. Schlosser RJ, Bolger WE (2003) Significance of empty sella in cerebrospinal fluid leaks. Otolaryngol Head Neck Surg 128:32–38
34. Schwartz TH, Fraser JF, Brown S, Tabaee A, Kacker A, Anand VK (2008) Endoscopic cranial base surgery: classification of operative approaches. Neurosurgery 62:991–1002; discussion 1002–1005
35. Spaziante R, de Divitiis E, Stella L, Cappabianca P, Genovese L (1981) The empty sella. Surg Neurol 16:418–426
36. Sternberg M (1888) Ein bisher noch nicht beschriebener Kanal im Keilbein des Menschen. Anat Anz 3:784–785
37. Tabaee A, Anand VK, Brown SM, Lin JW, Schwartz TH (2007) Algorithm for reconstruction after endoscopic pituitary and skull base surgery. Laryngoscope 117:1133–1137
38. Tabaee A, Placantonakis DG, Schwartz TH, Anand VK (2007) Intrathecal fluorescein in endoscopic skull base surgery. Otolaryngol Head Neck Surg 137:316–320
39. Tabaee A, Anand VK, Cappabianca P, Stamm A, Esposito F, Schwartz TH (2010) Endoscopic management of spontaneous meningoencephalocele of the lateral sphenoid sinus. J Neurosurg 112:1070–1077
40. Tsutsumi K, Asano T, Shigeno T, Matsui T, Ito S, Kaizu H (1999) Transcranial approach for transsphenoidal encephalocele: report of two cases. Surg Neurol 51:252–257

19 Man-to-Machine Interface in Neuroendoscopy: The Importance of Human Interface in the Development of Neuroendoscopy

Spyros Sgouros

19.1 Introduction

Neuroendoscopy was first employed in the surgical treatment of neurosurgical diseases early in the twentieth century by pioneers such as Walter Dandy, but it did not become an established practice for a long time, mainly because of poor technology and clinical results. We could call the 1910–1920s the invention phase. After decades of neglect, a kind of 'dark ages', neuroendoscopy is enjoying a sustained resurgence. After a slow timid reappearance in the 1980s, the 1990s saw an expansion of techniques and instrumentation. We could call the 1980s the reinvention phase and the 1990s the expansion phase. As it is common with many other 'inventions', there was an early phase of enthusiasm, which lasted several years. This was followed by crystallisation of indications and success rates. We could call the 2000s the era of consolidation. This does not mean that endoscopy will not expand any longer, in the contrary. But expansion will follow a mature course.

The history of neuroendoscopy is paralleled by the evolution of neuroendoscope design. The current design of neuroendoscopes dates back to the early days of cystoscopes, at the beginning of the twentieth century. Despite advances in other fields of medical technology and the wide use of computer and robotic technology, the neuroendoscopes which are in wide use today have an ergonomically disadvantageous design dating back to the early and mid-twentieth century, which in the author's experience at times hampers rather than enhances the skills of the neurosurgeon.

Still, neurosurgeons have moulded gradually their skills to the existing equipment, accepting its limitations and expending their energy in maximising its use. Nowadays that, with the routine use of neuronavigation, craniotomy flaps are smaller and microneurosurgery techniques have evolved, neuroendoscopy feels much less minimally invasive way to perform neurosurgical operations in comparison to 20 years ago.

A critical review of the endoscope design shortcomings will be presented, and possible means to overcome them will be discussed.

19.2 Brief History of Neuroendoscopy

In 1887, Nietze in Vienna operated for the first time using a glass lens cystoscope, with the help of an incandescent light source. In 1910, L' Espinasse used a cystoscope to perform a plexectomy [1, 5, 7, 16, 17]. In 1922, Dandy used a cystoscope to perform plexectomy as treatment for hydrocephalus [1, 5, 7, 12, 16, 18]. He inserted it in to the brain using a gynaecological speculum to retract the sides of a cortical incision. In 1923, Mixter is credited to have performed the first endoscopic third ventriculostomy [1, 5, 7,

S. Sgouros, MD, FRCS(SN)
Department of Pediatric Neurosurgery, Mitera Children's Hospital, Athens, Greece

University of Athens Medical School, Athens, Greece
e-mail: sgouros@med.uoa.gr, ssgouros@mitera.gr

S. Sgouros (ed.), *Neuroendoscopy*,
DOI 10.1007/978-3-642-39085-2_19,

16, 17]. Further developments came in 1931 by Burman, 1936 by Stern, 1938 by Pool, and later in 1960 by Ooi and Morosaki. A major step forward came in 1966 when Harold Hopkins utilised a solid rod lens in the construction of endoscopes, and this remains today in their current form [16, 18]. In 1973 Takanori Fukushima introduced the neurofibroscope in clinical practice [16]. Nevertheless, neuroendoscopy was held then in low esteem because of the poor outcome of the operated patients. The combination of crude non-specialist equipment and primitive neuroanaesthetic techniques conspired against the establishment of neuroendoscopy as mainstream technique at that early stage. Renewed interest was expressed in the 1980s by neurosurgeons who are now considered modern day pioneers. Dr Bernhard Bauer who practised at the time in Hannover, Germany, recalls that when he first discussed in meetings of the German Neurosurgical Society the use of the neuroendoscope, he was greeted by sincere scepticism (personal communication). It was the decade when the operating microscope was being established as mainstream prime neurosurgical instrument, and the comparison of the neuroendoscope with the small image of average quality to the microscope of the substantial illumination and large three-dimensional image, left the neuroendoscope wanting. After all, everybody was eager to learn to use the microscope, the new technological pride, which revolutionised neurosurgery, transformed operative outcome and brought neurosurgery in to a new era of increased surgical possibilities. It was not easy to have two technological revolutions at the same time. Nevertheless, in the late 1980s Huw Griffiths in Bristol, UK, used systematically the endoscope to perform choroid plexectomies for hydrocephalus [5] and Axel Perneczky in Mainz, Germany, used it in a variety of procedures as an adjunct to the microscope, creating the concept of endoscope-assisted neurosurgery. Neither of them are no longer with us, but most of us have fond memories of them presenting their work in international meetings. The 1990s saw a rapid technological improvement of the neuroendoscopic equipment, which paved the way for its increased use. Progress in the lighting source and camera systems has been particularly significant.

19.3 Knowledge Transfer

A quick overview of the development of neuroendoscopy identifies a transfer of 'know-how' from urology to neurosurgery, possibly facilitated by a common similar fluid medium (urine-CSF), which enabled the pioneers to embark on rather bold surgical experiments, which almost certainly would be impossible in today's climate of medicolegal practice.

There have been other examples of similar 'know-how' transfer between surgical specialities. A good example is the use of the Cavitron Ultrasonic Surgical Aspirator (CUSA). Developed originally for the removal of liver tumours, soon it migrated in to everyday neurosurgical practice. This transfer of 'know-how' takes a long time in surgery. The new invention needs to establish itself before it is propagated to another discipline, and this may take a while. The necessarily conservative approach of neurosurgeons towards 'progress' is probably related to the stark effect a surgical complication has on the psyche of a surgeon.

19.4 Reinvention of Neuroendoscopy

In the 1980s, the urological endoscopes were used again to revitalise interest in endoscopy, as there were no dedicated neuroendoscopes at the time. The modern day pioneers 'swam against the tide', enduring the criticism of their peers, in order to try again techniques that were first tried 70 years before! Only this time, in their favour was the evolution of neuroanaesthesia that could ensure better operating conditions and clinical results. The endoscope was used initially in the surgical management of hydrocephalus and gradually expanded to skull base and spinal procedures. In the 1990s, after the initial enthusiasm settled, the surgical techniques were crystallised and the indications for the use of the endoscope were set. It became obvious gradually that the endoscope was not panacea and a solution to all problems but yet another tool in the armamentarium of the neurosurgeon.

19.5 Scientific Evolution of Neuroendoscopy

Two axes of progress in neuroendoscopy could be identified, the scientific and the technical. The technological advance of the endoscopes influenced significantly the scientific progress that resulted from its use. Having said this, scientific progress has been comparatively bigger than technical progress.

The use of the endoscope gave us new insights on CSF physiology. The characterisation of aqueduct stenosis in its full form came only after the widespread use of endoscopic third ventriculostomy in its treatment. Prior to that, all forms of hydrocephalus were treated by shunting, with only occasional use of stereotactic third ventriculostomy guided by ventriculography. The use of the endoscope and in parallel the use of MR imaging to assess the result of endoscopy gave us the knowledge to differentiate between aqueduct stenosis and other forms of infantile hydrocephalus and greatly enhanced our understanding of CSF physiology [6, 8, 10, 11, 15]. So the use of the endoscope in the management of CSF circulation disorders has been pathophysiology driven. Following the introduction of the endoscope in the management of CSF disorders, the concepts of aqueductoplasty, septostomy and foraminoplasty of the foramina of Monro and Magendie emerged, which were previously unknown [8]. Similarly, the utilisation of endoscopic techniques in the surgical management of intracranial arachnoid cysts improved our understanding of their dynamic nature with respect to CSF movement in and out of them and the presence of a valve-like mechanism on their wall.

On the other hand, the use of the endoscope in the surgical treatment of skull base pathology has been approach driven, another instrument that would help us achieve the task at hand better, as it takes the illumination and magnification close to the point it is needed, for example, in pituitary surgery, in comparison to the microscope [9, 13–15]. Thus, the use of the endoscope in extended skull base tumour resections improved access to difficult areas and technically made possible extent of surgery that was previously either not possible or carried significant morbidity, and this is achieved with less complications and overall better clinical outcome.

19.6 Technological Evolution of Neuroendoscopy

The progress and the evolution of the technology of the endoscopes although important, overall could be seen as modest, at least in some aspects, in comparison to the scientific progress that this technical evolution sparked. The dedicated neuroendoscopes of today do not look in shape and handling too dissimilar to the cystoscopes of the 1920s that were used for neurosurgery (Fig. 19.1). A dramatic difference for the better is the presence of the rod lens since the late 1960s. Nevertheless, the rod lens has changed very little since its inception, and rod lenses are still hand polished today as they were then. Modern manufacturing techniques have allowed the creation of smaller diameter rod lenses, which enabled the reduction in size of the endoscopes. Now there are in the market endoscopes with external diameter of 4 mm that include a working channel (Fig. 19.2) and even narrower without a working channel. This makes them more suitable for work in children and overall less traumatic.

One small but important change has been the angle of the viewpiece. Originally in continuation to the long axis of the rod lens (straight vision), in many endoscopes today the viewpiece is at an angle to it with the use of a coupling prism (angled vision) (Fig. 19.3), giving arguably better handling of the whole system.

The light available at the operative field at the tip of the endoscope has improved significantly over the years with the advent of fibre-optic cables that 'conduct' the light from the 'cold'

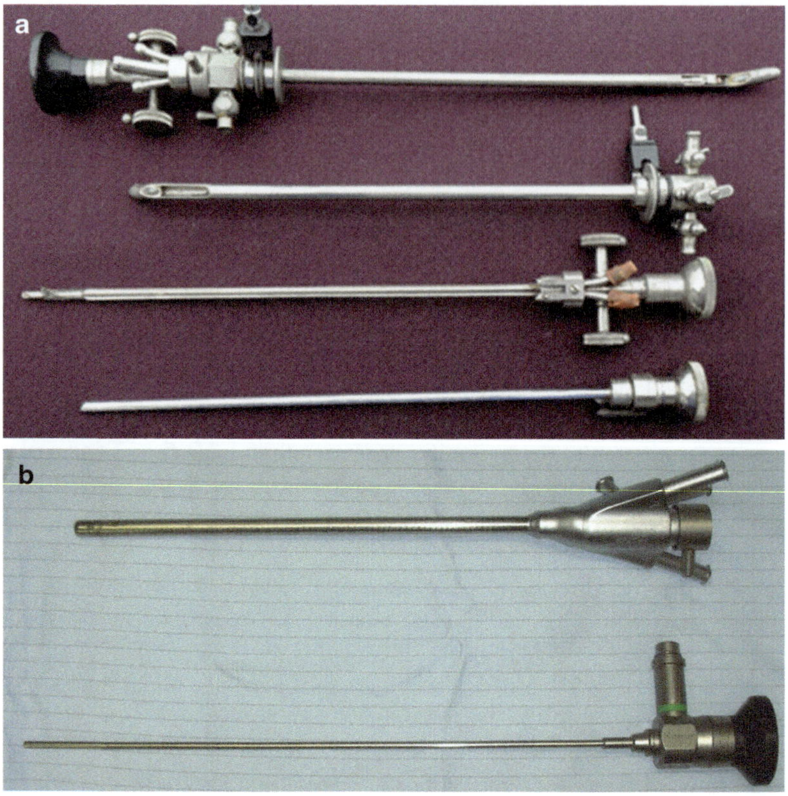

Fig. 19.1 Cystoscopes of 1920s vs. endoscopes of 2000s. (**a**) A collection of cystoscopes from 1923 (Image courtesy of Dr J.T. Goodrich, from his private collection) (**b**) 'Ventriculoscope'. Neuroendoscope that was commercially available from Aesculap, until the mid-2000s (Aesculap, Tuttlingen, Germany)

light source to the endoscope. The resulting improved illumination has made significant difference to the operating surgeon and is one of the main advantages of the endoscope over the microscope.

The biggest improvement though has been on the camera system. In the 1920s, and even in the reinvention of endoscopy in the 1980s, the surgeon had to look directly through the eyepiece at the end of the rod lens (direct vision). From the early 1990s there is a digital camera coupled to it (vision by proxy), and this has improved dramatically the quality of the image and the handling and ease of use of the whole endoscope system. The technological advance of the digital cameras, which goes hand in hand with the progress of computers and electronics, has made a dramatic change in neuroendoscopy [18]. Further improvement is expected to come from miniaturisation of the camera.

The development of the flexible endoscope has been less dramatic. Flexible endoscopes borrowed technology from the gastroscopes using flexible optical fibres, but their application in the small narrow confines of the brain has not been very successful. Their picture quality is inferior to the rod lens rigid endoscopes, their manoeuvrability is limited and not user friendly, and they have only one side port for all uses (Fig. 19.4). They were in vogue in the early 1990s. Although they are still used by many neurosurgeons, overall it would be fair to say that they have fallen out of favour and certainly they have not been developed any further. Flexible endoscopes available in the market today are more than a decade old designs.

Another field of progress has been the development of purpose-design surgical instruments for the neuroendoscopes (Fig. 19.5). The availability of suitable monopolar and bipolar diathermies can provide haemostatic control when working in the ventricular system. It has to be said though that this is limited in comparison to the microsurgical technique, and, often, intraoperative haemorrhage during a ventricular procedure leads to the premature ending of the

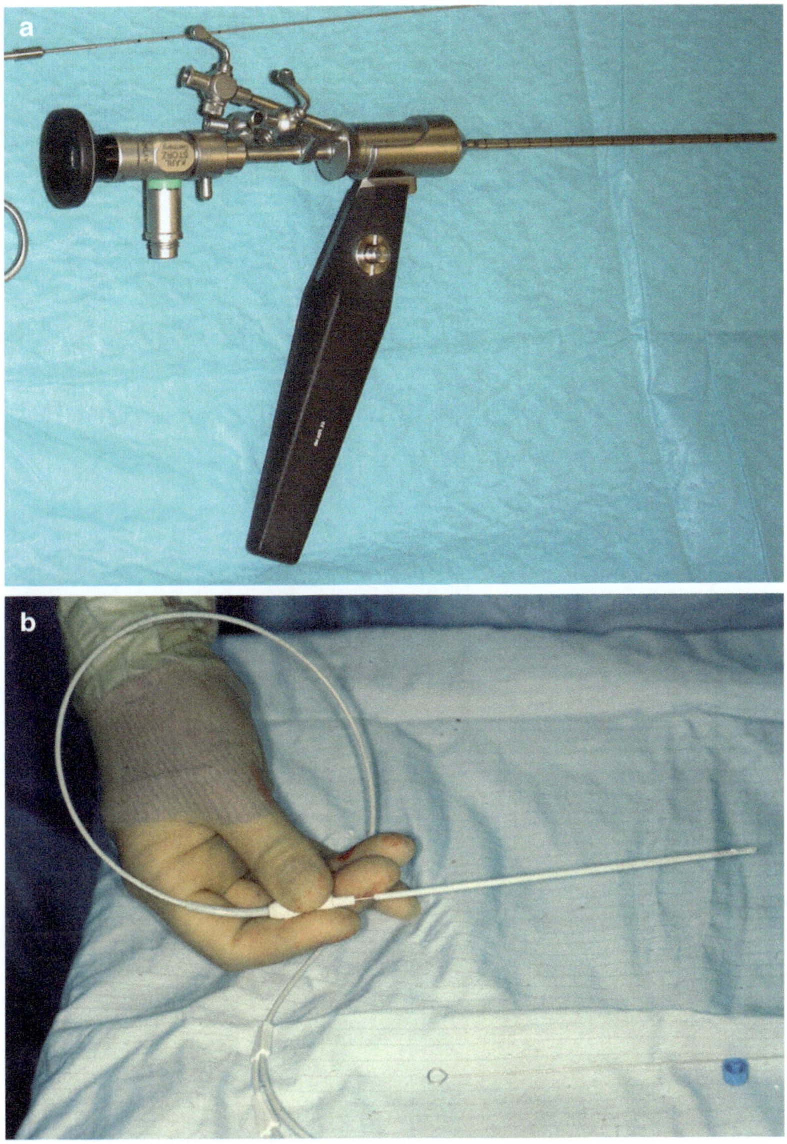

Fig. 19.2 Narrow neuroendoscopes (suitable for paediatric work). (**a**) Storz Oi endoscope system with external diameter 4 × 2 mm (Storz, Tuttlingen, Germany) (**b**) Neuropen, 1 mm fibre-optic endoscope in a rigid tube designed to go inside the lumen of a CSF shunt ventricular catheter with 'fish-mouth' opening, to aid visualisation of the final position of its tip

operation. Equally, suction through the endoscope is of limited power. In contrast, haemorrhage during transnasal skull base work is easier to control and has much less significance as it takes place in an open space extracranially. It is rare to have to abandon a transphenoidal endoscopic hypophysectomy because of bleeding, unless the intracavernous part of the internal carotid artery has been injured. The development of other equipment such as scissors, biopsy forceps and probes of various types gives the neuroendoscopist the ability to biopsy tumours or even remove them if they are not haemorrhagic (e.g. colloid cysts), divide adhesions and open cysts and in general perform a much wider spectrum of procedures, in comparison to what was possible 30 years ago [4]. It should be said though that the endoscopic biopsy forceps have small 'cup' and can only yield small samples, with a corresponding risk of false histology results.

A significant innovation, which has not materialised fully as yet, is the integration of the neuroendoscopes with image guidance systems (Fig. 19.6). This gives increased abilities to perform tasks that

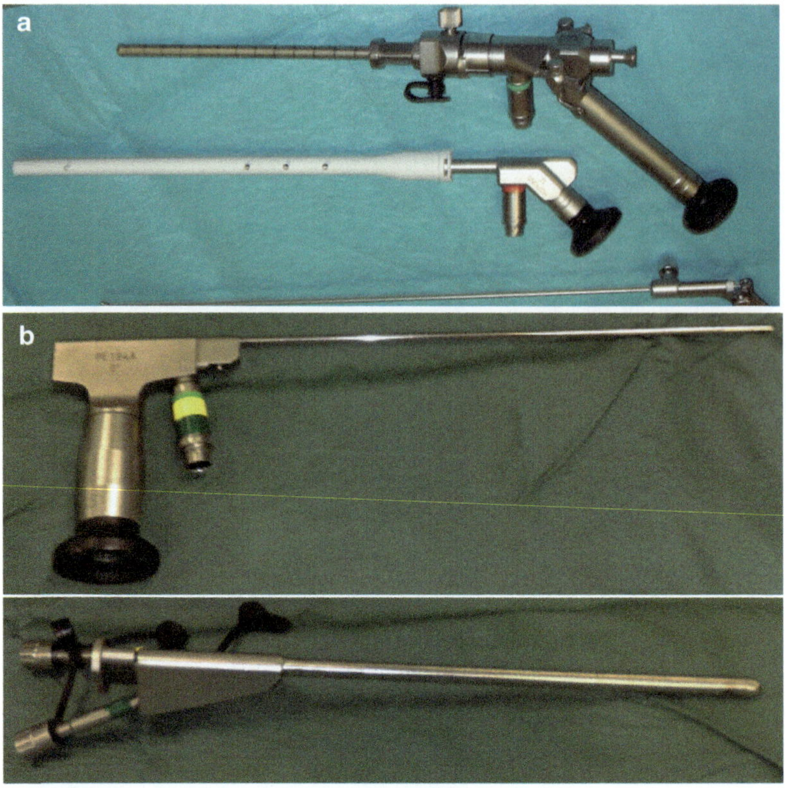

Fig. 19.3 Endoscopes with the viewpiece at an angle to the rod lens. (**a**) Storz Schroeder LOTTA endoscope system with the viewpiece at 45° to the rod lens. (**b**) Aesculap MINOP endoscope system with the viewpiece at 90° to the rod lens

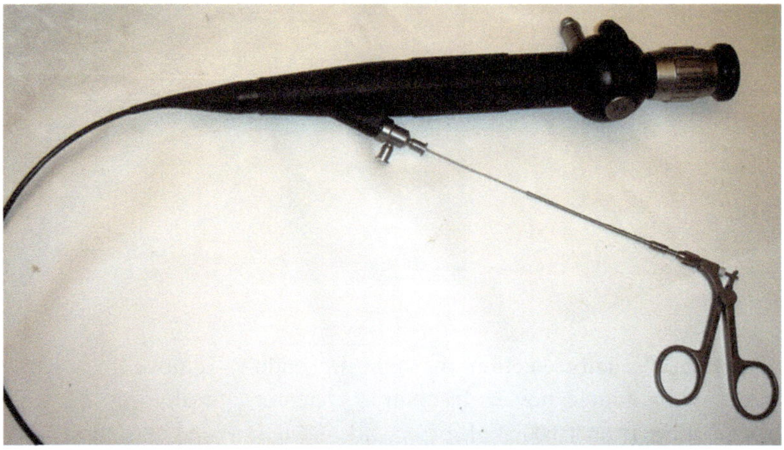

Fig. 19.4 Flexible fibre-optic neuroendoscope from Storz, with one working channel

otherwise would not be attempted, for fear of causing surgical damage. Multiloculated hydrocephalus is easier treated endoscopically with image guidance, which allows confidence of access in the presence of distorted ventricular anatomy. Equally, for extended skull base approaches image guidance is of paramount importance [13]. Further improvement is likely to come in this field as commercial image-guided systems develop further.

New developments such as robotic and 3D endoscopes are not in wide use yet; hence, one cannot comment on their contribution to neuroendoscopy. They are considered as the next frontiers of progress [18].

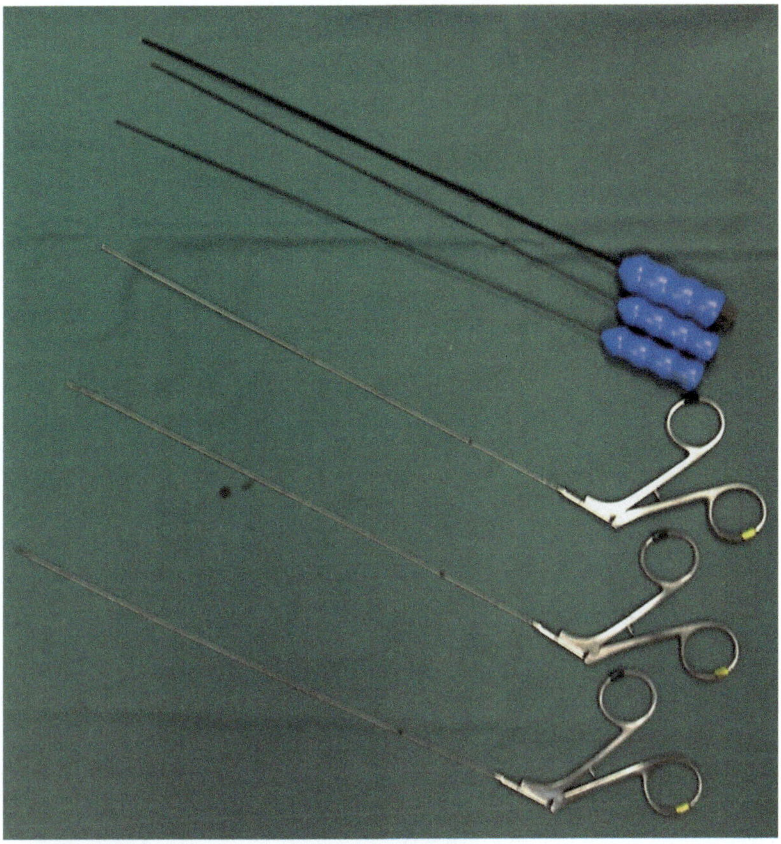

Fig. 19.5 Instruments for neuroendoscopes. (*Top three*) Bipolar diathermy for the Aesculap MINOP endoscope. (*Bottom three*) Biopsy forceps and microscissors used for ventricular surgery

19.7 Ergonomic Shortcomings of Neuroendoscopic Equipment

In its basic form the endoscope is ergonomically a fulcrum with disadvantageous biomechanical design from the operator's point of view (Fig. 19.7a). If one examines the use of the endoscope in a ventricular operation (e.g. ETV), the area of interest is approximately 1 cm from the tip of the rod lens, where only a few millimetres of movement is taking place throughout the surgical procedure. The corner of the fulcrum is at the point where the endoscope enters the skull through the burr hole. The part inside the head typically is a few centimetres (6–7 cm). On the other end of the fulcrum, 15–20 cm away from the corner of the fulcrum, a heavy camera lies 'hanging', reinforced by the traction that the camera and light cables exert. The operator is obliged to perform very fine manoeuvres of this heavy and ergonomically disadvantageous tail end in order to manipulate and move the front end for a few millimetres, and the region of the third ventricle is not forgiving at all. The avoidance of technical disaster is only a testament of how adaptable humans are, as they can learn very delicate and awkward manoeuvres and perform them without thinking. Certainly, if an engineer was requested to design a new endoscope today from a 'clean sheet' ('tabula rasa') perspective, ignoring all the technological inheritance of the past, it is unlikely that he would design such a difficult-to-manoeuvre ergonomically disadvantageous system.

The ergonomics of the modern neuroendoscope system are improved with the development of the digital camera but require familiarisation through training. The surgeon has a large computer screen directly in front of him with a big clear picture, but his line of vision is at right angle to the line of work of his hands (Fig. 19.7b). This ergonomically is quite different to the way

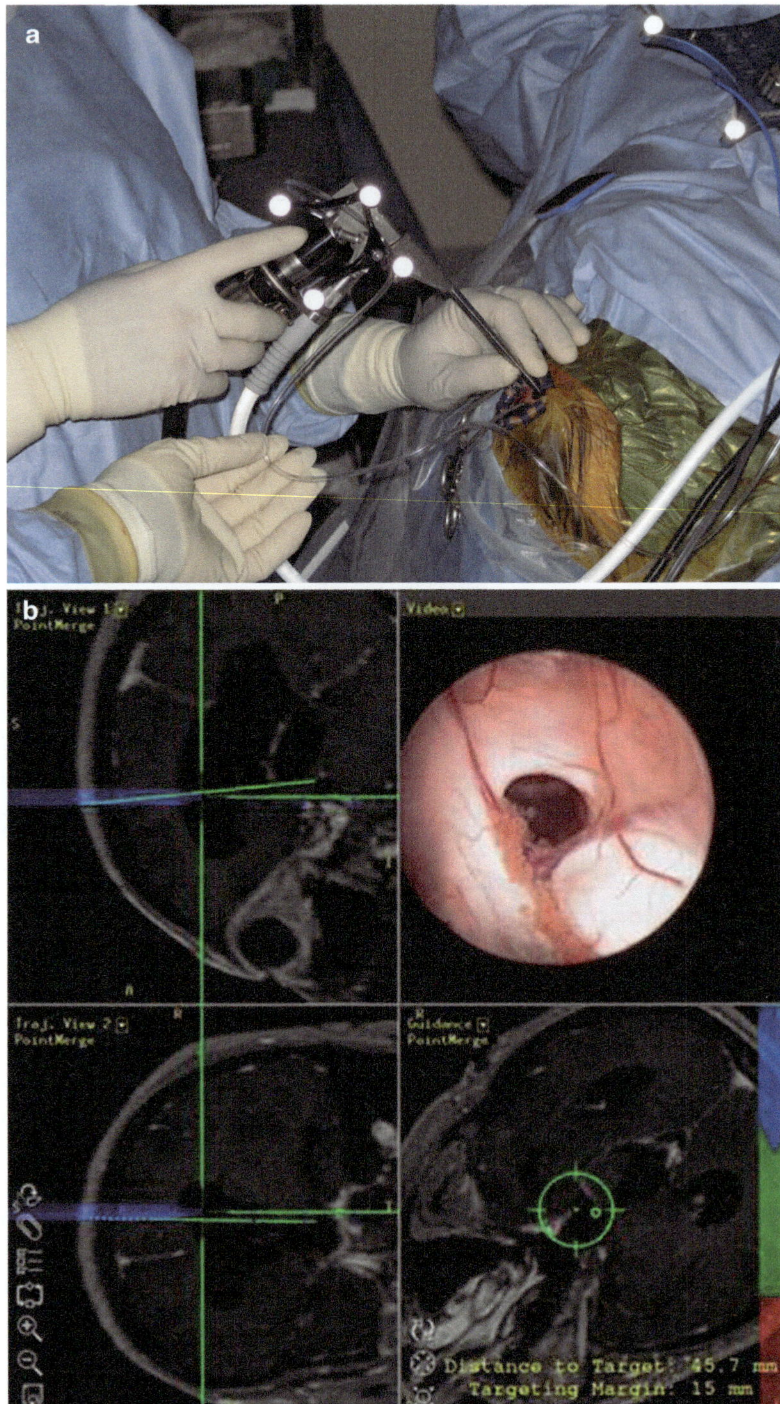

Fig. 19.6 Aesculap MINOP endoscope used in conjunction with the Brainlab neuronavigation system. (**a**) Reflective spheres attached to the endoscope make it "visible" by the cameras of the neuronavigation system. (**b**) Computer screen showing the simultaneous projection of the endoscope image and the reconstructed MR images annotated with the superimposed trajectory of the neuroendoscope, calculated by the neuronavigation software (Photograph courtesy of Dr A. Grotenhuis) (Brainlab, Munich, Germany)

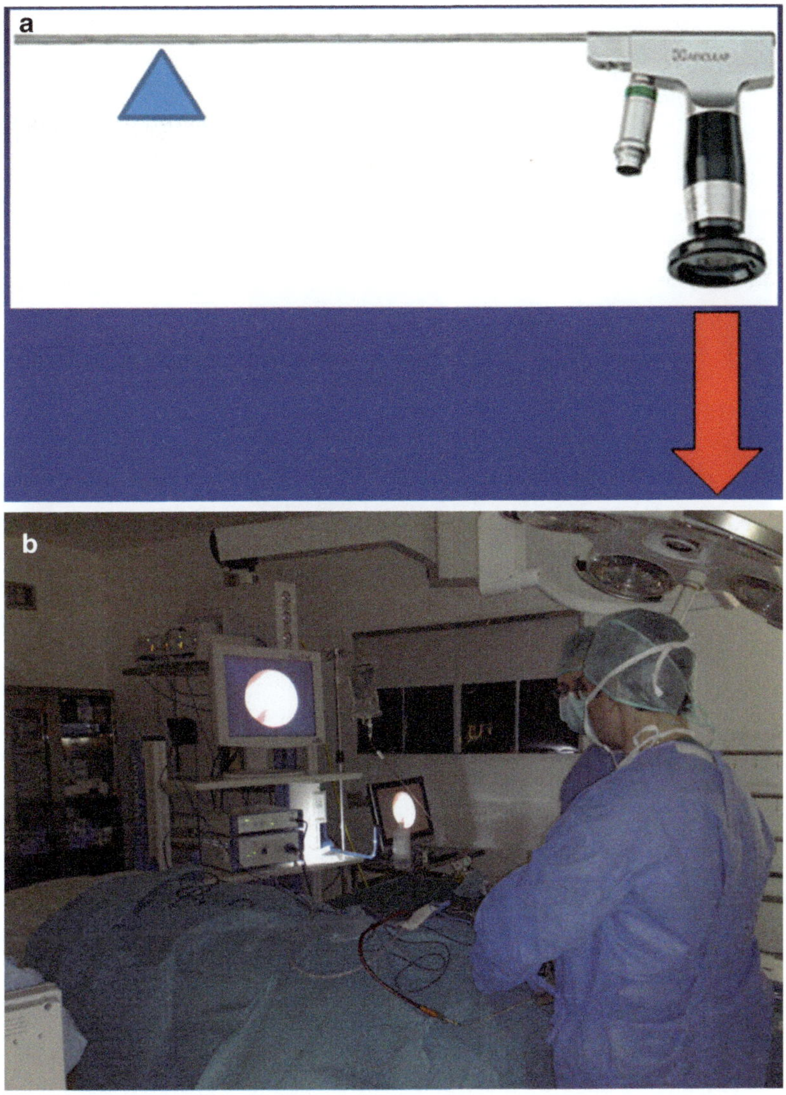

Fig. 19.7 Ergonomical disadvantage of endoscopes. (**a**) The heavy camera is situated too far posteriorly from the fulcrum point, the point where the endoscope enters the skull, making its manoeuvring difficult and open to errors. (**b**) Typical neuroendoscopic surgical setup. The surgeon is working with his line of vision at 90° degrees to his line of manual manipulation

we operate with the microscope, where the line of vision is parallel to the line of work of our hands. For this reason, a novice in neuroendoscopy has a learning curve to 'walk' before he can embark unassisted.

19.8 Minimally Invasive Techniques

Neuroendoscopy is commonly referred to as minimally invasive technique. Certainly, neuroendoscopic excision of ventricular tumours, such as colloid cysts, involves a much less traumatic approach in comparison to open transcortical excision [4]. Overall, compared to 'traditional' microneurosurgery techniques, neuroendoscopy offers a much less invasive approach to the ventricular system and the skull base. But by today's perceptions of safety, the word 'minimally' may be an exaggeration. Careful assessment of the MR scans of a child treated with ETV commonly reveals damage to the brain parenchyma in the area of insertion of the endoscope through the cortex, which looks at times impressive, especially when endoscopes of larger external diameter are used (Fig. 19.8). 'Slimmer' endoscopes have been developed, especially for use

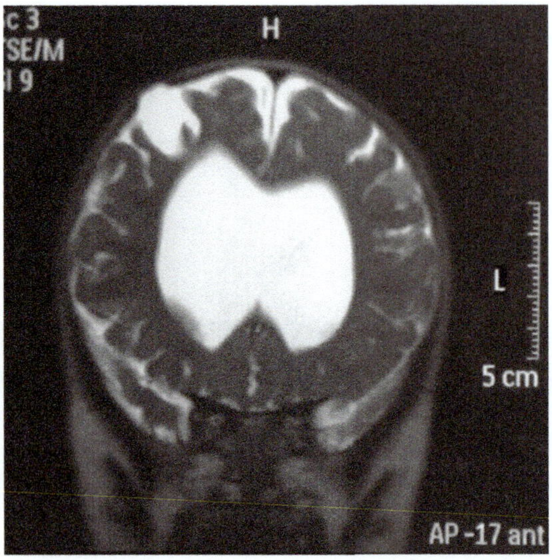

Fig. 19.8 Sagittal T-1-weighted MR scan of the head of a child obtained after realisation of a third ventriculostomy. A sizeable track is seen that has been created by the endoscope. This is a result of destruction of brain parenchyma

in children (see Fig. 19.3a), but they have some compromise in that they have limited capacity working channels only. Overall, if a lay person (non-neurosurgeon) looks at the front end of an endoscope, the part that enters the brain, cannot help but feel rather terrified about the seemingly large size of an instrument that has to penetrate the brain substance. The tip of the endoscope is twice as large as the tip of a ventricular catheter and much sharper. It is not known yet to what extent this damage to the frontal cortex at the endoscope insertion site becomes an epileptogenic focus in later years.

In addition, a small but appreciable risk exists of severe neurological damage after third ventriculostomy, damage to the basilar artery, the fornix, the basal ganglia or the hypothalamus [2, 3, 6]. The risk of such damage is smaller than that for most open craniotomy procedures, but it is uncertain if this merits the term 'minimally invasive'.

Equally, during skull base procedures a substantial part of the skull base has to be drilled in order to reach the target. The complication rate from endoscopic extended skull base approaches can be high, with CSF leak being the most frequent, but also risk of possible neurological damage of cranial nerves as they are exiting the skull base foramina [9, 13]. This hardly agrees with the perception of 'minimally invasive' procedure, at least how lay people perceive it, leaving aside the possible neurologic complications from damage to various anatomical structures.

19.9 Learning Curve

For most 'new' operative techniques, there is a so-called learning curve. Studies have shown that a considerable number of procedures, as many as 100, have to be performed by an individual surgeon before his results plateau at the lowest possible complication rate [14]. In neuroendoscopy, a major issue when it was introduced widely first was the migration from the 3-D vision of the microscope to the 2-D vision of a television screen; the ability to operate with your eyes at 90° to your hands, as opposed to being parallel as with the microscope; and the ability to operate with the limited functionality and ability to manipulation that the endoscopic instruments offer, in contrast to the complete freedom of movement of the microsurgical instruments and techniques. An objective observer would notice that a lot of the learning curve was devoted by the surgeon to learn to adapt to the design shortcomings of the instruments. This by engineering standards is unusual, and any new industrial design is commonly aiming to enhance the functional possibilities of its operator, not limit them. On the other hand, the fact that the endoscopes are rather basic designs has helped them to withstand the test of time.

19.10 Technological Challenge

With the exception of the electronic parts (camera, electronic image processing), most, if not all, commercially available endoscopes are at least 10-year-old designs, in fact mere evolutions of the 1920s and 1960s designs. Their cost is extremely high (tens of thousands of euros, the typical cost of an endoscopic system is at the order of 60,000 euros). By comparison, other technological goods which perform much less critical tasks (e.g. cars, DVD players), certainly not life saving, have evolved dramatically in the last decade, are infinitely more complex devices and cost considerably less than an endoscope (cars 1/3rd, DVD players 1/1,000th of an endoscope). This applies to most surgical instruments that commonly are manufactured by small companies (in comparison to companies that manufacture commercial goods) who perhaps do not have the ability to invest the large sums of money necessary to develop and test radically new ideas. And obviously it is related to the annual numbers of sales, which are very small for endoscopes and other surgical instruments and very high for commercial goods. Once a hospital has bought an endoscope system, that 'customer' 'disappears' for the manufacturing company for 10 years approximately (or more). It seems almost that society is willing to invest more in our entertainment and less in saving our lives!

Development of a new medical product of course is related to the ability of the end users, the doctors, to absorb new technologies. Doctors, surgeons in particular, are creatures of habit, prone not to attempt to use a new very radical device, over and above the fact that it is commonly very expensive and most hospitals would have difficulty in acquiring it. On the other hand, companies who manufacture surgical instruments typically perform 'market' research to identify how well a new design might be received, before investing millions of euros/dollars in the development of a new product, and during the development they use doctors as consultants. This situation produces an almost cyclical argument, the end result of which is slow progress, in comparison to other technological fields.

It is fair to say that the rod lens technology has reached its peak. It cannot be developed any further. With the rod lens as a standard, the only progress can come from improving the camera system using computer technology. And this progress is likely to be small, because the camera technology is reaching its peak. With today's technology, to improve the camera would require much bigger final device, which is impractical. Only significant improvement in miniaturisation will improve the handling properties of the camera. The tools currently in use could be described as simplistic, but it is difficult to see how they could be improved substantially. Any quantum leap has to come from a radically new design, possibly from the field of nanotechnology or robotics.

Having made all these criticisms, it would be unfair not to mention that the results of neuroendoscopy today are considerably better than the results of 20 or even 10 years ago and endoscopy is as safe as any other neurosurgical operation.

Conclusion

Considerable progress has been made in neuroendoscopy in the last 10 years, and this has made neuroendoscopic techniques safe and effective, but we need to keep striving for continuous improvement and radically new designs, rather than accept the current wisdom as a 'status quo'. Otherwise, in 30 years from now the endoscopes will still look like those of the 1920s, where the rest of the environment will have changed around us completely.

Acknowledgment The material of this chapter formed the core of the lecture of the Congress President of the 5th World Congress of Neuroendoscopy of the International Federation of Neuroendoscopy (IFNE), Athens, Greece, 2 June 2009.

References

1. Abbott R (2004) History of neuroendoscopy. Neurosurg Clin N Am 15:1–7
2. Bouras T, Sgouros S (2011) Complications of endoscopic third ventriculostomy. A review. J Neurosurg Pediatr 7:643–649
3. Bouras T, Sgouros S (2012) Complications of endoscopic third ventriculostomy. World Neurosurg. doi:10.1016/j.wneu.2012.02.014
4. Cappabianca P, Cinalli G, Gangemi M, Brunori A, Cavallo LM, de Divitiis E, Decq P, Delitala A, Di Rocco F, Frazee J, Godano U, Grotenhuis A, Longatti P, Mascari C, Nishihara T, Oi S, Rekate H, Schroeder HW, Souweidane MM, Spennato P, Tamburrini G, Teo C, Warf B, Zymberg ST (2008) Application of neuroendoscopy to intraventricular lesions. Neurosurgery 62(Suppl 2):575–597; discussion 597–598

5. Decq P, Schroeder HW, Fritsch M, Cappabianca P (2012) An history of ventricular endoscopy. World Neurosurg. doi:10.1016/j.wneu.2012.02.034
6. Di Rocco C, Cinalli G, Massimi L, Spennato P, Cianciulli E, Tamburrini G (2006) Endoscopic third ventriculostomy in the treatment of hydrocephalus in pediatric patients. Adv Tech Stand Neurosurg 31: 119–219
7. Duffner F, Freudenstein D, Wacker A, Straub-Duffner S, Grote EH (1998) 75 years after Dandy, Fay and Mixter – looking back on the history of neuroendoscopy. [Article in German]. Zentrabl Neurochir 59: 121–128
8. Enchev Y, Oi S (2008) Historical trends of neuroendoscopic surgical techniques in the treatment of hydrocephalus. Neurosurg Rev 31:249–262
9. Gruner P, Gaab MR, Hellwig D, Oertel JM (2009) German neuroendoscopy above the skull base. Neurosurg Focus 27(3):E7
10. Harris LW (1994) Endoscopic techniques in neurosurgery. Microsurgery 15:541–546
11. Hellwig D, Grotenhuis JA, Tirakotai W, Riegel T, Schulte DM, Bauer BL, Bertalanffy H (2005) Endoscopic third ventriculostomy for obstructive hydrocephalus. Neurosurg Rev 28(1):1–34; discussion 35–38
12. Hsu W, Li KW, Bookland M, Jallo GI (2009) Keyhole to the brain: Walter Dandy and neuroendoscopy. J Neurosurg Pediatr 3(5):439–442
13. Hwang PY, Ho CL (2007) Neuronavigation using an image-guided endoscopic transnasal-sphenoethmoidal approach to clival chordomas. Neurosurgery 61(5 Suppl 2):212–217; discussion 217–218
14. Jane JA Jr, Laws ER Jr (2001) The surgical management of pituitary adenomas in a series of 3,093 patients. J Am Coll Surg 193(6):651–659
15. Li KW, Nelson C, Sulk I, Jallo GI (2005) Neuroendoscopy: past, present, and future. Neurosurg Focus 19(6):E1
16. Stachura K, Libionka W (2007) An outline of the history of neuroendoscopy. [Article in Polish]. Przegl Lek 64:118–120
17. Walker ML (2001) History of ventriculostomy. Neurosurg Clin N Am 12:101–110
18. Zada G, Liu C, Apuzzo ML (2012) "Through the looking glass": optical physics, issues, and the evolution of neuroendoscopy. World Neurosurg 77(1): 92–102

Index

S. Sgouros (ed.), *Neuroendoscopy*,
DOI 10.1007/978-3-642-39085-2, © Springer-Verlag Berlin Heidelberg 2014

F

G

H

S

T

GPSR Compliance

The European Union's (EU) General Product Safety Regulation (GPSR) is a set of rules that requires consumer products to be safe and our obligations to ensure this.

If you have any concerns about our products, you can contact us on ProductSafety@springernature.com

In case Publisher is established outside the EU, the EU authorized representative is:

Springer Nature Customer Service Center GmbH
Europaplatz 3
69115 Heidelberg, Germany

Batch number: 10732758

Printed by Printforce, the Netherlands